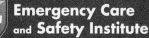
Wilderness First Aid

Emergency Care in Remote Locations

Fourth Edition

Howard D. Backer, MD, MPH, FAWM

Warren D. Bowman, MD

Bruce C. Paton, MD

Peter Steele, MD

Alton L. Thygerson, EdD, FAWM

Steven M. Thygerson, PhD, MSPH

Benjamin Gulli, MD
Medical Editor

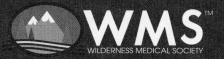

WMS™
WILDERNESS MEDICAL SOCIETY

D0112895

JONES & BARTLETT
LEARNING

World Headquarters
Jones & Bartlett Learning
5 Wall Street
Burlington, MA 01803
978-443-5000
info@jblearning.com
www.jblearning.com

Jones & Bartlett Learning books and products are available through most bookstores and online booksellers. To contact Jones & Bartlett Learning directly, call 800-832-0034, fax 978-443-8000, or visit our website, www.jblearning.com.

Substantial discounts on bulk quantities of Jones & Bartlett Learning publications are available to corporations, professional associations, and other qualified organizations. For details and specific discount information, contact the special sales department at Jones & Bartlett Learning via the above contact information or send an email to specialsales@jblearning.com.

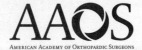

Editorial Credits
Chief Education Officer: Constance M. Filling
Director, Department of Publications: Hans J. Koelsch, PhD
Managing Editor: Barbara A. Scotese
Associate Senior Editor: Gayle Murray

Production Credits

Chief Executive Officer: Ty Field
President: James Homer
Chief Product Officer: Eduardo Moura
Executive Publisher: Kimberly Brophy
Executive Acquisitions Editor—EMS: Christine Emerton
Associate Managing Editor: Janet Morris

Production Editor: Jessica deMartin
VP, Sales, Public Safety Group: Matthew Maniscalco
Director of Sales, Public Safety Group: Patricia Einstein
VP, Marketing: Alisha Weisman
VP, Manufacturing and Inventory Control: Therese Connell
Composition: Cenveo® Publisher Services

Cover Design: Kristin E. Parker
Photo Researcher: Shaun Steele
Cover Image: © Hemera/Thinkstock
Printing and Binding: RR Donnelley
Cover Printing: RR Donnelley

Library of Congress Cataloging-in-Publication Data
Thygerson, Alton L.
  Wilderness first aid : emergency care in remote locations / Alton L. Thygerson, EdD, FAWM, Steven M. Thygerson, PhD, MSPH.—Fourth edition.
    pages cm
  "Emergency Care and Safety Institute."
  "American Academy of Orthopaedic Surgeons."
  "Wilderness Medical Society."
  Includes index.
  ISBN 978-1-4496-4218-1
  1. Mountaineering injuries. 2. Outdoor medical emergencies. 3. First aid in illness and injury. I. Thygerson, Steven M. II. Emergency Care and Safety Institute. III. American Academy of Orthopaedic Surgeons. IV. Wilderness Medical Society. V. Title. VI. Title: First aid.
  RC88.9.M6 T49 2014
  616.02'52—dc23
                              2013020772

6048

Printed in the United States of America
18 17 16 15   10 9 8 7 6 5 4 3

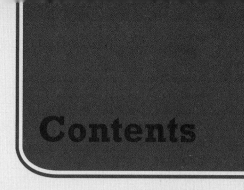

Contents

Chapter 7 Bone, Joint, and Muscle Injuries   104

Chapter 8 Specific Bone and Joint Injuries   117

Chapter 9 Circulatory Emergencies   148

Chapter 10 Respiratory Emergencies   155

Chapter 11 Neurologic Emergencies   171

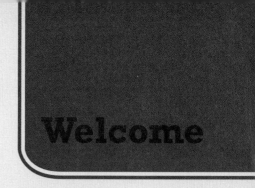

Welcome to the Emergency Care & Safety Institute

Welcome to the Emergency Care & Safety Institute (ECSI), brought to you by the American Academy of Orthopaedic Surgeons (AAOS) and the American College of Emergency Physicians (ACEP).

ECSI is an internationally renowned organization that provides training and certifications that meet job-related requirements as defined by regulatory authorities such as OSHA, The Joint Commission, and state offices of EMS, Education, Transportation, and Health. Our courses are delivered throughout a range of industries and markets worldwide, including colleges and universities, business and industry, government, public safety agencies, hospitals, private training companies, and secondary school systems.

ECSI programs are offered in association with the AAOS and ACEP. AAOS, the world's largest medical organization of musculoskeletal specialists, is known as the original name in EMS publishing with the first EMS textbook ever in 1971, and ACEP is widely recognized as the leading name in all of emergency medicine.

ECSI Course Catalog

Individuals seeking training from ECSI can choose from among various traditional classroom-based courses or alternative online courses such as:

- Advanced Cardiac Life Support
- Automated External Defibrillation (AED)
- Bloodborne and Airborne Pathogens
- Babysitter Safety
- Driver Safety
- CPR (Layperson and Health Care Provider Levels)
- Emergency Medical Responder
- First Aid (Multiple Courses Available)
- Oxygen Administration, and more!

ECSI offers a wide range of textbooks, instructor and student support materials, and interactive technology, including online courses. ECSI student manuals are the center of an integrated teaching and learning system that offers resources to better support instructors and train students. The instructor supplements provide practical hands-on, time-saving tools like PowerPoint presentations, DVDs, and web-based distance learning resources. Technology resources provide interactive exercises and simulations to help students become prepared for any emergency.

Documents attesting to ECSI's recognitions of satisfactory course completion will be issued to those who successfully meet the course requirements. Written acknowledgement of a participant's successful course completion is provided in the form of a Course Completion Card, issued by the Emergency Care & Safety Institute.

Visit www.ECSInstitute.org today!

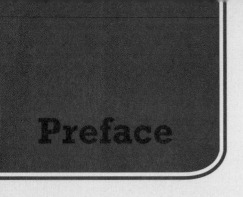

Preface

People who travel, work, recreate, or live in the wilderness and other remote areas must expect that, sooner or later, they will have to deal with an injury or medical problem. *Wilderness First Aid: Emergency Care in Remote Locations* provides comprehensive information about how to deal with medical emergencies when help is hours—even days—away.

This book is a must for outdoor recreationists (hikers, skiers, hunters, climbers, rafters, fishers), for people who work in remote places (farmers, foresters, linesmen, ranchers), for people who live in areas (small communities, ranches, and vacation homes) where the EMS system may not be able to respond immediately to an emergency, and for travelers in countries where medical care may be inadequate or difficult to reach.

This is not a wilderness survival book, although much of the information would help you survive if you were stranded unexpectedly. The information in *Wilderness First Aid: Emergency Care in Remote Locations* covers what to look for and what to do so that you can cope successfully with injury and illness.

The wilderness, national parks, and other remote areas of the United States are receiving more and more pressure from a population intent on using the "great outdoors" for fun, adventure, and travel. Rock climbing, river rafting, kayaking, and fly fishing are a few of the activities drawing millions into the wilderness. Unfortunately, many of these people are poorly prepared to deal with emergencies. Don't be one of the unprepared. Learn how to deal with emergencies before they happen.

Knowledge and understanding can prevent many accidents.

Much of the information in this book is different from what you might read in an urban first aid manual. Wilderness first providers must be prepared to treat problems that they would not be asked to deal with when an ambulance is only minutes away. Some of the procedures are tagged as "Advanced." You need to know about them, but don't use them without additional training.

Prepare yourself for wilderness emergencies by taking a Wilderness First Aid course taught by a qualified instructor. Courses vary in length, depending on how advanced you want your training to be. But when the time comes, the time and money you spend could be one of the best investments of your life.

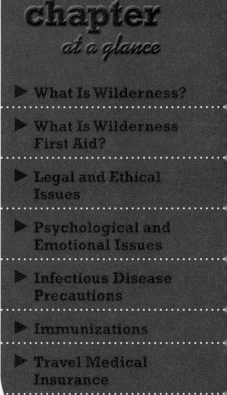

Introduction to Wilderness First Aid

1

▶What Is Wilderness?

Wilderness first aid is needed for activities in remote areas, such as hiking, climbing, camping, sailing, hunting, birding, or snowmobiling. Anyone living in, working in, traveling in, or just enjoying the wilderness should be prepared to manage a medical emergency. Broadly defined, wilderness is a remote geographic location more than 1 hour from definitive medical care **Figure 1-1**. Such locations include areas where outdoor occupations are conducted (farming, ranching, mining, commercial fishing, and forestry **Figure 1-2**), remote communities, developing countries, and urban areas after a disaster destroys infrastructure and overwhelms emergency medical services (EMS).

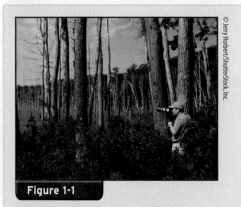

Figure 1-1

Wilderness is defined as any remote geographic location more than 1 hour from definitive medical care.

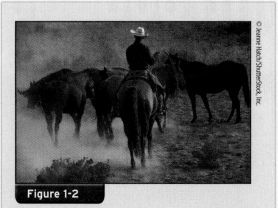

Figure 1-2

Many outdoor occupations occur in remote locations.

▶ What Is Wilderness First Aid?

Wilderness first aid is the immediate care given to an injured or suddenly ill person in a remote location. It does not take the place of definitive medical care. It consists only of providing assistance until a more advanced level of medical care, if needed, is obtained or until the chance for recovery without medical care is apparent.

Wilderness first aid has a distinct focus, because of the following factors:

- Injuries and illnesses occur outdoors, often in adverse conditions (such as heat, cold, high altitude, darkness, rain, and snow) that may affect both victims and rescuers.
- Definitive medical care may be delayed for hours or days by bad weather, a difficult location, and a lack of transportation or communication.
- Certain injuries and illnesses are more common in remote areas (such as altitude illness, frostbite, and wild animal attacks).
- Medical care beyond urban first aid may be needed (for example, reduction of some dislocations and wound management).
- First aid supplies and equipment are limited.
- Difficult decisions must be made (such as whether to start cardiopulmonary resuscitation [CPR] or whether it is necessary to evacuate a victim).

Most first aid books and training courses are designed for first aid providers who will have rapid access to EMS. In these cases, first aid providers usually help for a few minutes until an ambulance arrives, and then their job is finished. However, wilderness first aid may require extended skills, depending on the time and distance from, and the availability of, medical care **Figure 1-3**. A wilderness first aid provider may have to remain with a sick or injured person for many hours or days.

Table 1-1   **Simple Measures That Can Prevent Serious Medical Problems**
• Travel with a companion and let others know where you are going and when you expect to return.
• Do not use drugs or alcohol in the wilderness.
• Carry adequate food and water.
• Carry extra clothing and always anticipate a change in the weather.
• Learn route finding and avalanche avoidance for winter travel.
• Limit your rate of ascent at high altitudes and know the symptoms of altitude illness.
• Always ventilate a stove inside a tent or snow cave.
• Never approach or provoke wild animals.

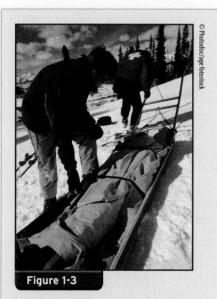

© Photodisc/age fotostock

Figure 1-3

Wilderness first aid may require skills that are not commonly needed in urban areas.

Skillful first aid may make the difference between life and death, rapid recovery and long hospitalization, or temporary disability and permanent injury. Above everything, wilderness first aid stresses prevention Table 1-1 . Prevention techniques are presented throughout this text, because it is much easier to avoid a problem than to manage an existing one.

You must also accept that, unfortunately, you cannot treat or save everyone. Tragic incidents do occur, especially with high-risk wilderness activities Figure 1-4 . Nature is beautiful, powerful, and impersonal, and it can overwhelm as easily as thrill the wilderness traveler. The risk of death increases in a remote area with no access to advanced medical care, and some injuries or illnesses are fatal despite first aid efforts or rapid access to a hospital.

The information in this text will help you manage many common, minor problems and recognize more serious ones. A few advanced first aid measures are discussed to allow you to perform some interventions in a desperate situation. Students interested in more advanced first aid skills, especially those students responsible for others in the wilderness, are encouraged to continue their training beyond this text Figure 1-5 .

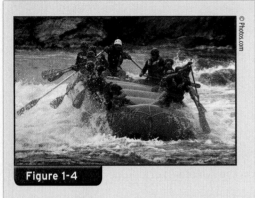

Figure 1-4

Some recreational activities can increase the risk of injury and death.

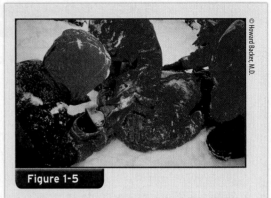

Figure 1-5

You can never have enough knowledge about what to do for injured or suddenly sick victims.

▶ Legal and Ethical Issues

Fear of a lawsuit makes some people wary of helping in an emergency. The following legal principles govern emergency care:

1. You are under no legal obligation to aid a stranger, unless your employment requires it (not only when on duty but sometimes when off duty) or a preexisting responsibility exists. The decision to help in an emergency is usually a moral one.
2. A contractual or legal obligation—a duty to act—applies to park rangers, law enforcement officers, fire fighters, and emergency medical personnel. It also applies to group leaders, guides, and designated health providers for a group.
3. In all instances, you are expected to follow accepted guidelines and act as a prudent person with similar training under the same circumstances would act. Good Samaritan laws do not protect against gross negligence in providing care.
4. You are not expected to give treatment or carry out procedures for which you have not been trained.
5. Many states have Good Samaritan laws that protect first aid providers from successful suits, provided that:
   - The aid is given during an emergency.
   - Treatment is unscheduled, unanticipated (an emergency), and given in good faith.
   - No monetary compensation is received for providing care.
6. You are not expected to place your own life and safety in jeopardy.
7. Once treatment has started, you are legally obligated to remain with the victim until care is turned over to an equally or better trained person or group. Unless your own safety is threatened, leaving a victim may be interpreted as negligent abandonment.

8. Obtain consent before touching a person. Usually consent is verbally expressed or implied. If a victim refuses help, try to persuade him or her to accept it. If a victim is mentally or medically incompetent (incapable of making a rational decision) and acting in a way that is detrimental to his or her health, you are legally justified in providing care. If a victim is a minor (younger than 18 years of age) and a parent or guardian is unavailable, consent is implied and treatment may be given. Most youth programs require signed consent from parents or guardians before minors are allowed to participate.

9. Explain any treatment you are about to give. If treatment involves a procedure such as reducing a dislocated shoulder, explain your training and experience.

10. Whenever possible, involve victims in discussions and decisions concerning their care.

▶ Psychological and Emotional Issues

In a wilderness emergency, first aid providers, as well as victims and bystanders, experience personal stress due to the isolation, absence of definitive medical care, pain, and difficulties of prolonged evacuation. Anxiety or panic may compromise safety and interfere with rescue and first aid. Personality traits often determine how a person reacts to such an emergency.

As a rescuer, you should provide comfort and reassurance to the victim. Reducing anxiety can decrease the pain and severity of injuries by reducing muscular spasm and tension. Try to provide the following support:

- Discuss the victim's condition calmly and honestly.
- Encourage the victim to express his or her feelings. Listen, but do not judge.
- Give realistic answers to the victim's questions, but try to be positive.
- Explain what you are doing and why you are doing it.
- Use stress management techniques such as slow, deep breathing; muscle relaxation; and imagining pleasant events or places to reduce pain and anxiety.
- Let the victim take part in the physical care and ask his or her opinion about decisions involving that care. This helps preserve the victim's dignity and self-esteem and reduces a victim's guilt that might later cause emotional disturbances.

Providing first aid is stressful for both you and the victim. You may feel frustrated by your inability to control the situation or to help, angry at the victim for interfering with your plans or at the dangers and difficulty of the rescue, or sickened by seeing serious injuries. If you feel overwhelmed, stop for a moment, calm yourself, and redirect your thoughts, or ask someone else to help you or (if he or she is equally trained in providing care) to take over.

After treating severe injuries, you may experience posttraumatic stress disorder, an emotional reaction that may include frustration, depression, and flashbacks. These reactions are now well recognized and addressed routinely by professional rescue personnel after difficult situations. To prevent later emotional problems, discuss your feelings with a trusted friend, mental health professional, or clergy member within 24 to 72 hours of helping at a traumatic incident. This brings out feelings quickly and may reduce personal anxieties and stress.

▶ Infectious Disease Precautions

First aid providers risk exposure to infectious diseases when caring for victims. The most serious diseases are bloodborne (caused by microorganisms present in blood). Wear fluid-barrier gloves (latex, vinyl, nitrile, or neoprene) and eye, face, and mouth protection to prevent contact with blood and body fluids **Figure 1-6**. Allergies to latex can be disabling and even life threatening, so caution should be taken to protect those who react when exposed to latex. Admittedly, such precautions may be difficult in many wilderness emergencies. Nonsterile protective gloves and a mouth-to-barrier device for rescue breathing should be carried in the wilderness first aid kit, as well as glasses or goggles to protect against splashing or spurting blood. A bandana can be tied over the mouth and nose to serve as a mask. However, do not delay control of serious bleeding or rescue breathing because protection is not available.

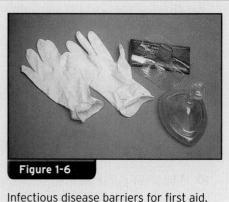

Figure 1-6

Infectious disease barriers for first aid.

Hepatitis B and the human immunodeficiency virus (HIV) infection that causes acquired immunodeficiency syndrome (AIDS) are serious viral diseases that are spread by contact with infected blood. Other infectious bloodborne diseases include hepatitis C and syphilis. Hepatitis B attacks the liver and causes jaundice, chronic illness, and occasional death. HIV disables the immune system, preventing the body from fighting off infections.

Vaccines are available to prevent hepatitis B infection, but not AIDS. People infected with HIV may be unaware that they are contagious. Because of the risk of these serious bloodborne diseases, first aid providers should treat blood and body fluids (since all body fluids may contain blood) as if they are infectious.

After giving first aid, vigorously wash your hands and exposed skin for 15 to 20 seconds with soap, especially if they have been in contact with the victim's blood. If your mouth and/or your eyes are exposed to blood, rinse or flush them with copious amounts of water. Alcohol-based hand sanitizers are also helpful and should be included in wilderness first aid kits.

If exposure to blood has occurred, and especially if there has been direct contact between a victim's blood and a wound on your skin, seek medical advice later. Requesting a test of the victim's blood for HIV may be desirable but is a complicated legal matter. In most cases, such testing cannot be done without the victim's consent.

Try to avoid infections that are spread through the air by coughing and sneezing (for example, tuberculosis) by using a mouth-to-barrier device for rescue breathing. Although the risk of infection while giving first aid is extremely low, and the risk of infection through blood splashing on a mucous membrane (eye, mouth) or contact with blood through minor scrapes on the skin is too low to be accurately measured, it is still important to implement any and all precautions available while you are providing care.

▶ Immunizations

No special immunizations are needed for wilderness activities in North America and other developed areas. Keep routine immunizations up to date. For remote travel in less-developed areas, some special vaccinations may be recommended **Table 1-2**. **Table 1-3** suggests resources for specific information.

Table 1-2   Immunizations

Routine	May Be Required at International Border	Commonly Recommended for International Travel	Special Needs
• Diphtheria, pertussis, tetanus (DPT)	• Yellow fever	• Typhoid	• Hepatitis
• Measles, mumps, rubella (MMR)		• Hepatitis	• Rabies
• Polio			• Japanese encephalitis
			• Meningococcal meningitis

Table 1-3   Resources for Foreign Travel Immunizations

- Current health care provider
- Local county or state health department
- U.S. Public Health Service Quarantine Stations: Chicago, Honolulu, Los Angeles, Miami, New York, San Francisco, Seattle
- The Centers for Disease Control and Prevention
  ◦ Provides detailed, current, printed fax information: toll free (888) 232-3299; http://www.cdc.gov
- The International Association for Medical Assistance to Travelers (IAMAT)
  ◦ Charts immunizations, malaria risk, and lists of doctors overseas: 1623 Military Rd. #279, Niagara Falls, NY 14304-1745; (716) 754-4883; http://www.iamat.org

Cholera immunization is not recommended for any international destination. Hepatitis B vaccination is now routinely given to infants. Tetanus, a serious infection acquired through contamination of wounds, is rarely seen in the United States, because all children are routinely immunized. Adults need a booster shot for tetanus every 10 years. Preexposure rabies vaccination is not needed for North America except for animal researchers or veterinarians, who are at a higher risk than the general public of being bitten.

▶ Travel Medical Insurance

Before traveling internationally, check your medical insurance coverage for illnesses and accidents that occur outside of the United States. Purchase appropriate travel/medical insurance, if necessary.

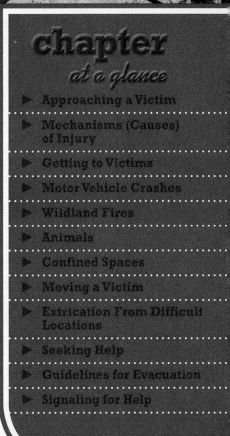

Action at an Emergency

2

Chances are, at some time you will have to decide whether to help another person in distress. Effective action is based on preemergency planning and training. Information about the incident may be sketchy and inaccurate, but it will probably contain something about the nature of the incident; it might have been a submersion, an avalanche, a burn, or a bad laceration. As you approach the scene, review what to do, as well as whom to call for help and how to contact them. You may be a member of a group going to the scene **Figure 2-1**. If so, talk with the other members of the group to decide about assigning responsibilities, because different people will have different skills. If you are not a member of a formal rescue group, choose a leader to make the decisions. Try to arrive at the scene of the incident with at least a basic plan, an understanding of how you can help, and a plan for a course of action if evacuation is necessary.

chapter
at a glance

▶ Approaching a Victim

When you first arrive at the incident scene, do a 10-second scene survey Figure 2-2A-C. Is the site safe? Is another avalanche or rockfall a possibility? Is there a dangerous animal to be avoided? Is there a spreading fire? Is the water too rough for a safe rescue? You cannot help if you become a victim!

In the first few minutes, try to determine the cause of any injuries. The mechanism of an injury may help you to determine its extent or if you should suspect hidden injuries. How many people are injured? There may be more than one victim; look for others.

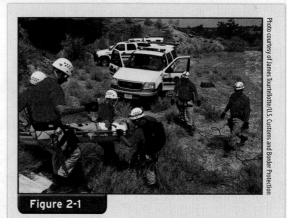

Photo courtesy of James Tourtellotte/U.S. Customs and Border Protection

Figure 2-1

It takes a major effort to evacuate a victim.

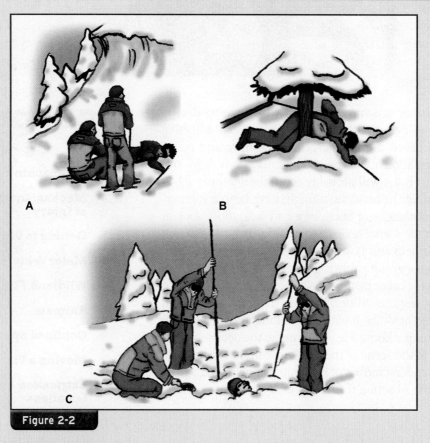

A
B
C

Figure 2-2

Scene survey. **A.** Assess hazards. **B.** Assess the extent and cause of injury. **C.** Determine the number of victims.

▶ Mechanism (Cause) of Injury

Consideration of the mechanism of injury will help you understand the injury and predict its severity. Most injuries involve an impact between a moving object and either another moving object or a stationary object. A moving object develops more energy in proportion to its speed than its weight. If the weight doubles, the energy doubles; but if the speed doubles, the energy increases fourfold.

At an injury scene when you are trying to reconstruct the event, consider the following:

- What was the distance of the fall or the speed of the moving object? Were the forces involved strong enough to produce serious injuries?
- In what direction and on what body part did the forces act?
- Where would you expect to find injuries?
- Are internal injuries likely?
- Is a spinal injury likely?

Suspect multiple, serious injuries, including internal injuries, in the following situations:

- A fall of two and a half to three times body height (this involves large mass and relatively low speed)
- A motorcycle, all-terrain vehicle, or snowmobile crash, especially if no helmet was worn (large mass and high speed are involved)
- A high-speed skier or snowboarder collision (large mass and high speed are involved)
- A gunshot wound of the head, neck, or trunk (small mass and very high speed are involved)

▶ Getting to Victims

Do not attempt a rescue unless it can be done without endangering the rescuers. Weather, the location of the victim, avalanche danger, fire, and entrapment of the victim may all pose hazards. Specialized rescue teams may be needed.

Water Rescue

Reach-throw-row-go is the sequence for attempting a water rescue **Figure 2-3**.

Reach
First, reach for the victim with a lightweight pole, a ladder, a long stick, a branch, or any other available object. Secure your footing. Hold onto a secure object or have a bystander grab your belt or pants for stability. Keep your weight low and back.

Throw
Throw anything available that floats—an empty picnic jug, an empty fuel can, a life jacket, a floating cushion, pieces of wood, an inflated inner tube, or a tire. If possible, tie a rope to the

object to pull in the victim. If you miss, you can retrieve the object and throw again. Few people can accurately throw an object farther than 50 feet.

Row

If the victim is out of range and there is a nearby rowboat, canoe, or motorboat, try rowing to the victim. Boat handling is dangerous and requires skill. Always wear a personal flotation device (PFD) such as a life jacket for your own safety. To avoid capsizing the boat, pull the victim in over the stern or bow, not over the side of the boat.

Go

Rescue a drowning victim by swimming only if you are a strong swimmer and trained in rescue techniques. A swimming rescue, even in calm water, is difficult and hazardous; frequently a would-be rescuer becomes a victim. If you enter the water, wear a life jacket, if available, and carry something (such as an extra life jacket or a plank) to place between you and the victim.

CAUTION
DO NOT try to rescue a drowning person by swimming unless you are trained in lifesaving.

Ice Rescue

If someone falls through ice near the shore, extend a pole or throw a line with a floating object attached. If the victim has fallen through ice far from the shore and cannot be reached with a pole or a thrown line, lie flat and push a ladder, plank, or tree limb ahead of you for the victim to grasp **Figure 2-4**. Another technique is to tie a rope anchored to the shore to a spare tire, lie flat, and push the tire ahead of you. Pull the victim ashore or to the edge of the ice.

Self Rescue

Victims who have fallen through ice should attempt to get their upper bodies onto the ice and pull themselves forward. Once onto the ice, they should keep as flat as possible to spread their weight to reduce the chance of falling through again.

CAUTION
DO NOT go near broken ice without supporting helpers.

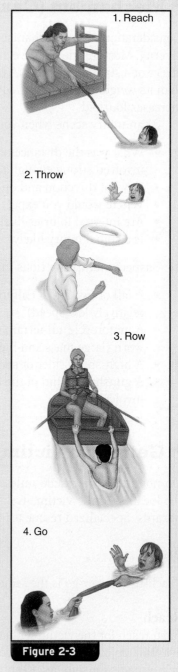

1. Reach

2. Throw

3. Row

4. Go

Figure 2-3

Water rescue rules. 1. Reach. 2. Throw. 3. Row. 4. Go.

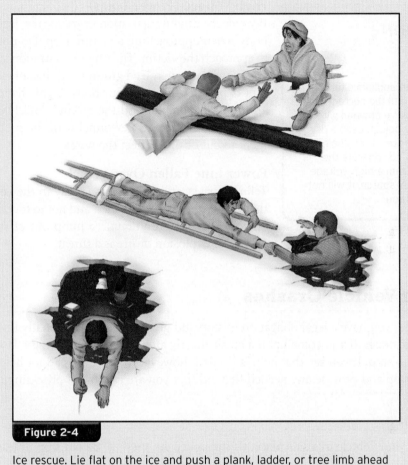

Figure 2-4

Ice rescue. Lie flat on the ice and push a plank, ladder, or tree limb ahead of you for the victim to grasp. Pull the victim to the edge of the ice. Keep as flat on the ice as possible and pull yourself forward.

Electrical Emergency Rescue

Even mild electrical shocks can cause serious internal injuries or death. A voltage of greater than 1,000 volts is considered high voltage, but even the 110 volts of household current can be deadly.

Electricity enters the body at the point of contact and travels along the paths of least resistance (nerves and blood vessels). Current traveling through the body generates heat and destroys cells.

Low Voltage (Inside Buildings)

Most indoor electrocutions are caused by faulty equipment or careless use of appliances. Before approaching the victim, turn off the electricity at the circuit breaker, fuse box, or outside switch box, or unplug the appliance.

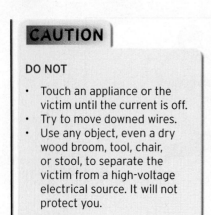

High Voltage (Power Lines)

If you feel a tingling sensation in your arms, legs, or lower body when approaching a victim, stop. Do not continue to approach the victim. The tingling sensation signals that you may be on energized ground and that an electric current is passing through your body. If this happens, turn around, raise one foot off the ground, and hop to a safe place. Wait for trained personnel with the proper equipment to cut or disconnect the wires.

Power Line Fallen Over Vehicle

Tell the driver and passengers to stay in the vehicle. Tell them to keep their arms folded and not to touch the vehicle. No one should attempt to jump out of the vehicle unless an explosion or fire is a threat.

▶ Motor Vehicle Crashes

In most states, you have a legal obligation to stop and give help when personally involved in a motor vehicle crash. If you come upon a crash shortly after it has happened, the law does not require you to stop. If you see that help is needed, however, you should call for help. Morally, you should stop and provide any needed first aid that you are capable of providing.

What to Do

1. Stop your vehicle in a safe place. (If the police are present, do not stop unless asked to do so.)
2. Turn on your flashing hazard lights and place warning reflectors or warning flares.
3. Direct someone to warn other drivers.
4. Try to enter the crashed vehicle through a door. If the doors are jammed, someone inside the car might be able to roll down a window. As a last resort, break a window. Once inside, place the vehicle in park, turn off the engine, and set the parking brake.
5. Stabilize the head and neck of an unresponsive victim or a victim who might have a spinal injury.
6. Look and feel for injuries. Treat life-threatening injuries first.
7. Whenever possible, wait for trained emergency personnel to extricate victims.

▶ Wildland Fires

Back-country travelers and people who live in the urban–wildland interface may encounter wildland fires. They should be aware of how fires spread, the causes of injury and death, and safety measures to avoid the hazards.

Fires have three requirements: heat, oxygen, and fuel . Therefore, fires most commonly occur in hot, dry climates; are fanned into greater intensity by wind; and use trees, bushes, and grass as fuel. Fire spreads by direct extension and spotting (the spread of fire by flying, burning debris).

Be aware of the fire hazards around you. The hazards in your camp include stoves and fuel. Hazards in the environment include dry grass, flammable trees, and bushes. Camp in safe places. Keep fire or stove sites clear of brush and dry fuel. The safest spots near a fire are along its flanks, behind the advancing fire (upwind), and downhill rather than uphill (fires spread rapidly uphill).

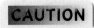

Heat

Oxygen   +   Fuel

Figure 2-5

How fires spread.

Safety during a fire depends on following the LCES principle—lookouts, communication, escape routes, and safety zones. Be constantly on the lookout for changes in the direction of the fire. Be able to communicate these changes to others. Plan your escape routes and potential safety zones.

NOTE

Heart attacks and heat stress are the most common causes of death among fire fighters. Internal trauma, burns, and asphyxiation account for most other deaths. Common injuries include burns and trauma from falling objects.

What to Do

1. Get all people out of the area quickly.
2. Call for help.
3. Use a fire extinguisher only if the fire is small and your own escape route is clear. Fighting a fire during the first 5 minutes is crucial.
4. Throw water over burn victims. Wrap a rug or blanket around the victim's neck and try to keep flames from the face. Flannel sleeping bags are safe wraps, but synthetic sleeping bags and clothing could melt and cause deeper burns if used to smother flames. Roll the victim on the ground to extinguish the flames. Restrain the victim from running, which fans the flames.
5. Remove burning clothing from the victim if possible to do so safely. Synthetic materials—polypropylene, polyester, and nylon—melt rapidly at high temperatures and cause deep, severe burns. Most of the high-tech materials used in outdoor clothing and tents are potentially very hazardous. Some are treated with fire retardants, but all should be regarded as dangerous in fires.

CAUTION

DO NOT
- Let a victim run with clothing on fire.
- Get trapped while fighting a fire. Always keep an escape route open so you can exit rapidly.

▶ Animals

Approach situations involving animals with caution. Large animals do not always retreat from humans and might attack rescuers **Figure 2-6** . Most smaller animals retreat from humans, but all wild animals are unpredictable and might attack even if not provoked. Be aware of the potentially dangerous animals in the area where you are traveling. Farm animals can also be dangerous.

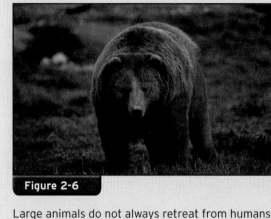

Figure 2-6

Large animals do not always retreat from humans and might attack rescuers.

When threatened by an animal, you should take the following actions:

- Do not stare at the animal. Instead, look down or away.
- Back away slowly.
- Speak quietly to reassure the animal.

If an animal has attacked another person, take the following actions:

- Use food to lure the animal away from the victim.
- It may back off after attacking. This affords you a chance to remove the victim.
- Animal attacks are rare but dangerous. In general, if you are attacked, fight back. An exception to this recommendation is an encounter with a grizzly bear or a mother black bear with her cubs. In these situations, you should lie down and play dead. In bear country, make noises as you travel, and be especially cautious if you see a mother bear with cubs.

▶ Confined Spaces

A confined space is an area such as a tank, vessel, vat, silo, bin, vault, cave, or mine shaft, and it might present a dangerous atmosphere. If a person becomes trapped in a confined space, take the following actions:

- Call for immediate help; activate the local emergency medical services (EMS).
- Do not rush in to help; the space could be filled with toxic gas.
- Try to rescue the victim without entering the space.
- If entry is necessary, trained and properly equipped rescuers must be the ones who enter the space to remove the victim.
- Administer first aid or CPR if necessary.

▶ Moving a Victim

Do not move a victim until he or she is in stable condition and ready for transportation. First provide all necessary first aid. Moving a victim in unstable condition should be done only if there is immediate danger from environmental hazards, if it is impossible to gain access to other victims (for example, in a vehicle) who need lifesaving care, or if the victim's heart has stopped. In any of these cases, you may move the victim to a flat, firm surface on which CPR can be carried out. Move the victim if it is impossible to administer first aid at the scene.

> **CAUTION**
>
> **DO NOT**
> - Move victims prematurely unless they are in immediate danger or must be moved to shelter while waiting for rescue.
> - Make an injury worse by moving the victim.
> - Move a victim who might have a spinal cord injury without first stabilizing the spine.
> - Move a victim unless you know where you are going to place him or her.
> - Try to move a victim by yourself if others are available to help.

Emergency Moves

Do not move the victim too quickly, because this could aggravate a spinal injury or other major injury. Place the victim supine (flat on his or her back with face and chest up). Protect the spine. If time and safety permit, stabilize all injured parts before and during the move.

Drags

To carry a victim a short distance over a rough surface, use a shoulder drag or blanket drag. For a shoulder drag, stabilize the victim's head with your forearms **Figure 2-7A**. For a blanket drag, roll the victim onto a blanket and pull from behind the head **Figure 2-7B**.

Nonemergency Moves

One-Person Moves

You can help a victim to walk by acting as a human crutch; if one leg is injured, the victim can walk on the uninjured leg while you support the injured side. Use a piggyback carry when the

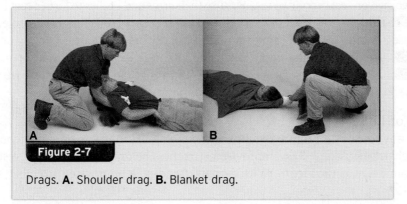

Figure 2-7

Drags. **A.** Shoulder drag. **B.** Blanket drag.

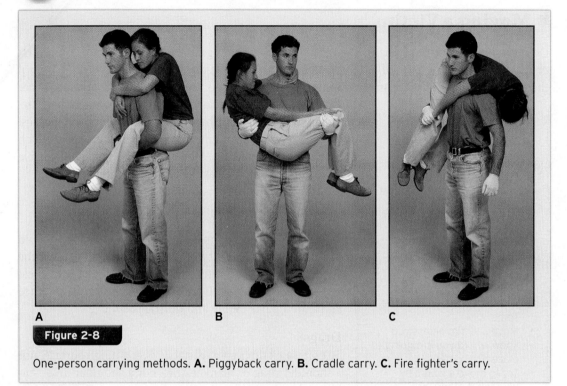

A   B   C

Figure 2-8

One-person carrying methods. **A.** Piggyback carry. **B.** Cradle carry. **C.** Fire fighter's carry.

victim cannot walk but can hang on to you **Figure 2-8A**. Use a cradle carry for children and lightweight adults who cannot walk and in whom spinal injury is not suspected **Figure 2-8B**. Use a fire fighter's carry if the victim's injuries permit; longer distances can be traveled if the victim is carried over your shoulder **Figure 2-8C**.

Two-or-More-Person Moves

Two or more people can help a victim to walk by using the two-person walking assist **Figure 2-9A**. With the two-person seat carry, two rescuers use their arms and bodies to form a seat for the victim **Figure 2-9B**. The four-handed seat carry is the easiest two-person carry when no equipment is available; use it when the victim cannot walk but can use his or her arms to hang on to rescuers **Figure 2-9C**. Use an extremity carry when the victim is located in a tight or narrow space **Figure 2-9D**. Use a hammock carry if three to six people can stand on alternate sides of the injured person and link their hands beneath the victim **Figure 2-9E**.

Stretcher or Litter

The safest way to carry an injured victim without a spinal injury is on a stretcher or impro-vised stretcher **Table 2-1**. Test improvised stretchers before use by lifting a rescuer who is about the same size as the victim. With a blanket-and-pole improvised stretcher, the victim's

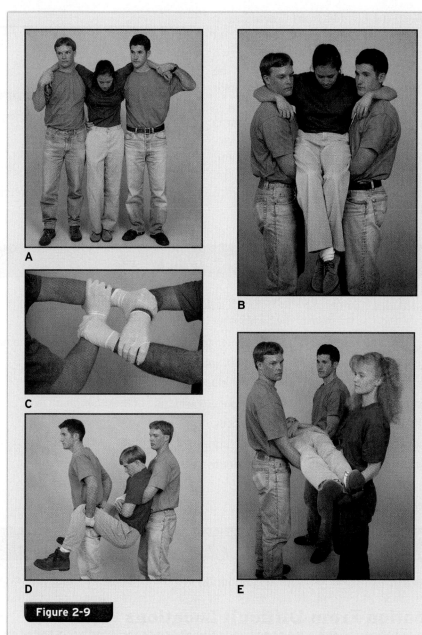

Figure 2-9

Two-person carrying methods. **A.** Two people assisting a victim to walk.
B. Two-handed seat carry. **C.** Four-handed seat carry. **D.** Extremity carry.
E. Hammock carry.

weight will keep the blanket from unwinding if it is properly wrapped **Figure 2-10**. Jackets and poles can also be used as a stretcher. Usually two jackets are required for adults. Button or zip up the jackets, invert the arms, and pass poles through the arm holes. An improvised board stretcher is sturdier than a blanket-and-pole stretcher but is also heavier and less comfortable. Secure the victim to the board. Skis, pack frames, sleds, and tree limbs can also be used to make stretchers. Pad stretchers well, using sleeping bags, clothing, or sleeping pads. Commercial stretchers are seldom available except with rescue groups.

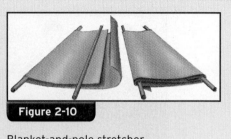

Figure 2-10

Blanket-and-pole stretcher.

Table 2-1   Principles of Lifting and Carrying
• Do not try to handle a load that is awkward or too heavy—seek help.
• Use a safe grip. Use the palm of the hand rather than the fingers.
• Keep your back straight **Figure 2-11**. Tighten the muscles of your buttocks and abdomen.
• Bend your knees to use the strong muscles of your thighs and buttocks.
• Keep your arms close to your body and your elbows flexed.
• Position your feet at shoulder width for balance, one in front of the other.
• When lifting, keep the victim close to your body.
• Do not twist your back; pivot with the feet.
• Lift slowly, smoothly, and in unison with other helpers.
• Tell the victim what you are about to do.
• Rest periodically.

▶ Extrication From Difficult Locations

An injured person might have been thrown or might have fallen into a site from which extraction is difficult. There are six positions in which the body can be trapped **Figure 2-12**.

Moving a victim from a position in which the body is distorted and crumpled requires skill and should not be attempted by untrained rescuers or by one person acting alone.

Four to six experienced rescuers are needed to move a victim safely. One person in the group is designated as the leader who gives all commands. The group must lift the victim as a unit, all working simultaneously and with a clear idea of what is being attempted.

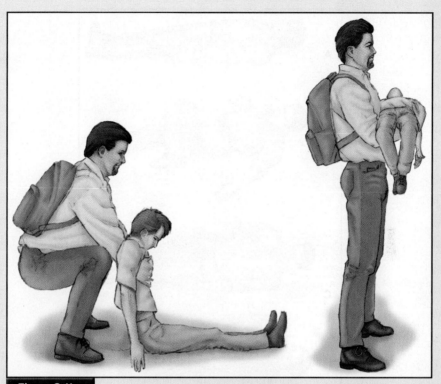

Figure 2-11

When lifting and carrying a victim, keep your back straight and bend your knees. Keep the victim close to your body.

CAUTION

DO NOT lift a victim with one person at the head and another at the feet (with the victim hanging like a U) unless you are certain there is no spinal injury.

The objective is to lay the victim flat on his or her back with the head and neck stabilized and the shoulders and hips at right angles to the vertebral column **Figure 2-12A** .

Concentrate on supporting the head and neck, the shoulders, and the hips. The victim does not have to be moved from the position in which he or she is found into the neutral, supine position in a single movement. Move the victim in stages.

The most difficult extraction is from a small space with limited access for rescuers. If there is any suspicion of a spinal injury, do not attempt to extract the victim, which could make matters worse. Wait for a rescue group with special equipment. You can help by keeping the victim warm and comfortable; providing food, drink, and encouragement; and getting help as quickly as possible.

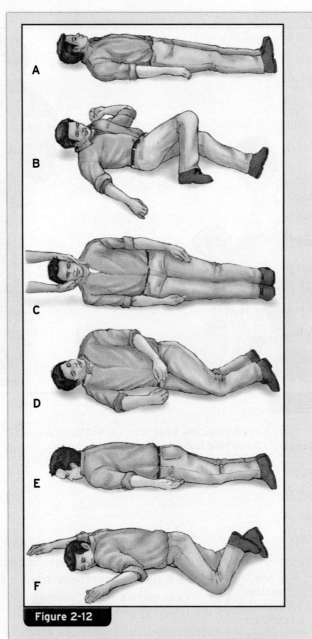

Figure 2-12

Basic body positions found in entrapment. **A.** Supine, neutral position, with all limbs aligned. **B.** Supine, but with head, back, or limbs out of alignment. **C.** On either side, neutral position, with limbs and back aligned normally. **D.** On either side, but with head, back, or limbs out of alignment. **E.** Prone, in neutral position, with limbs aligned. **F.** Prone, but with head, back, or limbs out of alignment.

▶ Seeking Help

Seeking help in the wilderness is always difficult, and it may be impossible when emergencies occur far from the nearest road or telephone. Before you go into a wilderness, know how to contact the local rescue group, sheriff, or police. Distance, weather, time of day, and the number of people available to go for help may limit what you do. In the face of an emergency, think of the mnemonic STOP **Figure 2-13** .

Stop and take a moment to calm yourself. Do not panic.
Think about the problem and the correct course of action.
Observe the situation. What has occurred? What are the conditions? What resources are available?
Plan your course of action and coordinate with the other potential rescuers **Table 2-2** .

If the situation is not an emergency, the victim may be able to walk out of the area. However, if in doubt, contact medical help. If you are with a group, send a member of the party to the nearest telephone, or, in very remote areas, try using signal mirrors, flares, or smoking fires. Many hikers now carry cellular phones, but these do not work in all areas, for example where mountains or ridges block the signals. Cellular phones and other electronic devices should be

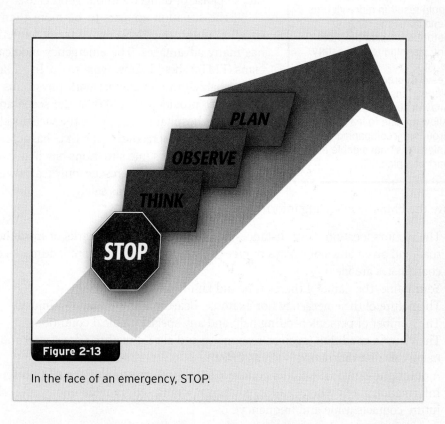

Figure 2-13

In the face of an emergency, STOP.

Table 2-2 Important Planning Questions

1. Can you handle the problem in the field and let the victim continue with the trip, such as a victim with a minor wound or injury or self-limited illness? Because you may be far from help, it is reasonable to wait and observe the victim before deciding to seek help.

2. Can the person walk unaided? This may be the fastest and safest means to reach medical care—despite a painful ankle or knee injury or after a venomous snake bite.

3. Does the victim need to be carried, and do you have the resources to do this? If not, how do you get help?

CAUTION

DO NOT

- Rush to rescue in a dangerous situation; this could result in more victims.
- Send someone for help before assessing the victim and planning for the safety of all.
- Leave injured or sick victims alone in the field, unless it is unavoidable.
- Allow anyone to leave the group unaccompanied unless it is unavoidable and part of a plan.

used sparingly and ethically. Rescue groups should not be summoned for minor injuries. Many rescue groups are composed of volunteers; they must not be put to unnecessary expense or danger without good cause.

If the situation appears to be more than you can handle, contact the EMS. Use of trained rescue groups has many advantages. The emergency medical technicians (EMTs) should know what to do. In addition, they are probably in radio contact with physicians at a hospital. Care provided by EMTs at the scene and on the way to the hospital can improve the victim's chances of survival and rate of recovery. The EMS has access to rapid transportation. In some situations, such as cave rescue and high-angle mountain rescue, only teams with special training can rescue victims safely.

Give the EMS the following information:

- The victim's location. Give distances from recognizable landmarks or from the nearest road and give names of valleys or creeks. Compass bearings from landmarks and map coordinates are ideal.
- Your name, the name of the victim, and family contacts.
- The nature of the emergency (for example, heart attack, submersion injury).
- The number of persons needing help and any special medical conditions.
- The victim's condition (such as responsive and alert, breathing, fractures) and what is being done for the victim (such as CPR).
- A description of local weather conditions if the information might affect rescue plans.
- Information about where, and if, you can be contacted; provide information about future contacts (time and frequency).

On the radio or phone, speak slowly and clearly. Ask the rescuers to repeat important information. Always be the last to hang up. If you send someone to make the call, have the caller report back to you to ensure the call was made.

▶ Guidelines for Evacuation

Each section in this text will consider criteria for evacuation of people with specific problems.

General Guidelines

The victim's health or survival may depend on your ability to move him or her from the scene. The following list describes conditions that may necessitate evacuation.

1. Deteriorating condition, increasing shortness of breath, altered mental status, shock, progressive weakness, persistent vomiting and/or diarrhea, inability to tolerate oral fluids, or fainting when attempting to stand
2. Severe pain
3. Inability to walk at a reasonable pace due to a medical problem
4. Severe or ongoing bleeding from any site, including wounds; blood in the vomit or stool
5. Signs and symptoms of serious high-altitude illness
6. Worsening infections
7. Chest pain that is not clearly musculoskeletal in origin—possible heart attack
8. Psychological disorder that impairs the safety of the person or group
9. Submersion injury
10. Large or serious wounds or burns or wounds with particular complications, such as fractures that break the overlying skin, gunshot wounds, deformed fractures, fractures with impaired circulation, impaled objects, or suspected spinal injury
11. Serious mechanism of injury (that at least warrants close observation) such as a fall from greater than 20 feet; a motorcycle, all-terrain vehicle, or snowmobile crash; a closed vehicle crash involving high speed, rollover, victim ejection, or death of another occupant; a high-speed skiing collision; or an injury by rockfall or avalanche

Travel may continue if it is toward medical care in the case of points 3, 4, and 8, or when descending in the case of point 5.*

---

*Adapted from the *Wilderness Medical Society Practice Guidelines for Wilderness Emergency Care*. Guilford, CT: The Globe Pequot Press, 2006.

▶ Signaling for Help

Many emergency conditions require a search for people in distress. Under such circumstances, it is always better if the people being sought know how to make their presence and their location conspicuous.

Signaling Aircraft

When you are creating a ground signal that people in an aircraft can see, remember that there are few straight lines or right angles in nature and that things are a lot smaller when viewed from the air. Bigger is almost always better. For ground signals, make a large "V" for immediate assistance or an "X" if medical assistance is needed. Make the lines of these signals as large as you can. Construct your signal so that each line is six times as long as it is wide, such as a "V" with each side 12 feet long and 2 feet wide. Contrast is another key to ground signals. Examples of materials to use include toilet paper, strips of plastic tarp, strips of tent material, tree branches, logs, and light-colored rocks. In snow and on open ground or sandy shores, signals may be tramped or dug into the surface using shadows to make the signals stand out.

Other Signals

A series of three of almost anything indicates "Help." Examples include three shouts, three shots, three blasts from a whistle, or three flashes from a light. Use smoke by day and bright flame by night if other signaling devices are not available. Add engine oil, rags soaked in oil, or pieces of rubber to your fire to make black smoke (best against a light background). Keep plenty of spare fuel on hand. If you are tending a fire as you wait for help, keep fuel handy and throw it on the fire when you hear an aircraft; do not wait, because it takes time for smoke to form and rise. Make sure to start the fire away from combustibles such as grass or trees.

A mirror is an effective means of sending a distress signal. On hazy days, aircraft pilots can see the flash of a mirror before survivors can see the aircraft, so it is wise to flash the mirror in the direction of a plane when you hear it, even when you cannot see it. Mirror flashes have been spotted by rescue aircraft more than 20 miles away.

To use a mirror, follow this procedure:

1. Hold the mirror up to the sun with one hand, and stretch your other hand out in front of you. Use your finger or thumb to block your view of your target.
2. Hit your extended finger or thumb with a reflection of the sun from the mirror.
3. Repeatedly flick the spot of light from the mirror across the finger or thumb and the target.
4. Try to hit the aircraft or rescuers with a flash as much as possible. Do not attempt to do series of three flashes—it is too difficult **Figure 2-14** .

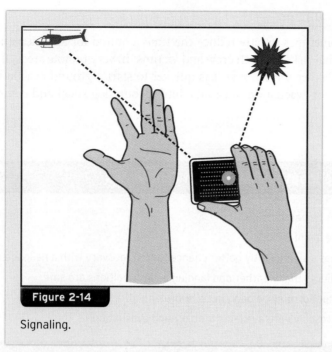

Figure 2-14

Signaling.

FYI

Survival Kit: The Bare Essentials

Minimal items	Purpose
One or two large plastic trash bags or an emergency blanket ("space blanket") made of Mylar	Protects against weather (wind, rain, snow). Wear one trash bag by cutting a hole in the bottom of the bag for your head; use the second bag to cover your legs.
Whistle (Mini Fox 40 or Windstorm)	Signal for help.
Signal mirror	Signal for help.
Metal match with striker (magnesium)	Start a fire.
Waterproof match case containing windproof and waterproof matches	Start a fire.
Waterproof match case or empty film canister containing several cotton balls smeared with petroleum jelly (such as Vaseline) or commercial tinder tabs	Petroleum jelly is flammable. Make tinder using cotton balls smeared with petroleum jelly. When using, open a cotton ball up to catch sparks from metal match.
Knife (multitool) and/or wire blade survival saw	Cutting
Food (such as energy bars and MREs [US military surplus meals-ready-to-eat])	Provides calories and a psychological boost

Helicopter Evacuation

Helicopters can sometimes greatly reduce the time required for an emergency transport, but they create additional risks for both crew and victims. In very remote areas, it may take so long to contact the helicopter service that it is quicker to start a ground evacuation. The decision to use a helicopter for evacuation must take into account logistical and environmental factors **Table 2-3**.

Table 2-3 Helicopter Evacuation Guidelines

Evacuate victims by helicopter if:

1. A victim's life might be saved.
2. The victim has a significantly better chance for full recovery with a helicopter evacuation.
3. The pilot believes that weather and landing zone conditions are safe.
4. Ground evacuation may be dangerous or prolonged.
5. Not enough rescuers are available for a ground evacuation.

Victim Assessment and Urgent Care

3

▶ Assessment

To find out what is wrong with a victim, you must be able to do a rapid, but accurate, examination, called an assessment. In wilderness first aid, help and other resources are limited, care for serious injuries and illnesses may be primitive, and the only first aid equipment available is what you have with you or can improvise. Unlike with urban first aid, there is often no way to call 9-1-1, there are probably no EMTs to take over for you, and there is often no ambulance available at all or not quickly accessible to transport the victim. The decision, however necessary, to transport a victim to medical care cannot be made lightly, because it takes time and manpower. Therefore, the ability to find out what is occurring and its significance through the development of good assessment skills is very important.

This chapter presents a detailed and systematic method for assessing a victim and giving urgent first

Table 3-1 Sequence of Victim Assessment

Injured Victim			Suddenly Ill Victim	
	Responsive			
Unresponsive	With Significant COI	Without Significant COI	Unresponsive	Responsive
• Primary check • Secondary check using the DOS parts of DOTS • SAMPLE history from others	• Primary check • Secondary check using DOTS • SAMPLE history	• Primary check • Examine chief complaint using DOTS • SAMPLE history	• Primary check • Secondary check using the DOS parts of DOTS • SAMPLE history from others	• Primary check • SAMPLE history • Examine chief complaint

COI = cause of injury; also known as mechanism of injury. DOTS = deformity, open wounds, tenderness, swelling. SAMPLE = symptoms, allergies, medications, pertinent history, last oral intake, and events leading up to the illness or injury

aid. Assessment must be learned well and practiced regularly to avoid missing important, life-threatening problems.

Assessment takes different forms, depending on whether the victim is responsive or unresponsive, injured or ill. The terms responsive and unresponsive are used instead of conscious and unconscious, because they identify what the first aid provider actually observes and do not require a diagnosis. Not all parts of the assessment process will apply to every victim, and the order of use of these parts may vary depending on the nature of the victim's problem(s). Most victims do not require a complete assessment. For example, a victim who cuts a finger while whittling a stick will not require a complete assessment, but a victim with a cut finger from slipping and falling 20 feet down a mountainside will, because other injuries might be present as well. Also, a victim might be injured and ill at the same time.

Victim assessment is divided into five parts: (1) scene size-up, (2) primary assessment, (3) history taking, (4) secondary assessment (vital signs and physical exam), and (5) reassessment. **Table 3-1** outlines the assessment sequences for injured and ill, responsive and unresponsive victims.

▶ Scene Size-up

The scene size-up gives you the first impression of what has happened and reveals hazards to the victim or to you **Figure 3-1**. Before beginning a scene size-up, always protect yourself if there is a chance of contact with blood or other body fluids. Put on medical exam gloves before entering the scene. In cold weather, put them over a thin pair of polypropylene or silk gloves to avoid chilling your hands.

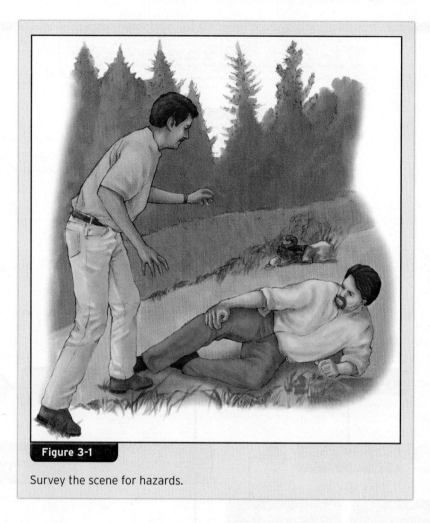

Figure 3-1

Survey the scene for hazards.

What to Look For

Look for the cause of the victim's condition and related problems at the scene. Ask yourself the following questions:

- Is the scene safe? Is there immediate danger to you and others?
- Is the victim injured or ill?
- If the victim is injured, what is the probable mechanism (cause) of injury?
- Is the victim obviously responsive or possibly unresponsive?
- As a general impression, does the victim appear critically injured or ill?
- How many victims are there?

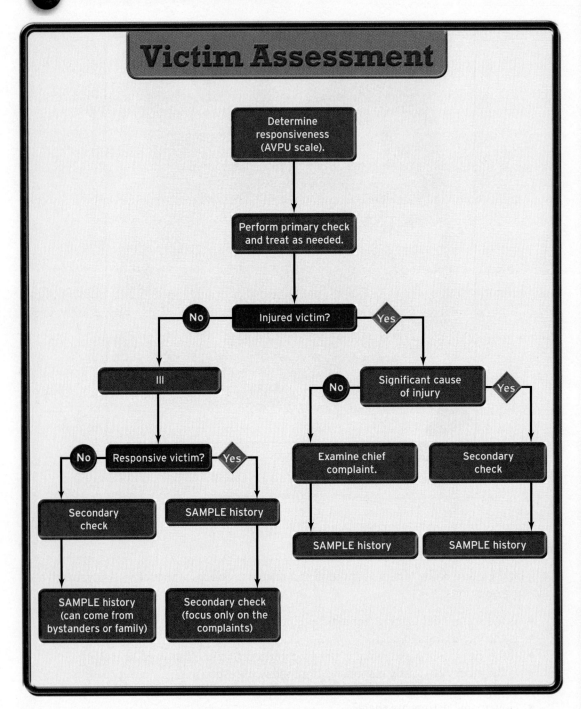

Victim Assessment

Determine responsiveness (AVPU scale).

Perform primary check and treat as needed.

Injured victim?

No → III

Yes → Significant cause of injury

III → Responsive victim?

No → Secondary check → SAMPLE history (can come from bystanders or family)

Yes → SAMPLE history → Secondary check (focus only on the complaints)

Significant cause of injury
No → Examine chief complaint. → SAMPLE history
Yes → Secondary check → SAMPLE history

▶ Primary Assessment

Do a primary assessment to detect any life-threatening conditions needing urgent care. It is important to know whether a victim is responsive or not. A responsive victim is alert, interacts with you, and knows his/her name and location. However, remember that in the wilderness it is not uncommon to lose track of the date or even the day of the week. If, by the time you reach the victim, you are unsure about the level of responsiveness, tap or gently shake the victim's shoulder and ask, "Are you okay?" If the victim does not answer or the answer is garbled or unintelligible, the victim is considered unresponsive. Start immediate preparations to evacuate the victim to medical care. If other people are nearby, call for help.

The primary assessment assesses breathing problems and bleeding, the two most immediate threats to life. If critical problems with breathing or massive bleeding are identified, attend to them immediately before proceeding further. Correct problems as you find them.

Assess the Airway

A responsive person who can speak in full sentences generally does not have an immediate breathing problem. If a responsive person cannot speak or cough, treat for an obstructed airway. Check breathing in an unresponsive victim.

Assess Breathing

Determine whether the victim is breathing normally, breathing inadequately, or not breathing. Look for rise and fall of the victim's chest.

What to Do

If the unresponsive victim is breathing normally, position him or her in the recovery position, which helps to keep the victim's tongue from falling back and blocking the airway. Vomit is also likely to be expelled if the victim is in this position. To position an unresponsive victim who is on his or her back, follow the steps in **Skill Drill 3-1**.

1. Bend the victim's left elbow to a right angle with the hand and arm still on the ground but above the head. Keep the victim's legs straight (**Step ❶**).
2. Place the victim's right hand against the left cheek with the palm facing outward. Put your right palm over the victim's right palm (**Step ❷**).
3. While keeping your palm against the victim's palm, grasp behind the victim's right bent knee and roll the victim toward you onto the left side. Keep the victim's head, shoulders, and torso moving together without twisting (**Step ❸**).
4. Keep the victim's right hand under the cheek to keep the head tilted and the top leg bent to prevent rolling (**Step ❹**).

If the victim is not breathing, give cardiopulmonary resuscitation (CPR), starting with chest compressions. See the appendix *CPR Basics* for detailed instructions. It is very difficult to assess or care for an unresponsive victim who is lying face down or on his or her side. Therefore, if

skill drill

3-1 Moving the Victim into the Recovery Position

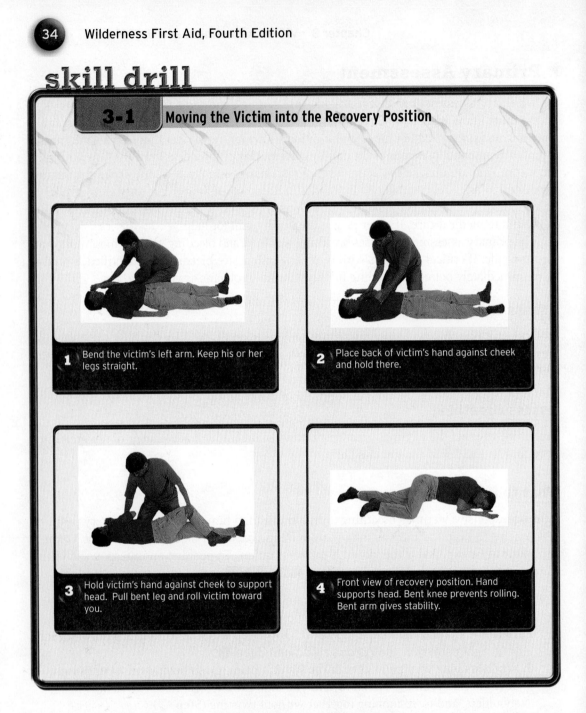

1 Bend the victim's left arm. Keep his or her legs straight.

2 Place back of victim's hand against cheek and hold there.

3 Hold victim's hand against cheek to support head. Pull bent leg and roll victim toward you.

4 Front view of recovery position. Hand supports head. Bent knee prevents rolling. Bent arm gives stability.

the victim is not lying face up, he or she must be rolled rapidly into that position. If help is available, use a log-roll maneuver **Figure 3-2**. If you are alone, roll the victim's body as a unit, with minimal bending or twisting of the back and neck:

1. With your hand that is nearest the victim's head, grasp the victim's neck just below the back of the head.

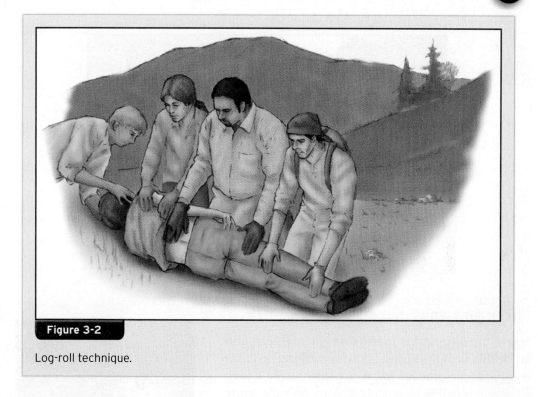

Figure 3-2

Log-roll technique.

2. With your other hand, grasp the edge of the victim's far hip or the clothing over the edge of the hip.
3. Gently roll the victim toward you.
4. After 30 chest compressions, give two rescue breaths.

To give rescue breaths, follow these steps:

1. Keep the airway open with the head tilt–chin lift maneuver.
2. Pinch the victim's nose shut.
3. To protect yourself against the victim's saliva, use a mouth-to-barrier device (face shield or face mask) if one is available **Figure 3-3A-B** .
4. Take a normal breath and seal your lips tightly around the victim's mouth or the mouthpiece of the barrier device.
5. Give two normal breaths, each lasting 1 second. Take a breath for yourself after each breath given to the victim.

If the first breath does not inflate the chest, reopen the airway and try another breath. If you are still unsuccessful, suspect a foreign body airway obstruction. After the two rescue breaths have been given (whether they were successful or not), if the victim is still not breathing, continue CPR.

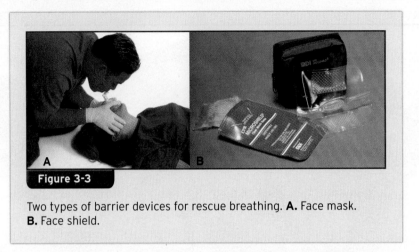

Figure 3-3

Two types of barrier devices for rescue breathing. **A.** Face mask. **B.** Face shield.

Check for Hemorrhage

Severe bleeding, either external or internal, can also be life threatening, because a victim can bleed to death within minutes from an injury to a large artery. Check for severe bleeding by quickly looking over the entire body for blood (blood-soaked clothing, blood spurting or flowing from a wound, and/or blood pooling on the ground). If you find blood, immediately expose the affected body area by moving, removing, or cutting clothing to find the bleeding source. Avoid contact with the victim's blood, if possible, by using vinyl or latex gloves or extra layers of cloth or dressings, and by wearing glasses or goggles and water-resistant clothing. To control bleeding, apply direct pressure over the bleeding area **Figure 3-4**.

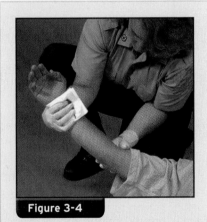

Figure 3-4

Most external bleeding can be stopped with direct pressure.

▶ History Taking

Use the mnemonic SAMPLE, which is explained in the following sections, to remember the steps in obtaining the victim's history. The best person to give the history is the victim. If the victim is unresponsive or unable to cooperate, some or all of the history can be obtained from companions. Also, ask about and check for an emergency medical identification tag. You should look for MedicAlert® emblems as an indication of the patient's medical history. The internationally recognized symbol is found on necklaces, arm bracelets, ankle bracelets, watches, rings, and wallet cards and is carried by people who have a medical condition that warrants special attention if they become ill or injured **Figure 3-5**. This is a victim directive that allows EMS personnel to access the victim's stored medical information by calling the MedicAlert Foundation. Each MedicAlert member has a unique, secure victim identifier engraved at the bottom of his or her emblem. By wearing this emblem, the victim has consented to the release of information to attending medical personnel. The stored information can include conditions, allergies, medications (and dosages), and implanted devices. If you find such a warning on a victim, it is your responsibility to give this information to the next person in the EMS system.

If you find no tags, check an unresponsive victim's wallet or purse for special medical alert cards (if possible, have a witness present before you do this).

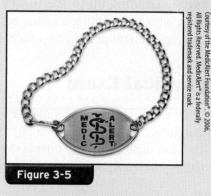

Figure 3-5

Medical identification is found on wrist and ankle bracelets, necklaces, watches, rings, and wallet cards.

SAMPLE Mnemonic

S: Symptoms
What symptoms accompany the present event? A symptom is a subjective problem that the victim notices and describes to you **Figure 3-6**. The symptoms of various injuries are given in detail in later chapters.

A: Allergies
Find out about any allergies to medicines, foods, insect stings, and so on. The problem might be related to an allergic reaction.

M: Medications
Is the victim taking any prescription or nonprescription medicines (or illegal drugs)? If so, find out why the victim is taking the medication(s).

P: Past Relevant Medical History
Find out about preexisting significant conditions, such as diabetes, heart disease, or high blood pressure. These conditions may be contributing to the current problem. Is the victim seeing a physician for any medical condition?

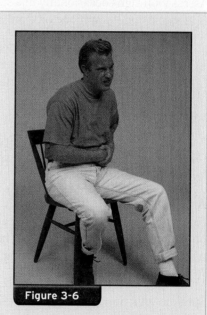

Figure 3-6

Symptom: a condition described by a victim, such as abdominal pain.

L: Last Oral Intake
When was the victim's last ingestion of food or drink? It is important to know if the victim's condition is related to dehydration, weakness from lack of food, or a complication of diabetes.

E: Events Leading up to the Injury or Illness

Find out whether anything unusual occurred before the victim became ill or injured. Finally, ask, "Is there anything else that I should know?"

▶ Physical Exam

The vital signs you assess include the victim's level of responsiveness, pulse, breathing, body temperature, and skin condition. Always check vital signs at the start of a physical exam. Assess vital signs frequently during the assessment and first aid of an unstable or seriously ill or injured victim. A victim is in unstable condition if one or more of the following is present:

- The victim's vital signs and/or mental status are abnormal and/or changing.
- The victim has obvious serious injuries and/or the mechanism of injury suggests that multiple and/or serious injuries might have occurred.
- The victim appears seriously ill.

Assess vital signs occasionally in a stable victim or one with a minor illness or injury. A victim is in stable condition if one or more of the following is present:

- The victim's vital signs and mental status are normal and unchanging.
- The victim has no obvious serious injuries or illness and the mechanism of injury does not suggest that multiple and/or serious injuries may have occurred.

Level of Responsiveness

A method commonly used to grade the level of responsiveness is called the AVPU scale. Record the letter (A, V, P, or U) that corresponds to the victim's condition each time you assess the level of responsiveness.

A: Awake and Alert

Talk to the victim. If he or she appears to be awake and alert, ask for his or her name, address, phone number, location, and what happened. Do not ask what day it is, since it is easy to lose track of the days when on vacations and excursions.

V: Responsive to Verbal stimuli

Speak to a victim appearing to be asleep or motionless. If the victim responds in some way to your voice (i.e., stirs, moans, or opens eyes), he or she fits into this category.

P: Responsive to Pain

A victim in this category does not react to your voice or your questions, but does react (i.e., moaning, stirring, or pulling away an arm or leg) to pain from a gentle but firm pinching of the muscle above the clavicle, pinching the victim's fingers, or rubbing your knuckle on the victim's sternum).

U: Unresponsive

A victim is classified as unresponsive when he or she fails to respond to your voice or when pain is inflicted.

Pulse

To find the radial pulse, place your index and middle fingertips 2" above the base of the thumb on the wrist **Figure 3-7**. Repeatedly practice finding the radial pulse on yourself and your companions until you can find it easily and quickly.

For unresponsive victims, lay rescuers do not use the carotid pulse (in the neck) to determine if CPR is needed. However, for severe hypothermic victims, all rescuers are advised to feel the carotid artery, found in the indentation next to the Adam's apple, for 30 to 45 seconds. Do not press on both of the carotid arteries at the same time.

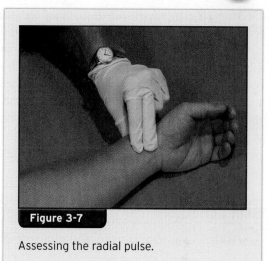

Figure 3-7

Assessing the radial pulse.

For extremity (arm, leg) injuries, check the blood flow (circulation). For an arm injury, feel for the radial pulse; for a leg injury, use the posterior tibial pulse (located between the inside ankle bone and the Achilles tendon). If there is no pulse, gently realign the extremity to try to restore the blood flow. A pulseless arm or leg requires surgical care within a few hours.

Breathing

Listen for abnormal sounds such as the following:

- Snoring or stridor (high-pitched noises when breathing in). If either is present, you need to recheck the airway—it may need repositioning.
- Wheezing (high-pitched noises when breathing out). This could indicate narrowing of the small air passages, as in asthma, bronchitis, or pulmonary edema. Inquire about a history of asthma, emphysema, or heart disease.
- Gurgling or rattling. Material in the airway, such as blood, mucus, or vomit, and the like, may be causing partial blockage.

Temperature

Body temperature may alert you to fever, heat illness, or hypothermia. Measure body temperature with a thermometer placed under the tongue for 3 minutes with the lips tightly closed or in the rectum for 3 minutes. In small children or disoriented adults, put the thermometer in the armpit for at least 5 minutes. Rectal temperatures are the most accurate but are difficult to take, especially in bad weather.

Normal body temperature is 98.6°F (range 97°–99°F) when measured by mouth. Normal rectal temperature is 99.6°F; normal axillary (armpit) temperature is 97.6°F. Carry a thermometer in your first aid kit; in cold weather, it should be a special low-reading one **Figure 3-8**.

Electronic thermometers are designed to measure the temperature in the ear canal, mouth, or rectum. If a thermometer is unavailable, you can estimate the victim's body temperature by putting the back of one hand (not the fingertips) on the victim's forehead (or, preferably, on the abdomen inside the shirt) and comparing it with your own skin temperature obtained at the same location. In a cold environment, the temperature of exposed skin is an unreliable indicator of body temperature.

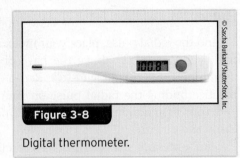

Figure 3-8

Digital thermometer.

Skin Condition

Assess the color, temperature, and moisture of the skin.

Color and Temperature

Skin color, especially in light-skinned persons, depends on the skin circulation and the amount of oxygen in the blood. In darkly pigmented people, changes might not be apparent in the skin; therefore, examine the linings of the mouth and eyelids (mucous membranes). In a hot environment, the skin becomes warm and pink, because blood flow to the skin increases in order to lose excess heat. Hot, red skin is also seen in people with fever and heatstroke. In a cold environment, the skin becomes cool, pale, or bluish, because blood flow to the skin decreases in order to conserve heat. Cool, cold, or pale, bluish skin is seen in hypothermia, shock, and severe injuries and illnesses without fever.

Moisture

Except when it is wet with water, moist skin is due to sweating. Sweating occurs when the body needs to lose excess heat by evaporation, as in exercise or hot weather, or due to serious illness or injury, pain, or strong emotion, which stimulate the nervous system to activate the sweat glands.

Physical Examination

After completing the primary assessment, attending to any life-threatening problems, obtaining the SAMPLE history, and checking the vital signs, make a thorough, systematic physical assessment of the victim. If possible, do this in shelter where clothing can be removed as necessary. You could discover additional problems that may not pose an immediate threat to life, but might if they remain uncorrected. Even minor injuries need care, but first they must be found.

Victims with minor injury or illness might not require a complete physical assessment. In these cases, you only need to examine the injured area.

Always assess the victim's body in the following order: head, neck, chest, abdomen, extremities, and back, so that you do not forget to check an area. In inclement weather, expose only a small area of the body at a time. Use your natural tools—your eyes, ears, fingers, nose, and voice—plus your brain to evaluate what you find.

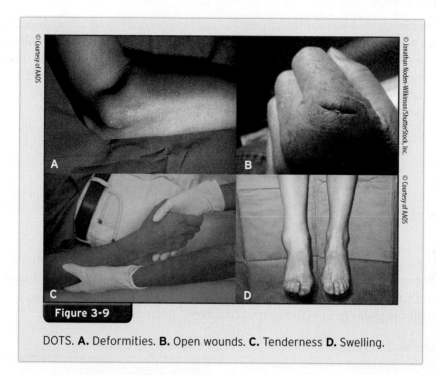

Figure 3-9

DOTS. **A.** Deformities. **B.** Open wounds. **C.** Tenderness **D.** Swelling.

The mnemonic DOTS helps you remember what to look and feel for **Figure 3-9A-D**.

- **D: Deformities.** Compare injured and uninjured parts.
- **O: Open wounds.** Open wounds include abrasions, lacerations, incisions, punctures, avulsions, and amputations. Bleeding might or might not be present.
- **T: Tenderness.**
- **S: Swelling.**

Head

Look for and use both hands to feel for DOTS on the face and scalp. Look for blood or clear fluid (cerebrospinal fluid) draining from the nose, ears, or mouth. Clear fluid can indicate a serious skull or spinal injury. Quickly look inside the mouth for wounds, bleeding, secretions, broken teeth, vomit, and dentures. Do not move the victim's head. Look at the pupils for reactivity and equal size **Figure 3-10**. Cover the victim's eye with your hand for 5 seconds and then uncover the eye to determine if the pupil constricts (gets

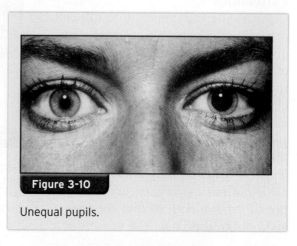

Figure 3-10

Unequal pupils.

smaller) in response to light or the shine of a flashlight beam. Unequal pupils occur normally in a small percentage of people. In a victim with a head injury, unequal pupils could mean bleeding or swelling inside the skull. Listen for abnormal noises in the nose or throat, such as gurgles, wheezes, and crowing. Smell the breath for unusual odors, such as alcohol or the fruity smell of diabetic acidosis. Any victim unresponsive due to an injury, especially a head injury, is assumed to have a spinal injury.

Neck

Look for and feel for DOTS and for the popping or crackling of air under the skin from an injury to the airway. Look for a medical identification tag on a chain around the victim's neck. Remember, if the victim is unresponsive due to injury or if you suspect spinal injury, do not move the victim's head and neck.

Chest

Look for and feel for DOTS. Place one hand on each side of the chest to see whether both sides are expanding equally with inhalation. Gently squeeze both sides of the rib cage together. If this causes the victim any pain, suspect a rib injury. If the victim is coughing up secretions, examine the coughed-up material for pus (yellow or green material) or blood.

Abdomen and Pelvis

Make sure your hands are warm. Using the pads of your fingertips, examine the four quadrants of the abdomen in a clockwise manner **Figure 3-11**. Look for and feel for DOTS, and feel gently for masses and tightening of the abdominal muscles as well as tenderness. The abdomen is normally soft. A hard or rigid area can indicate a problem.

Extremities

Compare the extremities. It is difficult to expose the thighs, legs, and arms adequately in victims wearing several layers of clothing, but these can be examined through the clothing and by pulling clothing up or down. Look for and feel for DOTS in all four extremities. Press gently with both of your hands around the victim's arm or leg along the entire length of each extremity. If abnormalities are found and a significant injury is suspected, remove clothing over the area to allow direct inspection. Use scissors or a

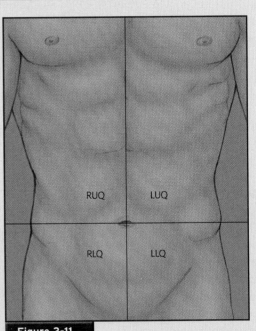

Figure 3-11

Gently press the four quadrants for firmness and softness. RUQ, right upper quadrant; LUQ, left upper quadrant; RLQ, right lower quadrant; LLQ, left lower quadrant.

knife if necessary, but in inclement weather, do not destroy clothing that will be needed later. Check each extremity for a pulse, sensation, and movement. Use the radial pulses for the upper extremities. Feel for a lower extremity pulse in the groove behind the inner ankle bone. Pulses are hard to find. Practice finding your own pulses. Pinch the skin of each forearm and leg to see if the victim reacts verbally, by moaning, or by withdrawing the extremity. Look for a medical identification bracelet.

Back

If the victim is found face down or on the side, check for a spinal cord injury before turning him or her face up. If found face up, the victim can be rolled to the side for back assessment. Look for and feel for DOTS. Feel the spine of each vertebra from above, moving downward. Tenderness and a step type of irregularity can mean a spine fracture.

After the Physical Exam

Once the primary assessment, history, and physical exam are completed, you will probably have a good idea of what is wrong with the victim. Suspect a spinal injury (as well as a head injury) in any unresponsive person injured in a high-velocity episode such as a motor vehicle crash; skiing, mountain-biking, or climbing incident; or a fall of greater than three times the victim's height. Such incidents frequently injure the neck and/or back. If you suspect such injury, do not move the victim without using proper techniques. Avoid twisting or bending the neck or back. If enough help is available, stabilize the victim's head and neck with your hands **Figure 3-12**. You can also kneel with your knees on either side of the victim's head (this prevents back cramps caused by bending over and holding the victim's head for a long period of time). If you are alone, pack available materials around the head and neck, for example, the victim's boots, large rocks padded with clothing, or backpacks.

To do a primary assessment of a responsive victim, survey the scene; approach the victim; make eye contact, and, if the victim is a stranger, introduce yourself, ask for the victim's name, and ask if you can be of help. If the victim assents, ask, "What happened to you?" The answer to this question will tell you whether the victim is injured or ill.

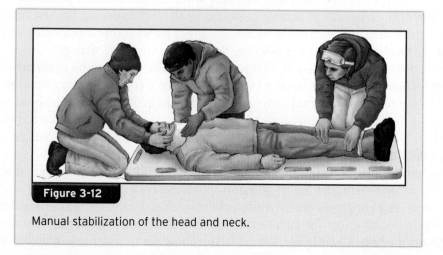

Figure 3-12

Manual stabilization of the head and neck.

In the case of an injury, ask, "Do you hurt anywhere?" Also ask the victim to describe what happened in detail so that you can consider the mechanism of injury. In the case of an illness, question the victim in detail regarding the signs and symptoms. The answer to the preliminary question is called the "chief complaint." After discussing the chief complaint, obtain a SAMPLE history from the victim.

For a responsive victim, determine whether the airway is open and if he or she is breathing.

- Airway Open?
  - If the victim is able to talk, the airway is open. If the victim is choking, use techniques for the obstructed airway.
- Breathing?
  - If the victim is having trouble breathing, or if there are abnormal sounds during breathing such as wheezes, gurgles, or stridor, have the victim sit up if possible. If this does not help to improve breathing, do a quick physical exam to look for such things as neck or chest injury and hemorrhage.

In the case of injury, after you have obtained the chief complaint and assessed the breathing, ask the victim these additional questions:

- Did you hit your head, neck, or back?
- Does your head, neck, or back hurt?
- Do you have any pain anywhere else?
- Can you feel me squeezing your toes?
- Can you move your feet?
- Can you feel me squeezing your fingers?
- Can you move your fingers?

Weakness or inability to perform the above actions might indicate an injury to the extremity or to the spinal cord **Figure 3-13A-F**. If you suspect a spinal injury, instruct the victim not to move while you are performing the rest of the primary assessment. Or, if help is available, the victim's head and neck can be stabilized manually while the examination proceeds.

Next, assess the chief site of trouble indicated by the victim during the chief complaint. Assess every body area indicated by the victim as a site of pain or other abnormality. When you think you are finished, always ask the victim, "Is there anything else wrong?"

If the victim appears seriously ill or injured, if the pulse or breathing is abnormal, if the mechanism of injury makes you suspect a serious injury, or if you are uneasy about the victim, proceed quickly to assess the vital signs and perform the physical exam. In good weather, remove the victim's clothing as necessary for an accurate assessment. In bad weather, assess the victim with his/her clothes on, pulling garments up or down briefly as needed. A more thorough examination can be done after the victim has been taken to shelter.

To summarize, in every body area, look for DOTS. Also check for closed wounds, discharges, and changes in skin color. Listen for coughing and abnormal breathing sounds, such as wheezes, crows, snoring, and gurgling. Feel for tenderness, swellings, lumps, depressions, deformities, the popping feel of air under the skin in the neck and chest, and the grating sensation at an injury site that may mean a fracture. Ask the victim about pain, tenderness, inability to move,

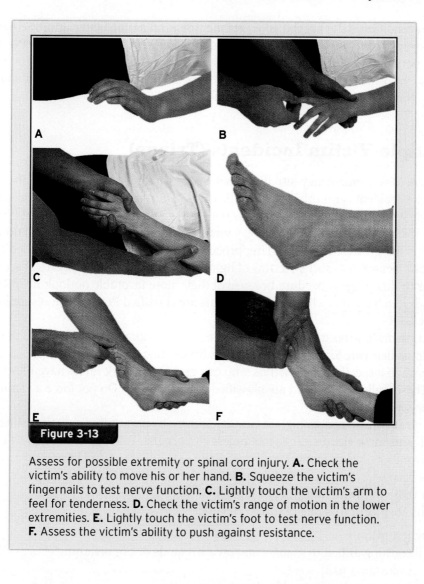

Figure 3-13

Assess for possible extremity or spinal cord injury. **A.** Check the victim's ability to move his or her hand. **B.** Squeeze the victim's fingernails to test nerve function. **C.** Lightly touch the victim's arm to feel for tenderness. **D.** Check the victim's range of motion in the lower extremities. **E.** Lightly touch the victim's foot to test nerve function. **F.** Assess the victim's ability to push against resistance.

numbness, or abnormal sensations such as pins and needles, and ask the victim to squeeze both of your hands simultaneously and to move all four extremities.

Compare each body area with the same area on the opposite side of the body to determine any differences. Think about the information you are gathering. What to do about what you find will be discussed in later chapters.

▶ Reassessment

The reassessment is used to monitor the victim's condition, which is very important when the victim is hours or days from medical care. In both injuries and illnesses, determine whether the victim's condition is staying the same, getting worse, or getting better, and whether any new signs and/or symptoms are developing. Reassess the breathing, mental status (AVPU scale), and vital signs periodically (every 15 minutes) in stable victims and more frequently (at least every 5 minutes) in unstable victims. Monitor the results of your first aid care. Calm and reassure the victim. If possible, keep a written record of what you find.

▶ Multiple-Victim Incidents (Triage)

You may encounter emergency situations with two or more victims. This is often the case in avalanche accidents and other natural disasters. After making a quick scene survey, you must decide who is to be cared for and evacuated first. When limited personnel do not allow everything to be done right away for every victim, be guided by the principle, "do the greatest good for the greatest number." This process of prioritizing victims is called "triage," a French word meaning "to sort." Victims of lightning strikes and other electrical accidents are exceptions to this triage procedure because of their more favorable outlook if CPR is started immediately. Such victims who are not breathing are classified Priority 1 and should be given immediate CPR.

Many systems have been used to identify care and evacuation priorities. To find those victims needing immediate care for life-threatening conditions, first tell all victims who can get up and walk to move to a specific area. Victims who can get up and walk rarely have life-threatening injuries. These walking wounded are classified lowest priority. Do not force a victim to move if he or she reports pain.

Find the life-threatened, or highest-priority, victims by performing only the primary assessment on all remaining victims. Go to motionless victims first. You must move rapidly (spend less than 60 seconds with each victim) from one victim to the next until all have been assessed. You should not become involved in treating victims at this point, but ask knowledgeable bystanders to care for those in the highest-priority category.

Victims are placed into one of three categories:

1. Highest priority:
   - Breathing difficulties (abnormal breath sounds or not breathing)
   - Severe chest pain
   - Uncontrolled or severe bleeding
   - Decreased mental status
2. Second priority:
   - Burns without airway problems
   - Major or multiple painful, swollen, deformed extremity injuries
   - Spinal injuries
3. Lowest priority:
   - Minor painful, swollen, deformed extremity injuries
   - Minor soft-tissue injuries
   - Death

Reassess victims regularly for changes in their condition. Only when those in the highest priority have received care should those with less serious conditions be given care.

Later, if higher-trained emergency personnel arrive on the scene, you may then be asked to continue giving first aid or help with evacuation.

This chapter introduced you to victim assessment. This process identifies information about the victim's condition, including the primary assessment, physical exam, vital signs, history taking, reassessment, and multiple-victim situations. Because there are four victim conditions—injured or ill responsive victims and injured or ill unresponsive victims—the sequencing of the assessment steps varies. Without an accurate victim assessment, such as the one explained in this chapter, inappropriate first aid results. Performing a good victim assessment is the mark of a good first aid provider.

4 Care of Bleeding, Wounds, and Burns

The objectives of first aid wound care are to control bleeding, prevent infection, and protect with appropriate bandaging. If kept clean, wounds are not likely to get infected, and a laceration can be closed several days later, if necessary. Minor wounds do not require immediate evacuation from the wilderness. Wounds that require evacuation are discussed on page 65.

Bleeding

▶ Controlling Bleeding

The first priority of wound care is to control bleeding. Major bleeding can lead to so much blood loss that blood pressure can fall to a dangerously low level, a condition known as shock (or cardiovascular shock). Shock occurs when the body's tissues do not receive enough oxygenated blood. Do not confuse this with electric shock or "being shocked," as in being scared or surprised. To understand shock, think of the circulatory system as having three components: a working pump (the heart), a network of pipes (the blood vessels), and an adequate amount of fluid (the blood) pumped through the pipes. Damage to any of the components can deprive tissues of oxygen-rich blood and produce the condition known as shock. Untreated cardiovascular shock is generally fatal.

To control bleeding, follow the steps in **Skill Drill 4-1**.

1. If possible, wash your hands with soap and water before caring for a wound.
2. Ask the victim to sit or lie down. Fainting reactions are common after any injury, even minor wounds. Treatment increases pain and the risk of fainting, which may be mistaken for shock. If there is excessive blood loss, anticipate shock and treat by laying the victim down. Keep the wounded person warm.
3. Expose the wound. Because clothing may be essential for protection, especially in cold, snowy, or rainy weather, do not cut garments unless absolutely necessary.
4. Put on medical exam gloves to protect against bloodborne infections. If gloves are unavailable, cover your hands with plastic bags or similar waterproof material (**Step ❶**). You can even have the victim put pressure on his or her own bleeding wound. After unprotected contact with blood and after removing gloves, wash your hands vigorously with soap and water.
5. Place a sterile gauze pad or clean cloth directly over the entire wound, and press evenly for 5 to 10 minutes. Direct pressure stops almost all bleeding (**Step ❷**). Wounds of the scalp, hands, and face bleed more profusely because of their rich blood supply.
6. If bleeding persists after you have maintained pressure on the wound for at least 10 minutes, press harder over a wider area.
7. Apply a pressure dressing. This will allow you to attend to other injuries or victims (**Step ❸**). Make a pressure dressing by covering the wound with a thick layer of gauze or the cleanest material available, and then tightly wrap a bandage over the

CAUTION

DO NOT

- Apply pressure bandages so tightly that they cut off blood flow. Pain, coldness, and color change beyond the dressing suggest the bandage is too tight.
- Apply a tourniquet. They are almost never needed. The only exception would be life-threatening hemorrhage that does not stop with direct pressure. If used, the tourniquet should be applied just above the bleeding site, between the bleeding site and the heart. It should be made of broad, flat material such as a scarf or wide belt and should not be released until the person is in the hands of a physician. Tourniquets shut off blood supply and can cause the loss of an arm or leg.
- Apply pressure to control bleeding from an eyeball injury (use pressure only on wounds of the eyelids or around the eye). Avoid using pressure on a wound with an embedded object or with bone protruding. In these cases, use a doughnut-shaped pad that applies pressure around the wound instead of directly on it.

dressing, extending above and below the site. If a pressure dressing is required, leave it in place for several hours to prevent further bleeding.

8. If the dressings become soaked with blood, place fresh dressings on top of the soaked ones rather than replacing the soaked ones (**Step ❹**).

skill drill

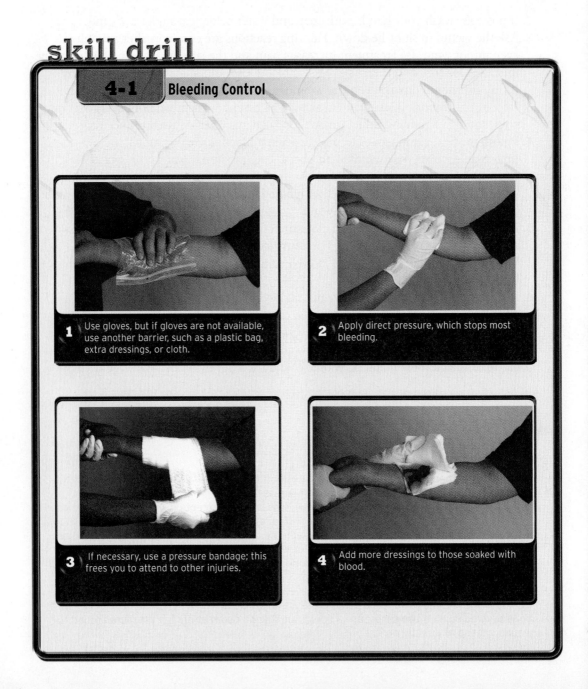

| **4-1** | **Bleeding Control** |

1 Use gloves, but if gloves are not available, use another barrier, such as a plastic bag, extra dressings, or cloth.

2 Apply direct pressure, which stops most bleeding.

3 If necessary, use a pressure bandage; this frees you to attend to other injuries.

4 Add more dressings to those soaked with blood.

Wounds

▶ Types of Wounds

Abrasions (scrapes, "road rash," and "rug burn") result in partial loss of the skin surface **Figure 4-1**. They usually produce little bleeding but are very painful. Lacerations are cut skin with jagged edges **Figure 4-2**. They can cause major bleeding and involve other structures below the skin such as tendons, nerves, and large blood vessels. Incisions are smooth-edged cuts **Figure 4-3**. Puncture wounds are produced by pointed objects such as nails or knives that leave small entry wounds, can extend deeply, and have the greatest risk of infection **Figure 4-4**. The object that produces the injury or other foreign matter might remain in the wound. Avulsions are tearing wounds that create a flap of skin and tissue still attached by a bridge of skin **Figure 4-5**. Amputations occur when a part of the body is completely separated from the body **Figure 4-6**.

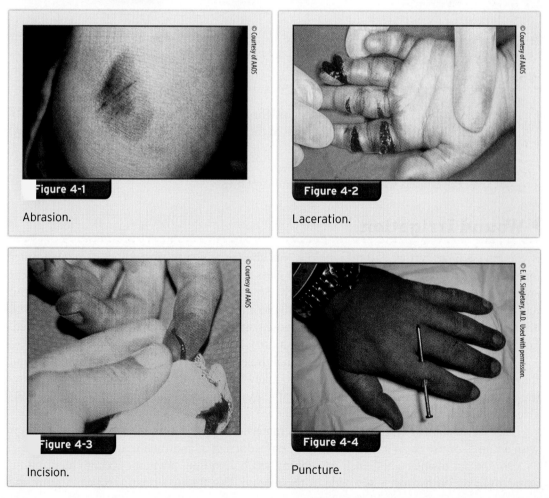

Figure 4-1
Abrasion.

Figure 4-2
Laceration.

Figure 4-3
Incision.

Figure 4-4
Puncture.

© Courtesy of AAOS

© Courtesy of AAOS

© Courtesy of AAOS

© E. M. Singletary, M.D. Used with permission.

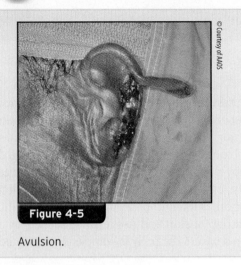

© Courtesy of AAOS

Figure 4-5

Avulsion.

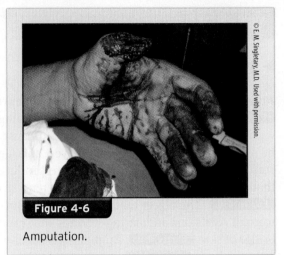

© E. M. Singletary, M.D. Used with permission.

Figure 4-6

Amputation.

▶ Cleaning a Wound

What to Do

1. Wash the wound. Although cleaning might restart bleeding, it is essential.
2. For a shallow wound, wash the inside of the wound and surrounding skin with soap and clean water.
3. Flush the wound with disinfected water.
4. Cover the wound with a sterile or clean dressing.

▶ Wound Irrigation

If you have a large syringe (20 mL), hold it just above the wound and squirt drinkable water forcefully into the depths of the wound. Wear glasses or shield your face with a hand to prevent splashing of blood into your eyes and mouth. Spread the wound open so that the fluid can reach the depths of the wound. Flush out small pieces of foreign matter. Continue irrigating well after all foreign material, clotted blood, and loose tissue fragments seem to have been removed. Forceful irrigation is painful but essential in a dirty laceration.

A bulb syringe or a plastic bag with a small hole in the corner can be used to irrigate but they are not as efficient as pressure irrigation. Likewise, pouring water on a wound or soaking the wound are not satisfactory substitutes for pressure irrigation, but may be all that are available and are better than doing nothing.

Remove remaining fragments of foreign material with tweezers (after sterilizing the tips with a flame) or use clean gauze to wipe out embedded dirt, and then irrigate again.

Do not put disinfectants, such as rubbing alcohol, iodine, povidone-iodine, merbromin, thimerosal, or 3% hydrogen peroxide in the wound. Use them to clean the skin around the

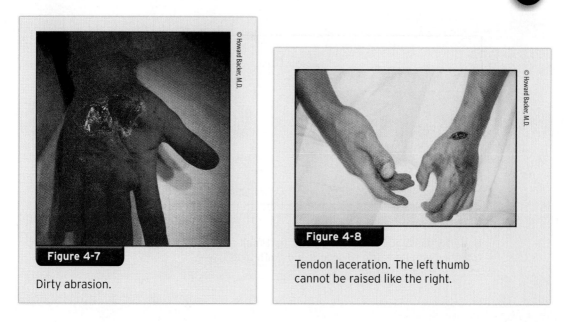

Figure 4-7

Dirty abrasion.

Figure 4-8

Tendon laceration. The left thumb cannot be raised like the right.

wound. Although they are commonly used, such agents are not needed; furthermore, they can harm tissue and delay healing.

If the wound is an abrasion, wash the affected area, rubbing gently to remove dirt **Figure 4-7**. Cover the wound with a thin layer of antibiotic ointment, a nonstick dressing, and a bandage or tape. Shallow wounds can be covered by a thin layer of antibiotic ointment.

In the event of a small puncture wound, clean only the surface, not the depths of the wound. Inducing bleeding is not beneficial.

▶ Evaluating Function

Check for normal movement and sensation beyond the wound, especially with wounds on or near the hands and feet or other joints. If a tendon in the hand is cut, the victim cannot move the finger **Figure 4-8**. Manage the wound in the same manner as you would for an uncut tendon, but splint the finger as well. The tendon can be repaired days later.

▶ Wound Closure

Close small, clean wounds with tape or "butterfly" strips if the edges can be pulled together easily. Do not suture wounds. For a forehead laceration, tie the hair across the wound and use tape strips to close. Pack large, gaping wounds and dirty wounds with sterile dressings held in place by a bandage; change dressings daily until the victim has been seen by a physician. Wounds can be sutured 3 to 5 days later.

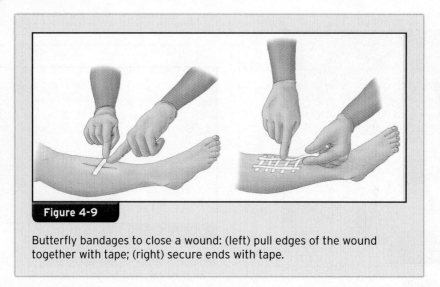

Figure 4-9

Butterfly bandages to close a wound: (left) pull edges of the wound together with tape; (right) secure ends with tape.

What to Do

Close a wound with strips of tape or "butterfly" bandages **Figure 4-9**.

1. Fashion strips by cutting the corners off a folded piece of 0.5" or 1" tape, or tear or cut the tape vertically to obtain strips about 0.25" wide.
2. Unfold and apply tape to one side of the wound. (If you have benzoin in the first aid kit, apply it to the skin first and wait about 30 seconds until it becomes sticky.) Squeeze the wound together and tape across the other side.
3. Apply strips 0.25" to 0.5" apart. Secure the ends with perpendicular strips of tape.

Cover all wounds with sterile or clean dressings and attempt to keep the dressings clean and dry. When possible, apply a nonstick dressing. Inspect the wound every 24 to 48 hours for signs of infection (see the following section). Change dressings every 24 to 48 hours or if they become wet or dirty.

▶ Wound Infection

All wounds can become infected **Figure 4-10**. Deep, dirty wounds; punctures; and bites have the highest risk of becoming infected. Dirt, gravel, and wood splinters left in a wound always produce infection. Animal and human bites also have a high risk of infection **Table 4-1**.

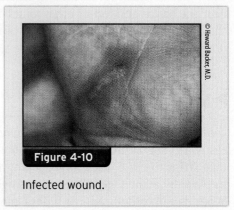

© Howard Backer, M.D.

Figure 4-10

Infected wound.

Table 4-1   Tetanus

Tetanus (lockjaw) causes spasm of the jaw muscles, as well as other symptoms. It is caused by a toxin produced by bacteria that enter the body through wounds. The bacterial spores are hardy and widespread in the environment, especially in areas with animal droppings. Neither the infection nor the toxin is spread from one person to another. Immunization is highly effective. In the United States, 96% of the population is immunized in childhood, but boosters are needed every 10 years. People who have had routine childhood vaccinations but no boosters within the past 10 years do not require immunization after a minor cut, scratch, or bite; however, they should seek medical advice after returning from a wilderness trip during which they've been wounded. Large and deep wounds contaminated with dirt may warrant earlier immunization, but the victim would usually be evacuated and immunized after such injuries.

Tetanus immunization is needed by:

- Anyone with a wound who has never been immunized against tetanus.
- Anyone with a wound received in the wilderness who has been immunized but has not received a tetanus booster in the past 10 years.
- Anyone who has a large and/or dirty wound or burn who has not had a booster for more than 5 years.

What to Look For

- Redness spreading from the margins of the wound. As infection spreads away from the wound, the surrounding redness enlarges and red streaks may appear, leading from the wound toward the heart.
- Warmth
- Swelling
- Increasing pain and tenderness
- Pus will appear only if the wound is open and drains. It may be thick and creamy yellow or white, or thin and watery with a pink or light green color.
- Swollen, tender glands in the groin, armpit, or neck (whichever is closest to the infected wound).
- Chills and fever, which indicate that an infection has spread into the blood and could become life threatening
- An abscess or boil (a collection of pus) might develop from a wound or in intact skin, starting as a pimple or small cyst (soft lump under the skin) and forming a whitehead (the natural drainage site) **Figure 4-11**.

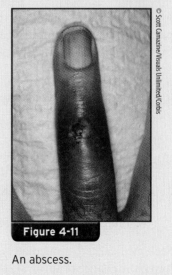

Figure 4-11

An abscess.

© Scott Camazine/Visuals Unlimited/Corbis

What to Do

1. Clean the area.
2. Separate the wound edges gently to allow pus or infected fluids to escape.
3. Soak the wound in warm water or apply a warm, wet compress (clean cloth dipped in bath-temperature water) for 15 minutes 4 times a day.
4. Change the dressings as often as needed to keep them clean and dry.
5. Elevate the infected part.
6. Give the victim aspirin, acetaminophen, or ibuprofen for pain. Do not give aspirin to children. It can cause a severe reaction called Reyes syndrome.
7. Evacuate the victim if the infection does not resolve or becomes worse, or if the victim has a fever or the chills.

ADVANCED PROCEDURE

Draining an Abscess

To treat an abscess, release the pus. Wait until a natural drainage site, the white area in the center of the tender swelling, has developed. The formation of this central whitehead can be encouraged by frequent warm soaks or compresses. Try to open this point with the tip of a sharp knife blade, sterilized over a flame or in boiling water. The point has diminished feeling, but the surrounding skin is very sensitive. Make an incision rapidly. Numb the skin with ice, if available. Insert sterile gauze in the incision made by the knife blade, and then apply a bandage **Figure 4-12** .

▶ Special Wounds

What to Do in the Event of an Amputation

Amputations are injuries in which parts of the body are completely cut off. Some amputated parts can be reattached surgically, so attempt to preserve the part. Whether or not you are able to preserve the severed part, take the following actions:

1. Control bleeding.
2. Treat the victim for shock.

If the amputated part can be found, take the following actions:

1. Rinse it with clean water to remove dirt and debris. Do not scrub it.
2. Wrap the part in sterile gauze or a clean cloth.
3. Put the part in a plastic bag or waterproof container, and then place it on ice or snow in a second container. Do not bury it.
4. Take the part to the hospital with the injured person.

Seek medical care immediately. Amputated body parts that are unchilled for more than 6 hours have little chance of survival; 18 hours is the maximum survival time for a properly cooled part.

CAUTION

DO NOT
- Wrap the amputated part in a wet dressing or cloth; the tissues will become waterlogged, soft, and more difficult to reattach.
- Bury the part in ice. Freezing results in unsuccessful reattachment.
- Cut small skin bridges, tendons, or other partial attachments. If the part is still attached, reposition it and wrap it firmly in a bulky, dry dressing.

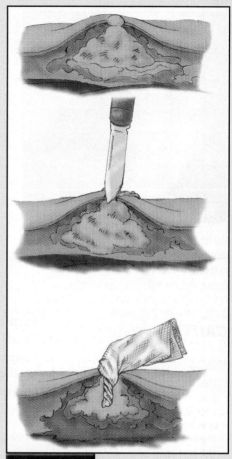

Figure 4-12

Fingertips amputated at the level of the nailbed or beyond cannot be reattached, but keep the tip, because it can be used as a skin graft. Skin and tissue lost through amputation at the end of a finger, not involving bone, will regrow and do not need reattachment. These injuries bleed for a long time; apply pressure and be patient.

▶ Blisters

Treatment of an abscess. Make an incision in the central whitehead of the abscess. Insert sterile gauze into the opening, and then bandage.

A blister is a collection of fluid beneath the skin caused by excessive friction. To prevent blisters from forming, tape susceptible areas like the backs of the heels with duct tape or adhesive tape, or cover with adhesive felt (moleskin) before blisters appear, especially when wearing new boots or shoes **Figure 4-13**.

What to Do

1. Cover a hot spot or an unbroken blister with tape, duct tape, or moleskin. Cover an area larger than the blister or hot spot to avoid peeling of the dressing.
2. Use several layers of moleskin or molefoam (thicker than felt) cut in the shape of a doughnut that fits around the blister to relieve pressure **Figure 4-14**.

© Howard Backer, M.D.

Figure 4-13

Blisters can be debilitating. Stop and tape over early hot spots before blisters like this form.

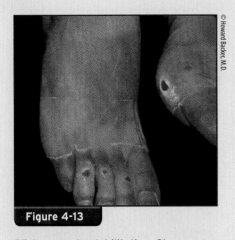

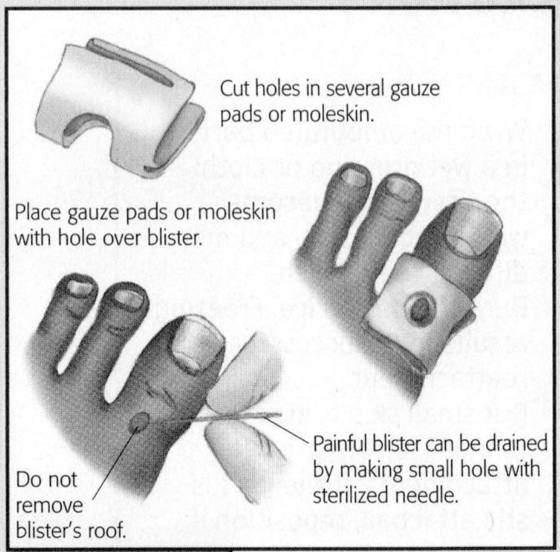

Cut holes in several gauze pads or moleskin.

Place gauze pads or moleskin with hole over blister.

Painful blister can be drained by making small hole with sterilized needle.

Do not remove blister's roof.

Figure 4-14

Blister care.

Painful, Unbroken Blisters

Clean the blister with soap and water or disinfectant. Puncture it several times around its edge with a needle sterilized over a flame. Gently press out the fluid. Do not remove the roof (blister covering), but cover it with a nonstick dressing or tape.

Broken Blisters

Clean the surrounding skin of a broken blister with soap and water. Washing the broken surface is painful, but sand or dirt must be removed. Cover small blisters directly with tape. Cover large blisters with a nonstick pad, and then apply tape or moleskin. It is more comfortable to apply several layers of moleskin cut in a doughnut shape on top of each other with the holes over the blister. Unroof the blister if you see dirt or sand under the skin and clean the area before applying a dressing.

Infected Blisters

Inspect painful blisters every 24 to 48 hours. Signs of infection include redness and tenderness extending beyond the edge of the blister, cloudy blister fluid, or pus. If a blister is infected, cut away the dead skin overlying the blister and begin warm soaks.

▶ Closed Wounds—Bruises

A bruise (contusion) is a collection of blood within or under the skin. Bleeding into deeper tissues can be extensive, especially in the thigh or buttock.

What to Look For

- Pain and discoloration
- Possible fracture; evaluate if the area is unusually painful or if moving the extremity is limited by pain
- Blood appearing beneath the skin as a purple or yellow discoloration within a few hours or days after a superficial bruise
- Over 5 to 10 days, a color change from purple/blue to yellow to green. The bruise spreads out under the skin, following gravity, to extend down the arm, leg, or face.

What to Do

1. Apply a cold pack, if available, for at least 20 minutes 4 times a day, or longer for major bruises.
2. If a cold pack is not being applied, wrap the bruised area firmly with an elastic bandage. Do not cut off circulation.
3. Evaluate the necessity of travel. A few hours after a severe bruise in the leg or hip, the injured tissues may become so stiff and sore that the victim cannot walk comfortably. If it is necessary to walk to a trailhead or continue to a safe campsite, this may take precedence over immediate immobilization and cooling.
4. Seek medical care for multiple bruises that appear spontaneously.

▶ Impaled (Embedded) Objects

Impaled objects come in all shapes and sizes, from pencils and screwdrivers to knives, glass, steel rods, and fence posts **Figure 4-15**. Proper first aid requires that the impaled object be stabilized because there can be significant internal damage.

Care for Impaled Objects

1. Expose the area. Remove or cut away any clothing surrounding the injury. If clothes cover the object, leave them in place; removing them could cause the object to move.
2. Do not remove or move the object. Movement of any kind could produce additional bleeding and tissue damage. Cheeks are one exception because the object or the bleeding could cause an airway obstruction. See the

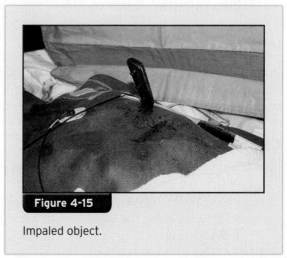

Figure 4-15

Impaled object.

following section on impaled objects in the cheek for more information. Small objects such as slivers (splinters) can be safely removed.

3. Stabilize the object with bulky dressings or clean cloths around the object. Some experts suggest securing 75% of the object with bulky dressings or cloths to reduce motion.

4. Control any bleeding with pressure around the impaled object. Apply pressure on the dressing surrounding the object. Do not press directly on the object or along the wound next to the cutting edge, especially if the object has sharp edges.

5. Shorten the object only if necessary. In most cases, do not shorten the object by cutting or breaking it. There are times, however, when cutting or shortening the object allows for easier transportation. Be sure to stabilize the object before shortening it. Remember that the victim will feel any vibrations from the object being cut away; also, the injury could be worsened by this action.

Impaled Object in the Cheek

The only time it is safe to remove an impaled object outside a medical setting is when the object is in the victim's cheek.

Care for Impaled Object in the Cheek

1. Examine the injury inside the mouth. If the object extends through the cheek and you are more than 1 hour from medical help, consider removing it.

2. To remove the object: Place two fingers next to the object, straddling it; then gently pull it in the direction from which it entered. If it cannot be removed easily, leave it in place and secure it with bulky dressings.

3. Control the bleeding. After you have removed the object, place dressings over the wound inside the mouth between the cheek and the teeth. The dressings will help control the bleeding and will not interfere with the victim's airway. Also place a dressing on the outside wound.

Impaled Object in the Eye

If an object is impaled in the eye, it is vital that pressure not be put on the eye. The eyeball consists of two chambers, each filled with fluid. Do not exert any pressure against the eyeball because fluid can be forced out of it, worsening the injury.

Care for Impaled Object in the Eye

1. Stabilize the object. Use bulky dressings or clean cloths to stabilize a long, protruding object. You can place a protective paper cup or cardboard folded into a cone over the affected eye to prevent bumping of the object. For short objects, surround the eye—without touching the object—with a doughnut-shaped (ring) pad held in place with a roller bandage.

2. Cover the undamaged eye. Most experts suggest that the undamaged eye should be covered to prevent sympathetic eye movement (that is, the injured eye moves when the undamaged eye does, thus aggravating the injury). Remember that the victim is unable to see when both eyes are covered and may be anxious. Make sure you explain to the victim everything you are doing.
3. Seek immediate medical care.

Care for Slivers

Small slivers of wood, glass, thorns, or metal can be painful and irritating and they also can cause infection. Because of their size, these slivers (also called *splinters*) can usually be easily removed with tweezers. Sometimes, it is necessary to tease one end of the object with a sterile needle to place it in a better position for removal with tweezers. After you have removed the sliver, clean the area with soap and water and apply an adhesive bandage.

Cactus Spines

Cacti are a part of the desert environment, and they also are used as ornamental plants. Infection from cactus-spine punctures is rare. Removing cactus spines is time consuming because they usually are acquired in groupings, are difficult to see, and are designed by nature to resist removal. Usually spines can easily, yet tediously, be removed with tweezers.

Another method for removing a large number of cactus spines is to coat the area with a thin layer of white woodworking glue or rubber cement and allow it to dry for at least 30 minutes. Slowly roll up the dried glue from the margins. Applying the glue in strips rather than puddles will make the rolling procedure go more smoothly. A single layer of gauze gently pressed onto the still-damp glue helps to remove it after it has dried. The combination of using tweezers and glue will remove most of the spines.

Using adhesive tape, duct tape, or cellophane tape, although quick and easy, removes only about 30% of the spines, even after multiple attempts. Do not use super glue (or other similar products) to remove cactus spines. Not only does it fail to roll up when applied to the skin, but it also welds the spines to the skin. In addition, there is the risk that the skin will permanently bond to anything it touches.

Care for Fishhooks

Tape an embedded fishhook in place and do *not* try to remove it if injury to a nearby body part such as the eye or an underlying structure such as a blood vessel or nerve is possible or if the victim (such as a young child) is uncooperative.

If the point of a fishhook has penetrated the skin but the barb has not, remove the fishhook by backing it out. Then treat the wound like a puncture wound. Seek medical advice for a possible tetanus shot.

If the hook's barb has entered the skin, follow these procedures:

1. If medical care is near, transport the victim and have a physician remove the hook.
2. If you are in a remote area, far from medical care, remove the hook using either the pliers method or the string-jerk method.

Use extreme care with the pliers method of fishhook removal because it can produce further severe injury if the hook is pushed into blood vessels, nerves, or tendons. Use pliers with tempered jaws that can cut through a hook **Figure 4-16** . The proper kind of pliers is often unavailable, or sometimes the barb is buried too deep to be pushed through. Test the pliers by first cutting a similar fishhook.

1. Use cold or use hard pressure around the hook to provide temporary numbness.
2. Push the embedded hook further in, in a shallow curve, until the point and the barb come out through the skin.
3. Cut off the barb, then back the hook out the way it came in.
4. After removing the hook, treat the wound and seek medical attention for a possible tetanus shot.

A better method to remove a fishhook is the string-jerk method.

1. Loop a piece of fishline over the bend or curve of the embedded hook **Figure 4-17** .
2. Stabilize the part of the victim's body in which the hook is embedded.
3. Use cold or use hard pressure around the hook to provide temporary numbness.
4. With one hand, press down on the hook's shank and eye while the other hand sharply jerks the fishline that is over the hook's bend or curve. The jerk movement should be parallel to the skin's surface. The hook will neatly come out of the same hole it entered, causing little pain.
5. After removing the hook, care for the wound and seek medical care for a possible tetanus shot.

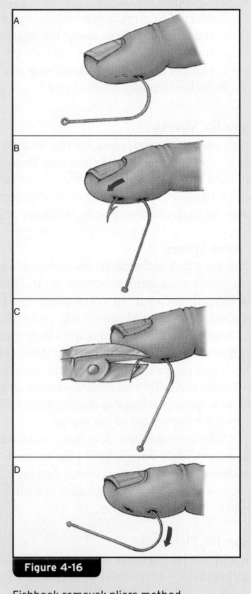

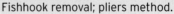

Figure 4-16

Fishhook removal; pliers method.

Sutures

If sutures (stitches) are needed, they usually should be placed by a physician within 6 to 8 hours of the injury. Suturing wounds allows faster healing, reduces infection, and lessens scarring. Some wounds do not usually require sutures, such as the following:

- Wounds in which the skin's cut edges tend to fall together
- Shallow cuts less than 1 inch long

Rather than close a gaping wound with butterfly bandages or elastic skin closures, cover the wound with sterile gauze. Closing the wound might trap bacteria inside, resulting in an infection. In most cases, a physician can be reached in time for sutures to be placed; if not, a wound without sutures will still heal but with scars. Scar tissue can be attended to later by a plastic surgeon.

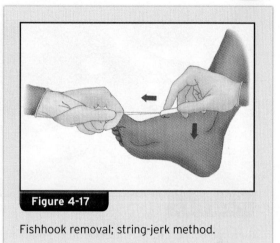

Figure 4-17

Fishhook removal; string-jerk method.

▶ Gunshot Wounds

Guns are abundant in the United States; it is estimated that about one half of all American homes have a firearm. There are two general types of firearms: low velocity, such as most civilian firearms, and high velocity, such as military weapons. Shotguns have low velocity but create severe tissue damage.

A bullet causes injury in the following ways, depending on its velocity, or speed:

- *Laceration and crushing.* When the bullet penetrates the body, it crushes tissue and forces it apart. That is the main effect of low-velocity bullets. The crushing and laceration caused by the passage of the bullet usually are not serious unless vital organs or major blood vessels are injured. The bullet damages only the tissues that it contacts directly, and the wound is comparable to that caused by weapons such as knives.
- *Shock waves and temporary cavitation.* When a bullet penetrates the body, a shock wave exerts outward pressure from the bullet's path. The shock wave pushes tissues away and creates a temporary cavity that can be as much as 30 times the diameter of the bullet. As the cavity forms, a negative pressure develops inside, creating a vacuum. The vacuum then draws debris in with it. Temporary cavitation occurs only with high-velocity bullets and is the main reason for their immensely destructive effect. The cavitation lasts only a millisecond but can damage muscles, nerves, blood vessels, and bone.

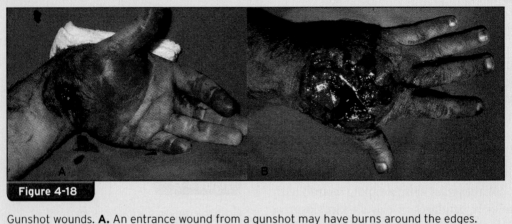

Figure 4-18

Gunshot wounds. **A.** An entrance wound from a gunshot may have burns around the edges. **B.** An exit wound is sometimes larger and results in greater damage to soft tissues.

In a *penetrating* wound, there is a bullet entry point but no exit. In a *perforating* wound, there are both entry and exit points. The exit wound of a high-velocity bullet is usually larger than the entrance wound; the exit wound from a low-velocity bullet is about the same size as the entry wound **Figure 4-18**. If the bullet was fired at very close range, the entrance wound may be larger than the exit wound because the gases from the gun's muzzle contribute to damage of the surface tissue.

Bullets sometimes hit hard tissue such as bones and may bounce around in the body cavities, causing a great deal of damage to tissue and organs. Moreover, bone chips can ricochet to other body areas and cause damage. Because a split or misshapen bullet tumbles and exerts its force over a larger area, it does more damage than a smooth bullet going in a straight line does.

Care for Gunshot Wounds

Regardless of the type of gunshot wound, initial care is roughly the same as for any other wound.

1. Monitor the victim's breathing.
2. Expose the wound(s). Make sure to look at all the skin, including hidden areas.
3. Control the bleeding with direct pressure.
4. Apply dry, sterile dressings to the wound(s) and bandage them securely in place.
5. Treat the victim for shock.
6. Keep the victim calm and quiet.
7. Seek immediate medical care.

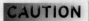
CAUTION

DO NOT try to remove material from a gunshot wound. The hospital emergency department personnel will clean the wound.

Legal Aspects

Because interactions with victims of gunshot wounds will involve contact with law enforcement agencies and possibly have you testifying in court, carefully observe the scene and the victim. Keep an accurate record of your observations. Preserve possible evidence, such as cartridge casings or shells, for the police. Do not touch or move anything unless absolutely necessary to treat the victim. All gunshot wounds must be reported to the police regardless of whether they are intentional (suicide, assault, murder, self-defense) or unintentional.

▶Wounds Requiring Evacuation

Consider evacuation for the following types of injuries:

- Uncontrolled or severe bleeding
- Deep incisions, lacerations, or avulsions that:
  - Extend into muscle or bone
  - Are located on or over a joint on the arm or leg
  - Gape widely
  - Contain a lot of dirt or debris
- Severe hand or foot wounds
- Large or deep puncture wounds
- Large or deeply embedded objects
- Human and animal bites
- Eyelid injuries with a break in the edge of the eyelid
- Infected wounds
- Amputations other than small areas of skin from the fingertips
- Open fractures

Most victims with wounds can walk and do not require helicopter or litter assistance.

Burns

Burns are caused by heat, electrical, or radiant energy and by certain chemicals. Although burns mainly involve the skin and underlying tissues, they can also affect the eyes and respiratory passages. In the wilderness, the most common causes of burns are campfires, stoves, lightning, and the sun.

▶ Burn Classification

The classification of a burn depends on its depth, extent, location, and severity.

Depth

First-degree (superficial) burns affect the skin's outer layer (epidermis). The skin is mildly swollen, red, tender, and painful. Blisters do not form. Second-degree (partial-thickness) burns extend through the epidermis into the inner skin layer (dermis) **Figure 4-19**. There is moderate to severe pain, swelling, and blister formation. Third-degree (full-thickness) burns extend into the underlying fat and muscle **Figure 4-20**. The skin is numb; looks charred, leathery, or pearly gray; and does not change color when pressed, because it is dead.

A burn may contain all three degrees of damage. A victim can have a third-degree burn in the center, surrounded by an area of second-degree burn with first-degree damage at the outermost edges.

Extent

Determine the extent of a burn by using the rule of nines, which assigns a percentage of total skin surface to each part of the body **Figure 4-21**.

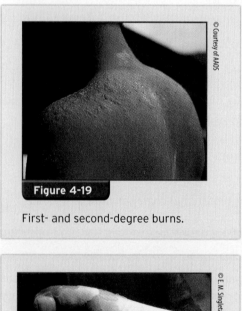

© Courtesy of AAOS

Figure 4-19

First- and second-degree burns.

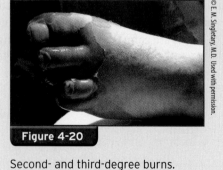

© E. M. Singletary, M.D. Used with permission.

Figure 4-20

Second- and third-degree burns.

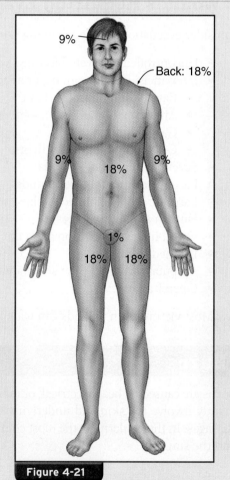

9%

Back: 18%

9%   18%   9%

1%

18%   18%

Figure 4-21

Rule of nines for calculating the extent of a burn. The entire head is 9%, each entire arm is 9% and each entire leg is 18%. The entire back is 18%. The entire front of the torso is 18%.

For small or scattered burns, estimate the surface area that has been burned by comparing it with the size of the patient's palm, which is rougly equal 1% of the victim's body surface area. This is known as the rule of the palms.

Location

Burns are serious if they:

- Involve the face, hands, feet, or genitals.
- Extend completely around the body or limb (circumferential burn), which may cause constriction of breathing or a tourniquet effect.
- Involve the respiratory tract, causing severe cough or shortness of breath; these burns will usually be associated with a burn of the face or mouth.
- Are associated with major injuries or illnesses.

Severity

Burns are classified as severe, moderate, or minor depending on their location, extent, and depth. Burns that cover a large area are more severe than small, localized burns. Deep burns are more severe than those that are superficial. Common sense will enable you to determine the severity of most burns.

Other Considerations

Particularly serious are major burns to children, the elderly, and those in poor health, and burns associated with other injuries.

Immediate Action

Stop the burning! Pour cold water onto the burned area immediately. If clothing is on fire and water is not available, tell the victim to roll on the ground, or wrap the person in a canvas tarp or wool jacket. Do not use polypropylene or nylon, which can melt and increase burn damage. Remove the victim from the flame or smoke-filled area. Cut off smoldering clothing immediately or soak it with water.

What to Do at First

1. Check the victim's breathing, paying special attention to breathing sounds.
2. For small burns (less than 20% body surface), immerse in clean, cold water or cover with a cold, wet, clean cloth; snow; or ice pack for about 10 minutes to relieve pain. When cooling extensive burns (greater than 20% of body surface area) monitor for hypothermia (shivering).
3. Estimate the depth and extent of the burn and note any circumferential burns or involvement of critical areas.
4. Check for additional injuries, especially if the victim was in an explosion or under falling debris.

5. Remove jewelry and watches from burned extremities before swelling occurs. Remove belts and clothing from burned areas.
6. Keep burned skin clean and prevent blisters from breaking. (Burned skin has been sterilized by the heat.) An intact blister filled with clear fluid minimizes infection.
7. If the burn is second or third degree, cover it with a dry, clean (preferably sterile) dressing. Cover a large burn with a clean sheet or blanket.
8. If the burn is on a hand or foot, put nonstick gauze pads between the victim's fingers or toes.
9. Evacuate the victim to medical care, unless the burn is minor in an otherwise healthy, uninjured adult. With moderate to severe burns, monitor the victim's airway and breathing at frequent intervals if there has been exposure to smoke or heat.
10. Encourage a large fluid intake in all victims except those with minimal burns.
11. Relieve pain and inflammation with aspirin or ibuprofen (acetaminophen relieves pain but not inflammation).

What to Do Later

First-Degree Burns

1. Apply a bland ointment or moisturizing cream (aloe vera) to the burned area to soothe the burn and keep skin soft.
2. Apply a dressing, which is not required but might reduce pain.

Second- and Third-Degree Burns

1. Wash the burn gently with lukewarm water and mild soap. Avoid breaking blisters.
2. Apply a thin layer of antibiotic ointment (such as Bacitracin).
3. Cover the burn with a nonstick dressing (preferably sterile but at least clean) held in place with a bandage.
4. If the burn is wet and oozing, remove the dressing daily (you may have to soak off old dressings with clean, lukewarm water). Wash the burned area, and then reapply antibiotic ointment and a nonstick dressing.

Third-Degree Burns

1. Keep the area covered with a dry, sterile dressing or clean cloth.

▶ Electrical Burns

Electrical burns are rare in the wilderness but can occur from lightning strikes (see the chapter *Physical and Environmental Hazards*), in remote households, or job sites supplied with electric power **Figure 4-22**. Sustained or high-voltage

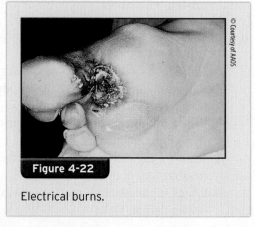
© Courtesy of AAOS

Figure 4-22

Electrical burns.

electricity produces entrance and exit burns on the skin. These can appear insignificant, but because the electric current penetrates deeply along the paths of least resistance (nerves and blood vessels), internal damage may be extensive. Respiratory and/or cardiac arrest might occur.

What to Do

1. Make sure the area is safe. Unplug the electric item, disconnect it, or turn off the power. If this is impossible, call the power company for help.
2. Check the victim's breathing. Be alert for possible fractures and/or head or spine injuries if the victim fell or was thrown to the ground by the electrical shock. Treat the victim for unresponsiveness, respiratory arrest, and cardiac arrest (see the chapter *Circulatory Emergencies*).
3. Care for entrance and exit burn wounds.
4. Evacuate to medical care unless the victim recovers rapidly and completely, the burn is minimal, and injuries do not interfere with the victim's ability to travel.

▶ Sunburn

Sunburn is caused by ultraviolet rays in the UVB wavelength. Prolonged exposure to the sun is dangerous, especially for children, and it increases the chances of skin cancer at a later age. The rays alter cells in the skin, causing cancer and premature aging. They also change pigments in the skin, increasing the amount of melanin (the golden tan). There is great variation in the tendency to become sunburned, but given enough exposure, all skin will burn **Figure 4-23**.

Sun reflects strongly off water, sand, and snow, and the effect is magnified by windburn. Ultraviolet rays penetrate hazy clouds, and though they are reduced by shadows, they are not eliminated. Preventing and reducing exposure of the skin is the cheapest, most effective way to avoid sunburn.

Clothing provides the best protection, but thin cotton clothes allow some rays to penetrate. Thicker, more opaque clothes can prevent exposure totally. Hats should have a wide brim in both the front and back. In environments with strong sun, long sleeves and pants are important.

Sun creams and lotions screen out the ultraviolet wavelengths that burn. The protective value of a sunscreen is indicated by its sun protection factor (SPF) number. The higher the SPF number, the more the protection; SPF 15 should be the minimum level of sun protection used by most people. Those with fair skin should use a sunscreen with an SPF of 25 to 30.

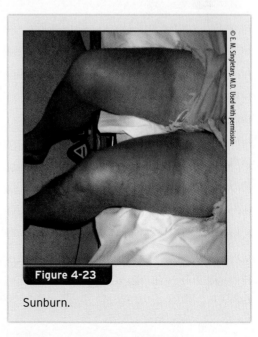

Figure 4-23

Sunburn.

Some sunscreens contain para-aminobenzoic acid (PABA), an effective sunscreen but one to which the wearer may be allergic. Alternative sunscreens do not contain PABA. In extreme sun exposure, an opaque sunscreen such as zinc oxide can be used.

Sweating and swimming will quickly remove most sunscreens. Waterproof sunscreens are available and are preferable if the wearer is going to be in and out of water. Most sunscreens should be reapplied every 2 to 4 hours.

What to Look For

- Bright lobster-red skin color.
- Blisters.

What to Do

1. Find shade if the victim's skin becomes pink and feels prickly and hot.
2. Soothe with cool compresses, baking soda compresses, or calamine lotion. Give antihistamine pills to decrease itching and ibuprofen to relieve the pain and inflammation.
3. Let burns heal. Most will do so in 2 to 3 days regardless of treatment.

▶ Emergency Care Wrap-up

What to Look For	What to Do
Bleeding	1. Ask the victim to sit or lie down. 2. Expose the wound. 3. Place a sterile gauze pad or clean cloth directly over the wound. 4. Apply direct pressure. 5. If bleeding continues for longer than 10 minutes, consider a pressure bandage. 6. If the dressings become soaked, place fresh dressings on top of the soaked ones.
Wound Infection • Redness • Warmth • Swelling • Increasing pain and tenderness • Pus • Swollen, tender glands in the groin, armpit, or neck • Chills and fever • An abscess or boil	1. Clean the area. 2. Separate the wound edges. 3. Soak the wound in warm water. 4. Change the dressings as often as needed. 5. Elevate the infected part. 6. Give the victim pain medication. 7. Evacuate the victim if the infection becomes worse.
Blisters	1. Cover with tape or moleskin. 2. Use several layers to relieve pressure.
Bruises • Pain and discoloration • Possible fracture • Purple or yellow discoloration	1. Apply a cold pack, if available. 2. Wrap the bruised area firmly with an elastic bandage. Do not cut off circulation. 3. Seek medical care for multiple bruises that appear spontaneously.

What to Look For	What to Do
Burns • Depth • Extent • Location • Severity	1. For small burns, immerse in clean, cold water or cover with a cold, wet, clean cloth. 2. Keep burned skin clean and prevent blisters from breaking. 3. Cover the burn with a dry, clean dressing. 4. Evacuate the victim to medical care.
Sunburn • Bright lobster-red skin color • Blisters	1. Find shade. 2. Soothe with cool compresses, baking soda compresses, or calamine lotion. 3. Let burns heal.

Dressings and Bandages

5

A dressing covers an open wound. Whenever possible, you should use a sterile, commercially prepared dressing, but in the wilderness, you might have to improvise. A bandage holds the dressing in place. Bandages can also be used to apply pressure over a dressing to control bleeding, prevent or reduce swelling, or provide support and stability for an injured joint or extremity.

▶ Dressings

A dressing is used to control bleeding, keep the wound clean, prevent infection, absorb blood and wound drainage, and protect from further injury. Because the dressing covers an open wound, it should be sterile. If a commercial or other sterile dressing is not available, use a clean cloth. The dressing should be larger than the wound; thick, soft, and compressible so that pressure is evenly distributed over the wound; absorbent (cotton is better than nylon or polyester); and lint free so that fibers do not stick to the wound. Do not use cotton balls as a dressing.

Types of Dressings

Use standard commercial dressings or improvise
Figure 5-1 . The following list provides examples
of commercial and improvised dressings:

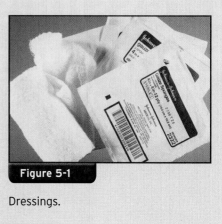

Figure 5-1

Dressings.

- Gauze pads are used for wounds requiring
  more than a small adhesive strip (such as
  a Band-Aid®). These are available in two
  common sizes (2" × 2" and 4" × 4") and
  are sold sterile in separately wrapped
  packages, or nonsterile in bulk. Nonstick
  dressings (see below) are especially useful
  for burns or oozing wounds.
- Adhesive strips come in many sizes and
  shapes. They can be improvised with a small piece of gauze and tape.
- Trauma dressings are large, thick, absorbent, and sterile.
- Nonstick dressings have a plasticlike coating or are impregnated with ointment to
  prevent adhering to wet wounds. To improvise, apply antibiotic ointment to the
  dressing or the wound.
- Improvised dressings can be any clean, absorbent, soft, and lint-free fabric. White
  cotton is optimal. Leaves, moss, and other natural products are not recommended.
  Paper is also not recommended because it sticks to wounds. If time allows, wash
  nonsterile cloth dressings in warm, soapy water and dry in the sun before using. To
  attempt sterilization, soak the dressing or cloth in a bleach solution, boil, or carefully
  heat over a flame.

▶ Bandages

A bandage is used with a dressing or to provide support for a joint or extremity injury. It should
be clean, but it does not have to be sterile.

Types of Bandages

Several types of bandages include the following:

- Adhesive tape includes white cloth athletic tape, which adheres even if it is wet. It can
  be used for taping sprains, blisters, and bandages, and it can be split lengthwise for
  narrower sizes. Duct tape is an excellent substitute. Other types of medical tape that
  can be used for wound dressings include those that feel like paper, silk, and plastic
  film (hypoallergenic) **Figure 5-2** .
- Roller gauze bandages are used to cover large wounds, to secure dressings, and to add
  extra layers. They come in various sizes (from 1" to 3" in width). Wider bandages can
  be folded as they are wrapped but are not as useful as conforming bandages.

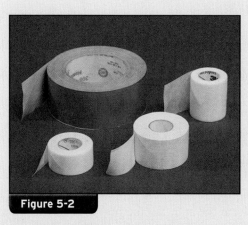

Figure 5-2

Several types of tape. Paper tape, athletic tape, hypoallergenic tape, and duct tape.

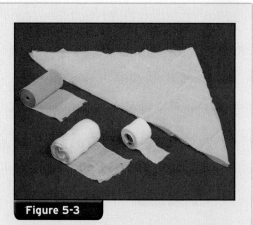

Figure 5-3

Bandage materials. Roller gauze, self-adhering roller bandage, elastic wrap, and triangular bandage.

- Self-adhering, conforming bandages are rolls of slightly elastic, gauzelike material. Two general styles are thin mesh and thicker, more absorbent mesh. The most useful widths for first aid kits are 2" and 4". If there is room in the first aid kit for only one size, take the 3" or 4" width. The self-adherent quality of these bandages makes them easy to use and to wrap around difficult areas such as joints.
- Elastic (rubberized) bandages are used for the compression of sprains, strains, and contusions. They provide good protection for wounds. Do not wrap them too tightly.
- When necessary, improvise a bandage with a bandanna or strips of cotton cloth. Other sources of improvised bandages include socks, rolled T-shirts, belts, towels, and pillowcases.
- Triangular bandages can be used as slings or to tie splints or hold bandages. They are available commercially or can be improvised from a 36" to 40" square of material. A sling can be improvised using safety pins **Figure 5-3** .

▶ Applying and Removing a Dressing

What to Do

1. Clean the wound. Wear gloves if there is any risk of blood contact.
2. Use a dressing bigger than the wound. Hold the dressing by a corner. Lay the dressing directly onto the wound; do not slide it on.
3. Tape over the dressing or secure it with a roller bandage.

4. Fasten the bandage with one of the following:
- Adhesive tape
- Safety pin(s)
- Clips provided with elastic bandage

To ensure the bandage remains in place, use the loop or split-tail method of bandaging. To perform the loop method, follow these steps:

1. Tie the bandage ends that encircle the body part from opposite directions  **Figure 5-4A** . If necessary, reverse the direction of the bandage by looping it around a thumb or finger and continue back to the opposite side of the body part.

2. Encircle the part with the looped end and the free end and tie them together **Figure 5-4B** .

CAUTION

DO NOT
- Touch the wound or the dressing that will be in contact with the wound.
- Bandage so tightly as to restrict blood circulation.
- Bandage so loosely that the dressing will slip. Bandages tend to stretch.

To perform the split-tail method of securing a bandage, follow these steps:

1. Split the end of the bandage lengthwise for about 12", then tie a knot to prevent further splitting **Figure 5-5A** .

2. Pass the ends in opposite directions around the body part and tie **Figure 5-5B** .

A square knot is preferred, because it will not slip and can easily be untied. If the knot causes discomfort, put a pad under it.

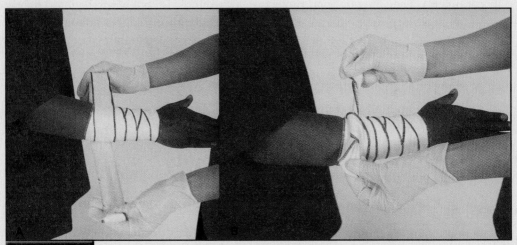

Figure 5-4

Loop method of bandaging. **A.** Tie the bandage ends that encircle the body part from opposite directions. **B.** Encircle the part with the looped end and the free end and tie them together.

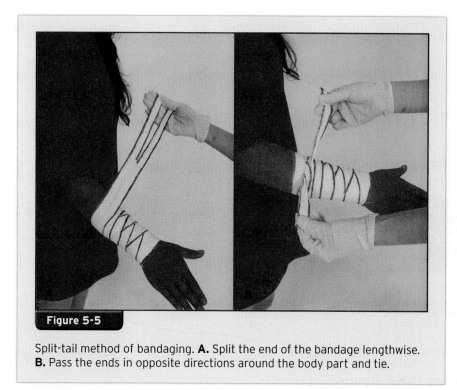

Figure 5-5

Split-tail method of bandaging. **A.** Split the end of the bandage lengthwise.
B. Pass the ends in opposite directions around the body part and tie.

A bulky wrap fashioned with a lot of turns will restrict most movement. If further immobilization is needed, add a splint or use a sling.

Removing Dressings

If a dressing is stuck to a wound, soak it in warm water for 10 to 20 minutes, and then gently peel it off. Burn used dressings in a campfire.

▶ Bandaging Techniques

Bandaging the Ear

If the bandage covers the ear, place strips of gauze or cloth behind the ear and the folds of the ear to maintain the ear's normal anatomic position and shape.

Bandaging the Head

For a wound on the forehead or back of the scalp, wrap the head with a cloth cravat or a roller gauze bandage. To avoid bandaging over the ears, wrap low on the forehead and place ties under the bandage in front of the ears **Figure 5-6A-B** .

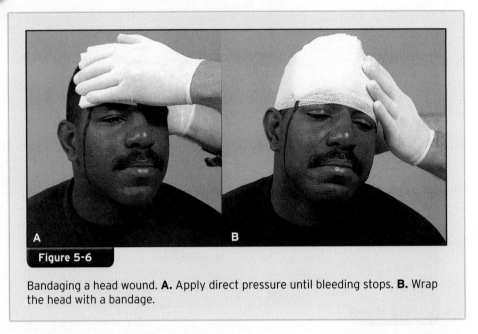

Figure 5-6

Bandaging a head wound. **A.** Apply direct pressure until bleeding stops. **B.** Wrap the head with a bandage.

Bandaging the Extremities

To bandage an arm or a leg, begin at the narrow part of the limb and wrap toward the wider part of the extremity. Start with two anchor turns, and then continue by overlapping each turn by one half to three fourths of the width of the bandage. Tape or tie the end **Figure 5-7A-C** .

Bandaging the Elbow and Knee

To apply a 4" or 6" roller bandage to the elbow or knee using the figure-8 method, follow these steps:

1. Bend the elbow or knee slightly and make two straight anchoring turns with the bandage over the elbow point or kneecap **Figure 5-8A** .
2. Bring the bandage above the joint to the upper arm or leg, and make one turn, covering one half to three fourths of the bandage from the first turn **Figure 5-8B** .
3. Bring the bandage just under the joint and make one turn around the lower arm or leg, covering one half to three fourths of the bandage from the first turn **Figure 5-8C** .

Bandaging the Wrist and the Hand

Use a figure-8 wrap for hands, too. Alternate encircling the hand, leaving the thumb free if it is uninjured **Figure 5-9A-C** .

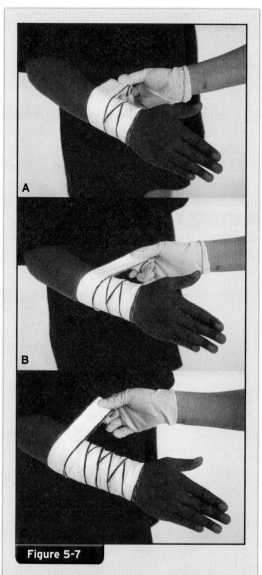

Figure 5-7

Spiral method of bandaging. **A.** Make two straight anchoring turns with a bandage. **B.** Wrap with criss-cross (figure-8) turns. **C.** Finish with two straight turns and secure the bandage.

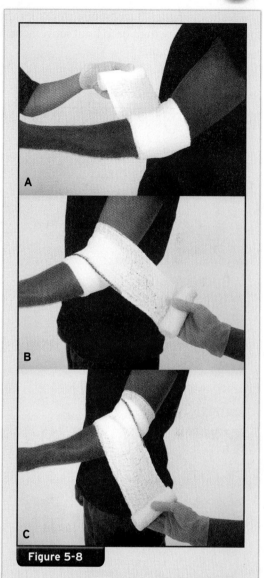

Figure 5-8

Figure-8 method of bandaging. **A.** Bend the elbow and make two anchoring turns. **B.** Bring the bandage above the joint and make one turn. **C.** Bring the bandage just under the joint and make one turn.

A similar figure-8 technique works for dressing the fingers when a bulky wrap is needed to cover the entire digit or to limit movement. Wrapping around the wrist anchors the dressing so it does not slip off.

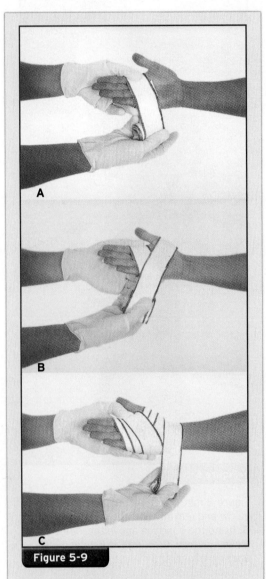

Figure 5-9

Bandaging the hand. **A.** Anchor the bandage with one or two turns around the palm. **B.** Carry the bandage diagonally across the back of the hand and then around the wrist. **C.** Repeat the figure-8 maneuver as many times as necessary to cover the dressing.

Bandaging the Palm of Hand

With deep wounds or injuries that might include tendons or bone, place a dressing on the wound; place a roll or wad in the palm of the hand with the fingers curled around it. Wrap the bandage around the victim's entire hand, anchoring and tying at the wrist **Figure 5-10A-B**. If the thumb and index finger are uninjured, they can be left out to maintain some use of the hand.

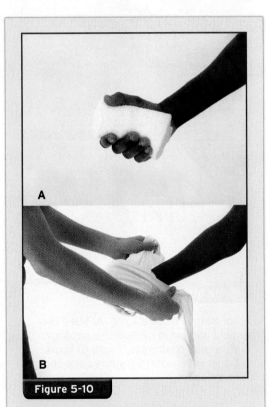

Figure 5-10

Bandaging the palm of the hand or to prevent movement of injured fingers. **A.** Fill the palm with a bulky dressing or pad. **B.** Wrap the bandage, crossing over the fingers and around the wrist.

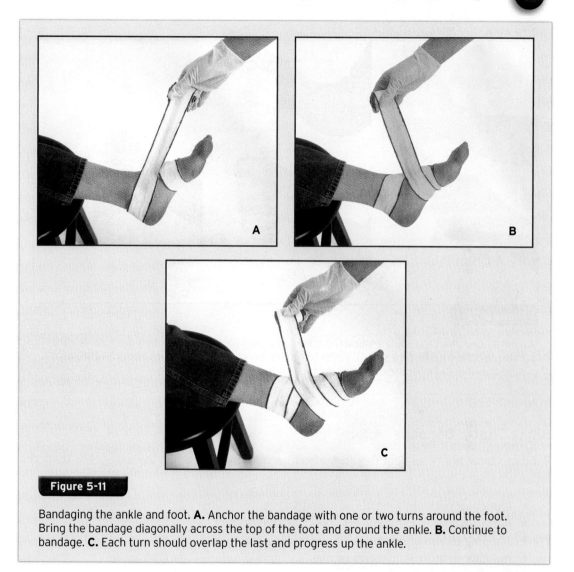

Figure 5-11

Bandaging the ankle and foot. **A.** Anchor the bandage with one or two turns around the foot. Bring the bandage diagonally across the top of the foot and around the ankle. **B.** Continue to bandage. **C.** Each turn should overlap the last and progress up the ankle.

Bandaging the Ankle and Foot

For ankle and foot injuries, use a figure-8 wrap. Alternate encircling the foot and the ankle **Figure 5-11**. The same technique is used for a dressing or compression wrap for an ankle sprain.

Applying Indirect Pressure

Use a doughnut-shaped object to avoid pressure on a wound with a suspected skull fracture, for an open fracture, or in the event of an embedded foreign body object like glass or gravel that cannot be removed in the field **Figure 5-12**.

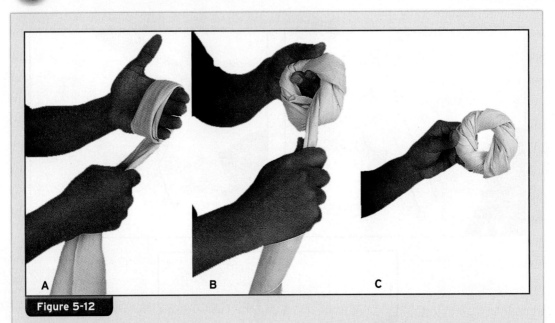

Figure 5-12

Making a "doughnut" to apply around the edges of a skull fracture or an open fracture. **A.** Wrap a cravat around your fingers several times to create a ring. **B.** Wrap the remainder of the roll around the ring. **C.** Finish the doughnut by tucking the end into a fold.

Signs That a Bandage Is Too Tight

Bandages must not be so tight that they affect normal circulation. If a bandage is too tight, the following might occur:

- Blue tinge of the fingernails or toenails
- Blue or pale skin color and coldness of the extremity
- Tingling or loss of sensation
- Inability to move the fingers or toes
- Pain beyond the bandage

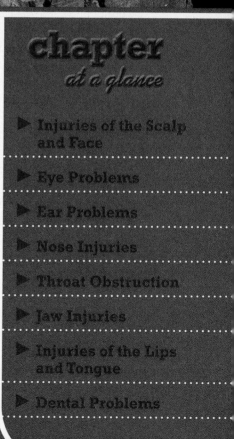

© Tomasz Laplaszynski/iStockphoto/Thinkstock

Head and Facial Injuries

6

Injuries of the face and head are common. Severe injuries may damage the airway by breaking the nose or jaw and causing swelling inside the mouth. Because of the mechanism of injury, all victims with face or head injuries should be assumed to have a brain or spinal injury until proven otherwise. In some instances, the injury will be so superficial that it is obvious that the spine and brain are undamaged. In other injuries, there may be doubt about the integrity of the brain and spine, increasing the danger and complexity of these cases. The ability to differentiate between serious head and neck trauma and minor injuries is important.

Injuries of the Scalp and Face

▶ Scalp Wounds

What to Look For

- Profuse bleeding, because of the generous blood supply of the scalp. Extensive bleeding does not necessarily imply a brain or skull injury.
- Signs of neck or brain injury, such as neck pain, paralysis, or altered level of responsiveness
- Exposed bone, indicating a deep, severe wound, possibly associated with a skull fracture

What to Do

1. Evaluate for head and spinal injury.
2. Control bleeding with pressure.
3. When bleeding has been controlled, remove dirt, blood clots, and hair from the wound, and then wash the wound with soap and water. Cover the wound with a sterile dressing.
4. If medical care will be delayed and the wound is gaping, twist small bundles of hair and tie them across the wound, drawing the edges snugly together. Make sure there is no dirt or debris in the wound before it is closed.
5. If oozing continues, do not remove the first blood-soaked dressing, but add another dressing over it.
6. Monitor the victim for brain injury using the AVPU scale.
7. Evacuate the victim if:
   - The laceration is extensive.
   - Infection is likely because of wound contamination.
   - There is significant involvement of the face.
   - The injury is associated with signs of brain injury.

▶ Facial Wounds

What to Look For

In the event of facial wounds, look for extensive bleeding. The bleeding might be superficial or it might involve the cavity of the mouth, the eyelids, or the ears.

What to Do

1. Clean the wound with soap and water.
2. If the wound is large, restore the skin flaps as best as you can, and apply a dressing.
3. Evacuate all but trivial injuries. Helicopter evacuation is not necessary for a simple laceration; wounds may be safely closed several days later.

▶ Facial Fracture

A blow to the head can cause a facial fracture. The bony ring around the eye socket might be broken and deformed.

What to Look For

- An eyeball that is protruding outward or sunken inward
- Double vision or abnormal eye movements (eyes that do not point in the same direction, or one eye that does not move in all directions)
- A cheek on one side that is tender and flatter than on the other side
- A step in the smooth lower rim of the orbit
- Pain on opening the mouth widely or chewing

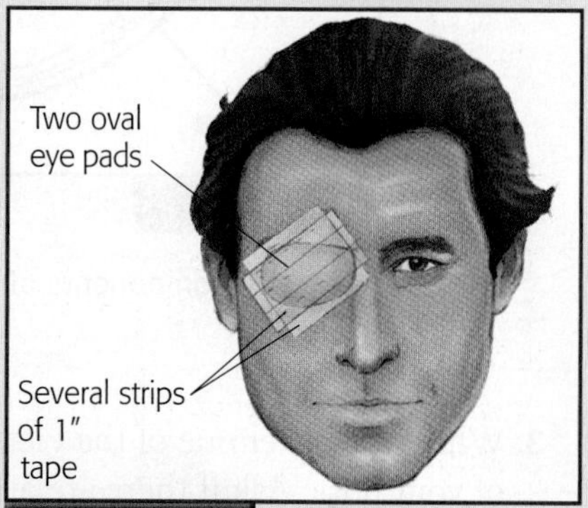

Two oval eye pads

Several strips of 1" tape

Figure 6-1

Method for patching an eye. Use a double eye patch held in place with several strips of 1" tape.

What to Do

1. Patch one eye to correct double vision **Figure 6-1**.
2. Evacuate to a surgeon.

Eye Problems

Eye problems are common in the wilderness. Many are mild and can be treated in the field, but some are very serious and require evacuation. Accurate assessment and treatment of eye problems requires careful observation and a basic understanding of eye anatomy **Figure 6-2**.

What to Look For

1. Observe the eyes. Are there any obvious problems, such as foreign bodies, redness, blood, pus, or unequal pupils? Do both eyes move in the same direction?
2. Test the vision in each eye separately, covering one eye at a time. Ask the victim to read normal print or to count fingers.

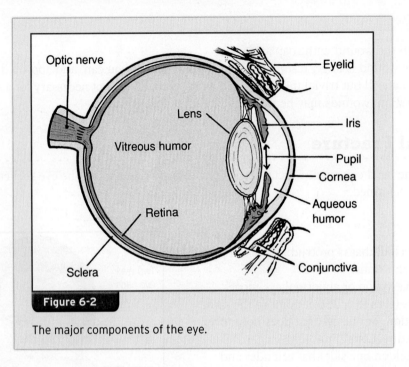

Figure 6-2

The major components of the eye.

3. While you cover one of the victim's eyes, ask the victim to look straight at the bridge of your nose. Ask if there are any blind spots or dark areas. Repeat while covering the other eye.

What to Do

1. If the victim has any new changes in vision, seek medical care as soon as possible.
2. Evacuate the victim.

▶ Contact Lenses

Contact lenses can cause severe problems, especially if they are worn for longer than recommended, or if they are improperly cared for. Contact lens wearers should always bring proper supplies and a pair of glasses into the wilderness. Treat problems from overuse by having the wearer remove them and use glasses, if possible. Do not replace the lenses until eye discomfort has resolved. If it is not possible to remove the lenses, try putting a few drops of lens rewetting solution (not cleaning solution) into the eye, and using sunglasses. Should an eye injury or infection occur, remove the lens.

Two methods for removing soft and hard lenses are as follows: (1) slide the lens over to the white area away from the nose; (2) while keeping the eye slightly open, put one finger at the outer edge of the lower eyelid and pull the eyelid tight causing the lens to be squeezed off the eyeball. Another removal option for a soft contact lens is to pinch the lens gently between your thumb and index finger forming the lens into the shape of a taco shell.

▶ Dry Eye

Dry eye is caused by increased tear evaporation, usually in very dry climates, windy conditions, or dusty or smoky environments. Symptoms may be described as itchy, scratchy, stinging, or tired eyes. Pain and redness may occur.

Treatment includes blinking more often and resting the eyes. Rubbing the eyes can irritate them further. Applying artificial tears every few hours can provide temporary relief. Avoid environments that might exacerbate the condition. Wearing wraparound glasses can help reduce the drying effects of wind.

▶ Infection

Eye infections can result from injury, foreign bodies, or transmission from another person. The most common eye infection is conjunctivitis or "pinkeye." Pinkeye is a highly contagious viral infection that is uncomfortable, but rarely causes long-term problems. Foreign bodies in the eye and infection may have a similar appearance. If you suspect infection, also look for foreign objects.

What to Look For

- Red, possibly itching, eye
- Lids stuck together with pus, especially in the morning after waking up

What to Do

1. Wash the eye frequently with warm water.
2. Apply antibiotic eye drops or antibiotic ophthalmic eye ointment in both eyes three to four times a day.
3. Avoid spreading the infection to other people. The victim, other members of the victim's party, and the first aid provider should wash their hands frequently. Remember, frequent hand washing is the best way to prevent communicable diseases.

▶ Nonpenetrating Injury

Subconjunctival bleeding (blood over the white part of the eye) can occur after a blow to the eye or often without a history of significant injury. Although a subconjunctival hemorrhage appears serious, it usually is not, and it normally requires no treatment. Blood visible in the clear part of the eye, over the iris, represents a serious injury and requires evacuation to medical care immediately. Injury to the eye can also cause a retinal detachment, which is a serious injury to the retina (the light-detecting membrane of the eye). Retinal detachment usually causes visual changes. Any change in vision should receive medical care immediately **Figure 6-3** .

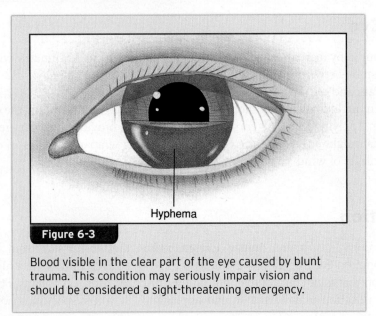

Hyphema

Figure 6-3

Blood visible in the clear part of the eye caused by blunt trauma. This condition may seriously impair vision and should be considered a sight-threatening emergency.

What to Look For

- Change in vision
- Blood over the white of the eye, with no change in vision
- Blood in the clear part of the eye

What to Do

1. If blood is seen under the cornea, or if visual changes are present, evacuate the patient.

▶ Foreign Body

A small foreign body, such as dirt, a wood chip, or a metal fragment, may become embedded in the cornea or lodged under an eyelid. Injury to the eye may cause a scratching feeling, pain, watering of the eye, redness, and discomfort in bright light.

What to Look For

- Look on the surface of the eye for foreign material.
- Check under both upper and lower eyelids for a foreign body. Pull down the lower eyelid. Turn the upper eyelid over a smooth, clean object such as a cotton swab or matchstick **Figure 6-4** .

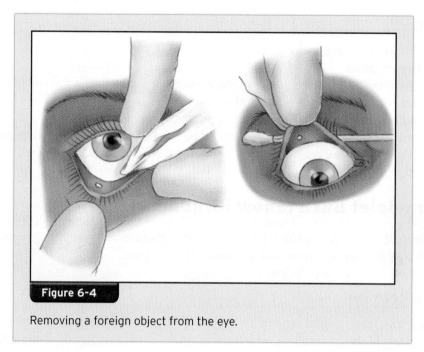

Figure 6-4

Removing a foreign object from the eye.

What to Do

1. If the foreign object is visible, carefully remove it with a clean, preferably damp, cotton swab or corner of gauze or cloth.
2. Have the victim pull the upper eyelid down over the lower eyelid and blow his or her nose on that side. This helps flush tears over the eye and may wash out a loose piece of foreign material.
3. Wash the eye with clean water or eye wash solution. Repeat as necessary.
4. Reexamine the eye and remove any visible debris.
5. If the object is metal, seek medical care. Evacuation is not necessary, but the victim should see an eye doctor as soon as possible, even if the symptoms resolve. Metal can become permanently embedded and cause problems later.

▶ Scratch

A foreign object can scratch the eyeball. The painful scratchy feeling usually heals within 24 to 48 hours. It may feel like the foreign object is still present, even if it is not.

What to Look For

- Symptoms are similar to those of a foreign body. A severe scratch or abrasion may be visible.
- Changes in vision

What to Do

1. Treat as for a foreign object.
2. Try sunglasses.
3. Use pain or anti-inflammatory medications such as acetaminophen or ibuprofen. A damp cloth over the eyes can provide some relief.
4. If pain persists, patch the eye until symptoms improve.
5. If pain or visual changes last beyond 48 hours, signs of infection develop (such as pus), or a visible ulcer develops on the cornea, seek medical care immediately.

▶ Ultraviolet Burn (Snow Blindness)

Ultraviolet radiation from the sun reflecting strongly off of snow, dry sand, light-colored rocks, or a body of water can burn the cornea, causing intense pain.

What to Look For

- Redness, tearing, light sensitivity, slight clouding of the cornea soon after exposure
- Swelling of the conjunctiva, which causes the eyes to close tightly, leading to temporary blindness
- Blistering of the cornea, which blurs vision

To prevent snow blindness, wear dark glasses or goggles. In an emergency, cut horizontal slits or punch multiple pinholes in a piece of cardboard or duct tape doubled on itself, and tie it around the head with string **Figure 6-5**. Cut side shields to prevent glare.

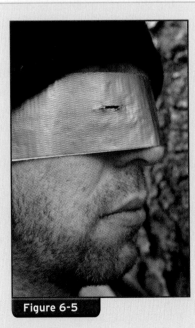

Figure 6-5

Improvised goggles.

What to Do

1. Give the victim painkillers.
2. Lead or carry the victim to safety.
3. After reaching safety, treat both eyes as if they have suffered a severe corneal scratch. The pain and swelling should subside in a day.

▶ Chemical Burn

Acid burns (eg, from battery acid) usually heal quickly, like an abrasion or ultraviolet burn. Alkali burns (eg, from lime) are severe and need urgent medical care.

What to Do

1. Find out what entered the eye. Was it acid or alkali? Give this information to medical professionals. Do not try to neutralize the chemicals with other chemicals.
2. Irrigate the eye with water immediately, continuously, and gently for 20 minutes. Remove any chemical particles.

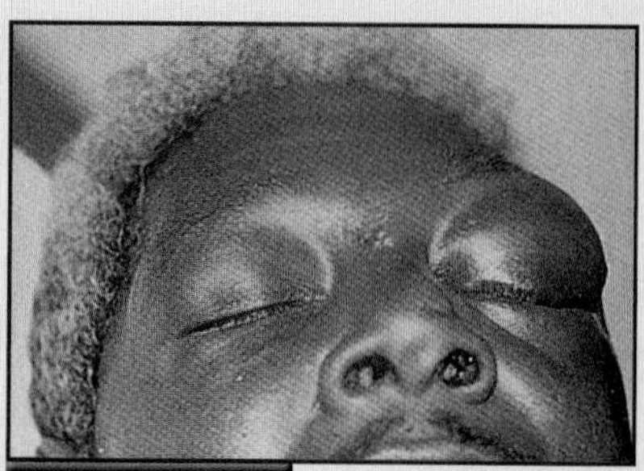

Figure 6-6

Swelling around the eye caused by a blow to the area.

▶ Bruising

A black eye is the blue or purple discoloration of the tissue around the eye. Causes vary, and include a blow to the area or blood that settles into the area from a broken nose, skull fracture, or forehead wound **Figure 6-6** .

What to Look For

- Decreased vision. You might need to hold the eye open to evaluate vision if the lids are swollen shut.
- Blood in the clear part of the eye
- After a few hours, the blood settles by gravity; a level of blood can be seen in the front of the eye, and vision clears.
- Increasing pain, redness, tearing, and light sensitivity 1 to 3 days after a blow to the eye (indicating inflammation inside the eye or iris)

What to Do

1. Apply a cold pack for about 15 minutes. Do not press the pack on the eye.
2. Evacuate the victim as soon as possible if there is any alteration in vision or blood in the clear part of the eye over the iris.

▶ Frozen Eyelashes

During a blizzard, eyelashes can become frozen together so that the eye cannot be opened. Warm the eye with a hand to melt the ice. No harm will come to the eye.

▶ Open Injury (Penetrating)

An open injury of the eyeball is an injury that penetrates through to the inside of the eye, possibly allowing eye contents to spill out, and causing serious damage to the eye. Open injuries can be obvious, such as from a large object like a stick or ski pole, or less obvious, such as from a flying piece of debris like fragment from a metal axe. Often the wound in the cornea is tiny and seals over, disguising the injury.

What to Look For

- Red, painful eye with tearing and light sensitivity
- Damage to the iris, causing an irregularly shaped pupil
- Impaired vision
- Extrusion of the contents of the eyeball

What to Do

1. Protect the eye with a cardboard shield or a doughnut-shaped rolled bandage (this depends on the length of the penetrating object).
2. Administer painkillers.
3. Evacuate to an eye surgeon immediately.

▶ Impaled Object

Objects may become caught or embedded in the eyeball. Do not push the object further into the eye by applying a patch. Evacuate the victim as soon as possible.

Protect the injured eye with a paper cup, cardboard folded into a cone, or a doughnut-shaped pad made from roller gauze bandage or a cravat bandage.

▶ Eyelid Injury

If an eyelid is infected or lacerated, always check the globe of the eye for associated injury **Figure 6-7**.

▶ What to Look For

- A cut in the eyelid margin, creating a notch
- A cut in the corner of the eye near the nose where the tear ducts lie

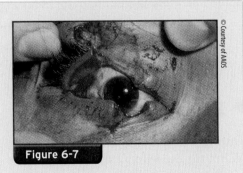

Figure 6-7

Laceration of the upper and lower eyelid.

▶ What to Do

1. In the event of an eyelid injury, protect the eye with a cardboard shield or a doughnut-shaped rolled bandage.
2. If medical care is delayed, use butterfly strips to reapproximate the skin. Patch the eye if more protection is needed, or to keep the eye from drying out.
3. Keep the victim reclining at 45°; cover the damaged eye with a soft, sterile dressing.
4. Evacuate the victim to a surgeon.

▶ Lost Eyeglasses

All persons who wear eyeglasses should take an extra pair on a wilderness trip. A cheap pair of drugstore glasses might be sufficient to allow the person to function adequately if necessary. Nearsighted people who lose or break their only pair of glasses can increase the acuity of their vision by looking through cardboard or duct tape goggles punched with multiple pinholes.

Ear Problems

Generally, ear problems do not threaten a person's life. But in the wilderness, small objects or insects may lodge in the ear canal and damage hearing if not treated.

▶ Foreign Body in the Ear

What to Do

1. Pull the earlobe upward and backward to straighten the canal. Lubricate the inside of the ear with vegetable or mineral oil. Have the victim turn his or her head to one side to drain the oil.
2. Flush the ear with clean, warm water using a syringe. Use moderate pressure, but do not block the ear canal with the syringe. Vegetable objects, such as beans, might swell in contact with water, so try an oil lubricant (not motor oil) first if such an object is in the ear.

3. Insects are best removed by first drowning them with water or a drop of mineral or vegetable cooking oil. If the insect can be seen, remove it carefully with tweezers; otherwise flush the ear with warm water.
4. Remove visible foreign bodies from the ear canal carefully with tweezers.

> **CAUTION**
>
> DO NOT probe the ear with matchsticks or twigs; this can damage the eardrum.

Nose Injuries

▶ Nosebleed

Bleeding usually stops after a few minutes with pressure alone. On rare occasions, an uncontrollable nosebleed may threaten the victim's life. Bleeding typically comes from a spot that cannot be seen on the center divider (septum) of the nose.

What to Look For

- Bleeding from one or both nostrils

What to Do

1. Have the victim lean slightly forward, with his or her head bowed.
2. Squeeze the nostrils together for 5 minutes.
3. If bleeding continues, have the victim blow his or her nose gently or sniff to remove clots. If available, spray the nose four times on both sides with nasal decongestant spray (such as Afrin or Neo-Synephrine).
4. If bleeding continues, squeeze the nose again for 5 minutes.
5. Place a cold pack, preferably made of ice or snow wrapped in a damp cloth, across the bridge of the nose.
6. Encourage breathing through the mouth.
7. Instruct the victim to avoid picking at clots, rubbing, or blowing his or her nose other than when attempting to stop the nosebleed as described in step 3 above.

▶ Broken Nose

What to Look For

- A swollen, tender, and possibly misshapen nose
- Bleeding and difficulty in breathing through the nostrils
- Black eyes, which usually appear 1 to 2 days after the nose has been broken
- Check for an eye injury by testing the vision of both eyes.

What to Do

Apply ice or a cold pack to reduce the swelling and bleeding. Treat a nosebleed as described previously.

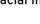

CAUTION

DO NOT try to straighten a crooked nose.

A nasal fracture and two black eyes may look bad, but, without deformity, they need no treatment. Even with some deformity, this is not an urgent problem. A surgeon can deal with a deformed fracture up to a week later.

Throat Obstruction

▶ Swallowed Foreign Body

A small bone or piece of food can become stuck in the throat or esophagus. Objects stuck in the throat require immediate action.

What to Look For

- Meat or food stuck in the esophagus is painful and can cause vomiting, but the victim can breathe and speak normally.
- A piece of meat or other food stuck in the throat or at the vocal cords causes choking, and the victim cannot speak or breathe.

What to Do

1. For obstructed breathing, use abdominal thrusts (the Heimlich maneuver).
2. For food stuck in the esophagus, have the victim sip liquids to try to wash the piece down. It may be possible to regurgitate the food, but this can take several hours. Try to see a small bone in the throat by pushing the tongue down with the handle of a spoon. Bones commonly lodge at the base of the tongue or around the edge of the tonsil. If you can see the bone, grasp it with tweezers or rub it off with a cotton tip. If you cannot see the lodged bone, have the victim swallow dry bread to dislodge it.

Jaw Injuries

▶ Fracture

What to Look For

- Injury to the jaw or face
- Uneven, loose, or missing teeth

- Inability to chew or clench the teeth; the jaw does not close properly
- Pain and tenderness along the jawbone (feel along the lower and inner edge to avoid causing simple bruises) or at the joint in front of the ear (there are often two areas of fracture)
- Double vision, a flattened cheek, or numbness on one side of the nose and lip, which indicate other facial bone fractures

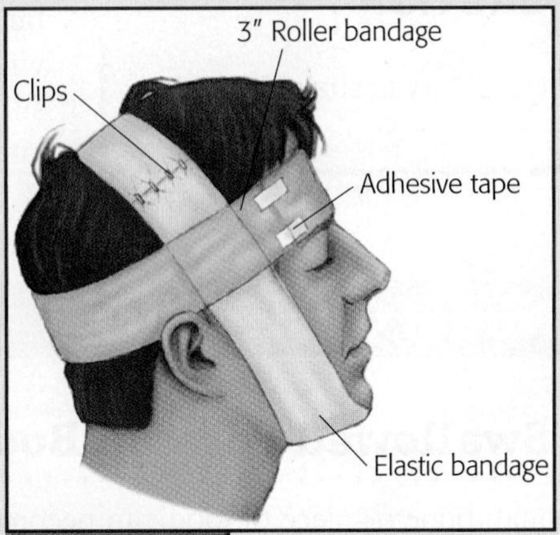

What to Do

1. Guide the lower jaw into position against the upper jaw and secure with a cravat bandage tied around the head and under the jaw **Figure 6-8**. Be sure the cravat bandage can be removed rapidly if the victim begins to vomit.
2. Feed the victim a fluid diet until the jaw can be seen by a dentist or oral surgeon.

Figure 6-8

Method of bandaging a fractured jaw.

▶ **Dislocation**

What to Look For

- The jaw popped out of place with a yawn, wide opening of the mouth, yelling, or a blow to the jaw.
- Inability to close the jaw
- Misalignment
- Pain in front of the ears (temporomandibular joint, or TMJ) but no tenderness in the lower arch of the jaw
- Prominence of the jaw bone in front of the ears and below the cheekbones

What to Do

1. Stand in front of the seated victim. Place the fingers of both hands under the lower jaw. The classic method is to place your thumbs into the mouth over the lower molars (pad your thumbs to protect from biting), and then push steadily downward and backward **Figure 6-9**. Hold steady firm pressure until the jaw slides back into position. A newer method is to push down and back on the prominent bone in front of the ears and below the cheekbones, from outside of the mouth.

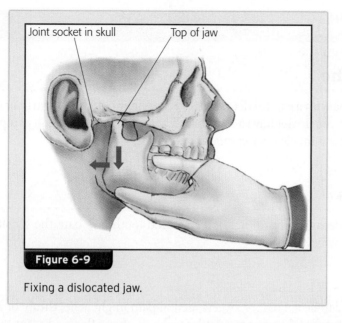

Joint socket in skull   Top of jaw

Figure 6-9

Fixing a dislocated jaw.

Injuries of the Lips and Tongue

Cuts to the tongue and lips are usually caused by the teeth. Bleeding is the major problem because of a rich blood supply. The laceration may be on one side or all the way through, in the middle, or at the edge.

▶ Cuts on the Lips and Tongue

What to Do

1. Control bleeding by applying direct pressure with a gauze pad or cloth pinched with the fingers.
2. Apply ice, if available.
3. Soak gauze or cloth with nasal decongestant spray or drops, and then apply it to the wound.
4. Have the victim avoid crumbly foods.
5. Have the victim rinse well after eating.
6. Evacuate the victim in the event of:
   - Full-thickness lacerations of the tongue, longer than ½".
   - Significant-sized flaps of the lips or the edge of the tongue that do not stay in place.
   - Cuts of the lip that extend through the junction of the lip and facial skin wounds that extend through the lips.

Dental Problems

▶ Toothache

Prevent toothache with a careful dental check, especially before a long trip or expedition. Clean teeth regularly. If you do not have a toothbrush, rub your teeth with salt or a peeled green stick. Chewing sugarless gum cleans the mouth and gums.

▶ Cavities

A cavity due to decay, a lost filling, or a fractured tooth lays bare the sensitive dentin under the enamel.

What to Look For

- Sensitivity to heat, cold, or sweets; dental pain might ache, throb, or sear, and it might be difficult to localize to a particular tooth. It often affects adjacent teeth and can spread from the upper jaw to the lower and vice versa, but never across the midline.
- Sensitivity to touch. Tap the teeth gently with something metal (such as a spoon handle) on the top and side. A diseased tooth will hurt.

What to Do

1. Rinse and flush the mouth.
2. Apply oil of cloves (eugenol) on a cotton swab to the cavity to deaden the pain.
3. Apply a temporary filling of synthetic tooth cement (such as Cavit), if available. Push the dressing paste into the cavity with a finger and press it down with a matchstick. Have the person with the toothache bite it into place before it sets. Other options that could be applied include sugarless gum, ski wax, or candle wax.
4. Give aspirin, ibuprofen, or acetaminophen for pain. Do not place an aspirin directly on the painful tooth; it should be swallowed.

▶ Abscess

What to Look For

- Swelling of the gums around the diseased tooth
- Swelling of the jaw visible in the face
- Foul breath
- Pain that is exacerbated by tapping the tooth

What to Do

1. Have the victim rinse his or her mouth with warm water to soothe, cleanse, and encourage pus to discharge into the mouth.
2. Give the victim aspirin or ibuprofen for pain. If the person has antibiotics available, the best choices are amoxicillin or erythromycin, 500 mg 4 times a day; the next best choice is penicillin. See the appendix *First Aid Equipment and Supplies* for use of antibiotics.
3. See a dentist after leaving the wilderness.

▶ Avulsed (Knocked-Out) Tooth

What to Do

1. Handle the tooth only by the crown, not the root.
2. If the tooth is dirty, rinse the tooth gently with clean water or milk.
3. Give the victim a warm salt mouthwash if it is immediately available (1 teaspoon of salt to 1 quart of water).
4. Replace the tooth immediately into the socket **Figure 6-10**. Do not delay this step. Survival of the tooth depends on prompt replacement. Have the victim hold the tooth in place by holding the jaws gently clenched together with enough pressure to keep the tooth in place. If the tooth cannot be replaced in the socket, have the victim hold the tooth in the mouth between the cheek and gums (this should not be done if there is a risk of choking, such as in young children or with altered level of responsiveness). If the victim cannot keep the tooth in the mouth, transport the tooth with the victim while keeping the tooth covered with saliva or cold milk.
5. Evacuate to a dentist immediately.

CAUTION
DO NOT
• Pull the tooth out.
• Probe with a needle.

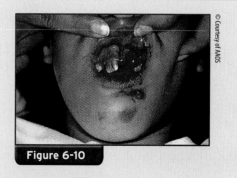

© Courtesy of AAOS

Figure 6-10

A tooth knocked from the upper jaw.

▶ Emergency Care Wrap-up

What to Look For	What to Do
Injuries of the Scalp and Face	
Scalp Wounds • Profuse bleeding • Blood pooled under the neck • Exposed bone	1. Evaluate for head and spinal injury. 2. Control bleeding with pressure. 3. Remove dirt, blood clots, and hair from the wound. 4. Wash the wound with soap and water. 5. Cover the wound with a sterile compress. 6. Twist small bundles of hair and tie them across the wound. 7. Monitor the victim for brain injury using the AVPU scale. 8. Evacuate the victim.
Facial Wounds • Extensive bleeding	1. Clean the wound with soap and water. 2. If the wound is large, restore the skin flaps and apply a dressing. 3. Evacuate all but trivial injuries.
Facial Fracture • An eyeball that is displaced inward • A tender cheek • Double vision • Eyes that look in different directions or do not move together • Painful chewing or opening the mouth	1. Patch the eye on the injured side 2. Evacuate to a surgeon.
Eye Problems	
Eye Infection • Red eye • Lids stuck together with pus	1. Wash the eye with warm water. 2. Apply antibiotic eye drops or antibiotic ophthalmic eye ointment.
Foreign Body in Eye • Inspect the cornea with magnification • Look under both eyelids. Pull down the lower lid; turn the upper lid over a matchstick or cotton swab	1. Wash the eye with water; reexamine and wash again if a foreign body is still present, or 2. Carefully remove the speck with a folded corner of a damp gauze, cloth, or cotton tip.

What to Look For	What to Do
Scratched Eye • Tearing • Blurred vision • Indications of pain	1. Give the victim painkillers and apply a damp cloth over the eye. 2. Patch or pad the eye if pain is severe.
Ultraviolet Burn (Snow Blindness) • Redness, tearing, light sensitivity, slight clouding of the cornea • Swelling of the conjunctiva • Blistering of the cornea	1. Give the victim painkillers and apply a damp cloth over both eyes. 2. Lead or carry the victim to safety. 3. After reaching safety, treat both eyes as if they have suffered a severe corneal scratch. The pain and swelling should subside in a day. If it has not resolved in 24–48 hours, evacuate for medical care.
Chemical Burn	1. Try to determine what entered the eye. 2. Irrigate with water for 20 minutes.
Bruising Around Eye • Decreased vision • Blood filling the front of the eye • Increasing pain, redness, tearing, and light sensitivity	1. Apply a cold pack for about 15 minutes. 2. Evacuate the victim if there is decreased vision or blood in the clear part of the eye.
Open Injury (Penetrating) • Red, painful eye with tearing and light sensitivity • Pear-shaped pupil • Impaired vision	1. Protect the eye with a cardboard shield or a doughnut-shaped rolled bandage. 2. Administer painkillers. 3. Evacuate to an eye surgeon immediately.
Impaled Object	1. Do not push the object further into eye. 2. Protect the eye with a cardboard shield or a doughnut-shaped rolled bandage. 3. Evacuate the victim to an eye surgeon immediately.
Eyelid Injury • A cut in the lid margin • A cut in the corner of the eye near the nose where the tear ducts lie	1. Protect the eye with a cardboard shield or a doughnut-shaped rolled bandage. 2. Recline victim to 45° and cover injured eye with sterile dressing. 3. Evacuate the victim to a surgeon.

What to Look For	What to Do
Nose Injuries	
Nosebleed • Bleeding from one or both nostrils	1. Have the victim lean slightly forward. 2. Squeeze nostrils together for 5 minutes. 3. If available, spray the nose with nasal decongestant spray. 4. If bleeding continues, squeeze the nose again for 5 minutes. 5. Place a cold pack across the bridge of the nose. 6. Encourage breathing through the mouth. 7. Instruct the victim to avoid picking at clots, rubbing, or blowing his or her nose.
Broken Nose • A swollen, tender, and possibly misshapen nose • Bleeding and difficulty in breathing through the nostrils • Black eyes	1. Apply ice or a cold pack to reduce the swelling and bleeding.
Throat Obstruction	
Swallowed Foreign Body • Choking • Cannot speak or breathe	1. For obstructed breathing, use abdominal thrusts. 2. For food stuck in the esophagus, have the victim sip liquids to try to wash the piece down.
Jaw Injuries	
Jaw Fracture • Uneven, loose, or missing teeth • Injury to the jaw or face • Inability to chew or clench the teeth • Pain and tenderness • Double vision, a flattened cheek, or numbness on one side of the nose and lip	1. Guide the lower jaw into position against the upper jaw and secure with a cravat bandage tied around the head and under the jaw. 2. Feed the victim a fluid diet until the jaw can be seen by a dentist or oral surgeon.

What to Look For	What to Do
Jaw Dislocation • History of the jaw popping out with a yawn or wide opening of the mouth • Inability to close the jaw • Misalignment • Pain in front of the ears but no tenderness in the lower arch of the jaw	1. Support the lower jaw with the fingers of both hands, place your thumbs over the person's lower molars, and then push steadily down and backward. 2. Secure with a cravat for a few days and feed the victim liquids.

Injuries of the Lips and Tongue

Cuts on the Lips and Tongue	1. Control bleeding. 2. Apply cold pack. 3. Soak gauze or cloth with nasal decongestant and apply to wound.

Dental Problems

Cavities • Sensitivity to heat, cold, or sweets • Sensitivity to touch	1. Rinse and flush the mouth. 2. Apply oil of cloves on a cotton swab to the cavity. 3. Apply temporary dressing of synthetic tooth cement.
Abscess • Swelling of the gums • Swelling of the jaw • Foul breath • Pain exacerbated by tapping the tooth	1. Have the victim rinse his or her mouth with warm water. 2. Give the victim aspirin or ibuprofen for pain. 3. See a dentist after leaving the wilderness.
Avulsed Tooth	1. Give victim a warm salt mouthwash. 2. Rinse the tooth gently in clean water and replace it immediately. 3. Evacuate the victim to a dentist as soon as possible.

7

Bone, Joint, and Muscle Injuries

Sprains, strains, contusions, fractures, and dislocations of the extremities are among the most common injuries in the wilderness. How these injuries are treated depends on the expertise of those in the party and the distance from medical help.

Common sense, diagnostic skills, and sensitivity are needed to manage these incidents. When you are confronted with a knee injury, determine the victim's ability to walk, the availability of transportation, the distance from help, and the conditions of the terrain before making any decisions. Encourage the injured person to carry on without calling for outside help. Provide whatever physical and emotional support is necessary. In the face of deteriorating environmental conditions, walking on an injured knee may be better than remaining exposed to the elements.

A fracture is a break or crack in a bone. Important distinctions are whether a fracture is deformed or not and whether it is closed or open. In a closed fracture, the skin has no wound near the fracture site. In an open fracture, the skin overlying the fracture is broken by bone protruding through the skin or by the blow that produced the fracture.

Bones are connected together at joints by ligaments. Sprains result in partially or completely torn ligaments, and are caused by partial and temporary separation of the bone ends. A dislocation is where the bones are completely separated at a joint, and are out of alignment, creating a deformity. True dislocations usually do not go back into position by themselves. Dislocations are associated with severe sprains **Figure 7-1**.

Strains are injuries to muscles. Strains occur when a muscle is stretched beyond its limits or from overuse. A severe strain may result in complete rupture of the muscle with loss of function. Muscle cramps are uncontrollable contractions (spasms, charley horses) that can cause severe pain and loss of mobility. Tendons connect muscles to bones; they can be partially or completely torn or become inflamed and painful from overuse.

Contusions (bruises) result from a direct blow, and can affect skin, muscle, and even bone. They can often be very painful, but usually are not serious injuries.

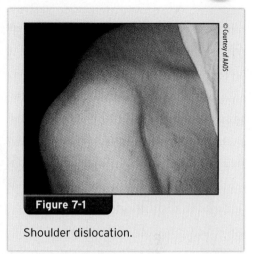

Figure 7-1

Shoulder dislocation.

Bone Injuries

▶ Assessment

It may be difficult to tell if a bone is fractured. Signs and symptoms of a fracture may include deformity, an open wound, tenderness, and swelling. Dislocations, severe strains, sprains, and even contusions may cause swelling and pain that mimic fractures. When in doubt, treat the injury as a fracture. Use the sequence "ask, look, and feel" to examine an extremity with a possible fracture.

Ask how the injury occurred. What was the mechanism of injury? Severe impact accidents or falls are more likely to cause a fracture. Also ask the victim where it hurts and how severely. Can the victim use the injured part? A snapping sound can be heard with fractures and with ligament or muscle tears (sprains and strains).

Look at the injury for deformity, open wounds, and swelling.

- Deformity is not always obvious. Compare the injured side to the uninjured side. Severe deformity (angulation), shortening, or rotation of the extremity when compared with the opposite extremity indicates a bone injury **Figure 7-2**.
- An open wound (such as a puncture or laceration) overlying an obvious deformity or unstable bone is considered an open fracture. The bone is not always seen in the

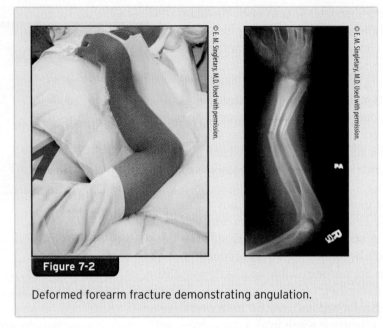

Figure 7-2

Deformed forearm fracture demonstrating angulation.

wound. Persistent oozing of blood despite pressure on the skin wound is another clue to an open fracture. An abrasion or a clearly superficial cut does not imply an open fracture.

- Swelling and bruising caused by bleeding from the bone or overlying muscle damage occur rapidly after a fracture. Swelling and bruising also occur with contusions and strains.
- There can be loss of use in which pain and muscle spasm restrict movement of nearby joints. Ask the victim to move the injured limb. Support the injured area and gently move the involved joints for the victim. If this causes severe pain or grating/cracking (crepitus), a fracture is likely. Grating with no history of injury indicates possible tendinitis.

PEDIATRIC NOTE

Children's bones are more elastic but not as strong as bones in adults because they are still growing. In adults, a fracture is usually a complete break in the continuity of a bone. A child's fracture, however, might be incomplete. It might be a greenstick (partial) fracture, a gentle but distinct bending of the bone called plastic deformity, or a buckling of the bone. The ligaments that join bones together at joints are relatively stronger than the bones they connect, and in some injuries, segments of bone might be pulled away, attached to a ligament that remains untorn. Therefore, a child should be presumed to have a fracture rather than a sprain if there is localized pain and swelling near a joint.

Feel for tenderness and the grating sensation of broken bone movement. Tenderness and pain are found at the site of injury. Feel gently along the bone; a fracture will be tender when felt from either side of the bone, whereas a bruise will be tender only on the side of impact (**Figure 7-3**). Abnormal movement is associated with crunching sounds or grating sensations and causes severe pain.

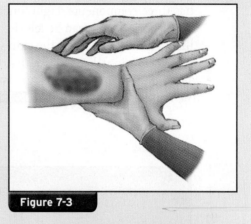

Figure 7-3

Feel along surface of the injured bone opposite from the bruise and swelling. If there is no tenderness, a fracture is unlikely.

▶ Treatment

What to Do

1. Control bleeding. Treat the victim for shock as needed.
2. Expose the injury. Gently remove clothing that covers the injured area. Cut clothing at the seams if necessary to avoid excessive movement and pain. In cold environments, remove as little clothing as possible to examine the person.
3. Check damage to blood vessels and nerves. A serious complication of a fracture is decreased blood flow (circulation) to the extremity. Major blood vessels lie close to bone, so a fracture or dislocation that causes a marked deformity of the bone may stretch, compress, or pinch adjacent blood vessels and nerves. Rarely are vessels or nerves actually torn by bone fragments.
   - Check circulation. Without blood, the tissues of the arms and legs cannot survive for more than 2 or 3 hours. Deformity and swelling can reduce the blood flow significantly, but circulation is rarely blocked or disrupted completely. Numbness and bluish color indicate decreased circulation. Splinting or wrapping too tightly can also obstruct blood flow.
     Compare the color of the hand or foot on the injured and uninjured sides. A blue or pale limb beyond an injury may indicate diminished circulation. Press on the tip of a nail or the pad of a finger or toe to blanch the skin. The pink color should return as quickly on the injured as on the uninjured side. Check the pulse at the wrist or the ankle (**Figure 7-4A-B**). Feel the uninjured side first to locate the pulse. Swelling over the injured area will make the pulse difficult or impossible to feel. If you locate the pulse, mark the spot with a pen so it can be found again quickly.
   - Assess sensation. Major nerves and blood vessels can sustain damage from direct injury or can be compressed by swelling. Numbness can result from nerve damage or from poor circulation. Numbness is not an urgent problem unless it is associated with impaired circulation.

Ask the victim whether the hands and feet have normal sensation. Sensation has three components: Light touch, pressure, and pain. Touch the victim's skin lightly and ask if it can be felt (light touch). Squeeze the victim's fingers and toes firmly (pressure). Touch the skin with a sharp object, such as a pin or pine needle (pain sensation), but be careful not to puncture the skin **Figure 7-4C-D**.

- Assess movement. If the victim can wiggle his or her toes or fingers, the nerves to the muscles are working **Figure 7-4E-F**. Pain can restrict movement, however.

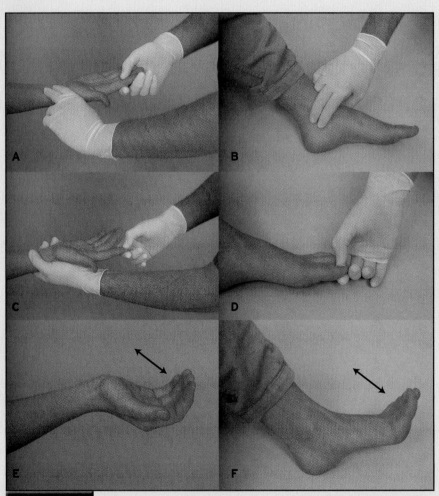

Figure 7-4

Checking circulation: **A.** Radial pulse. **B.** Posterior tibial pulse. **C.** and **D.** Sensation: squeeze one or more fingers or toes. **E.** and **F.** Movement: have the victim wiggle his or her fingers or toes. Movement might be decreased due to pain.

4. Realign deformities if medical care will be delayed   **Table 7-1** . This differs from first aid in less remote areas, where injuries should be splinted in the position in which they are found ("splint as it lies").

- If there are signs that circulation is impaired, realign the deformity immediately   **Figure 7-5** .

- The deformity of a limb should be corrected gently but firmly to eliminate the major deformity and allow placement of a splint. It is not necessary to completely correct a deformity. In general, deformities of long bones should be straightened, but injuries around the joints are often best treated in a position of function (the position in which a person normally uses the joint. For example, the elbow is in a bent position, the wrist is straight, and the ankle is in a position normally used for walking.)

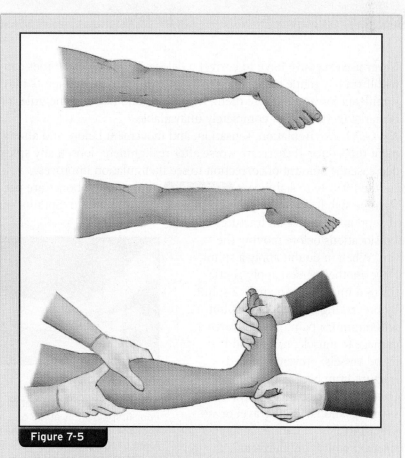

Figure 7-5

Correct major angulation and deformities by applying traction along the normal axis of the bone. The goal is to improve alignment, not to achieve the optimal position for healing.

Table 7-1   How to Apply Traction to Deformed Fractures

1. Explain to the victim that straightening the fracture may cause pain, but the pain will decrease when the fracture is straightened and splinted.

2. Grasp an injured limb firmly with both hands—one hand above the injury site and the other below it. Pull, gradually increasing pressure to exert steady, firm traction along the long axis of the bone. For a leg, pull with both hands below the injury site while the victim's body acts as an anchor or another person holds the upper leg in place. Compare the injured side with the normal side to see what the straightened extremity should look like. Traction might not pull the limb back into perfect alignment, but that can be achieved later in the hospital.

3. Stop pulling if the victim feels intolerable pain or if firm but gentle traction fails to improve the position.

- Never use excessive force to correct a deformity. Most deformities can be corrected with firm but gentle traction and manipulation. Dislocated joints may require significant force to relocate them, but this should not be done unless medical care is markedly delayed or completely unavailable.
- Always check circulation, sensation, and movement before and after any realignment procedure. If these are worse after realignment, loosen any splints and/or decrease the amount of correction to see if circulation improves.

5. Splint the fracture to stabilize it 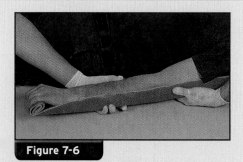 **Figure 7-6**. Most broken bones are not displaced and can be stabilized in the position in which they are found. Sprains and strains also need support. Stabilize all fractures and dislocations before moving the victim. When in doubt, apply a splint.
   - Have another person apply gentle traction until you can apply a splint.
   - By preventing movement, a splint will minimize pain; prevent further damage to muscle, nerves, and blood vessels; prevent a closed fracture from becoming an open fracture; reduce bleeding and swelling; and facilitate travel or evacuation.

   For maximum immobilization, stabilize the joint above and below the injury. For example, a fractured fore-arm requires a splint long enough to

Figure 7-6

A SAM splint, a good splint to carry in your first aid kit, is made of a malleable sheet of aluminum sandwiched between foam padding. It weighs very little and can be rolled or folded flat to carry. It can be molded to any part of the body. Forming a longitudinal fold or groove in the splint adds strength.

secure the wrist and the elbow. If you stabilize the wrist only, the forearm bone (radius) can still move whenever the elbow turns. If the injury is near a joint, splinting only that joint might provide adequate comfort while allowing better function. For an injured joint, stabilize the bone above and below the injury. For example, for a knee injury, secure the splint at both the thigh and lower leg. Balance adequate immobilization with the need for comfort and function. Place splint materials on both sides of the injured part (creating a "sandwich splint") to prevent the part from turning or twisting.

You may have to improvise splints with clothing, foam sleeping pads, backpack stays, pillows, branches, or ski poles. Splints should be padded for comfort and rigid for safety. The victim will tell you if the splint works. Monitor circulation and sensation before and after applying the splint and periodically while the splint is in place to ensure that it is not too tight. Ask the victim to tell you if pain increases or sensation changes.

Techniques of splinting are described under the individual injuries.

6. Limit swelling and pain with rest, ice, compression, and elevation (RICE).

Rest, Ice, Compression, and Elevation

The acronym RICE is used to remember first aid procedures for contusions (bruises), strains, sprains, dislocations, and fractures.

R: Rest. Stop or decrease use of the injured part with the aid of splints, wraps, slings, and periods of rest.

I: Ice. Apply an ice pack frequently during the first 48 hours after the injury has occurred. In the wilderness, use snow or cold water if ice is unavailable. Skin treated with cold passes through four states: cold, burning, aching, and numbness. When it becomes numb (in about 20 minutes), remove the ice pack. Cold constricts the blood vessels in the injured area, which reduces swelling, dulls pain, and relieves muscle spasm. The sooner cold is applied, the better. Apply the ice pack directly on the injured area. Be careful not to use ice or snow that is very cold directly on the skin for a prolonged period, or frostbite can result. A thin cloth or a paper towel placed over the skin prevents freezer burn.

C: Compression. Compression of the injured area may limit internal bleeding around the injury. Less bleeding or bruising means less soreness, less limitation of movement, and a faster recovery time, especially for muscle or ligament injuries. Apply cold about every 2 to 3 hours; maintain compression at other times using an elastic bandage. At night, loosen, but do not remove, the elastic bandage.

- Use an elastic bandage or wrap the injured area snugly with strips of cloth.
- Start the elastic bandage several inches below the injury or at the base of the fingers or toes and wrap in an upward, overlapping spiral, starting with even and somewhat tight pressure and then gradually wrapping more loosely above the injury.
- Do not apply an elastic bandage too tightly; it can restrict circulation. Stretch the elastic bandage to about half its maximum length for adequate compression.

- Leave fingers and toes exposed to see color changes. Compare the color and movement of the toes or fingers of the injured extremity with those of the uninjured extremity.
- If there is pale skin, numbness, tingling, or increased pain, remove the elastic bandage and rewrap the area less tightly.

E: Elevation. Elevating the injured limb helps limit bleeding and minimizes swelling. Elevate to the level of the heart or 5" to 10" higher.

▶ Open Fractures

As previously indicated, if a fracture is associated with broken skin (either caused by the broken bone or by the blow that produced the fracture), it is considered to be an open fracture. Minor lacerations are not indicators of open fractures.

What to Do

1. Clean off dirt and debris and irrigate the bone end.
2. Do not push the bone end back under the skin. Gently try to correct deformities, as described previously. This will sometimes return the bone end to its correct position below the skin.
3. Cover all open fracture wounds with a dry, sterile dressing before applying a splint.
4. Make a written note of how much bone is protruding and if there is debris on the bone or in the wound before immediate evacuation to an orthopaedic surgeon.
5. Splint and wrap the extremity.

Joint Injuries

▶ Dislocations

A dislocation occurs when a joint comes apart and stays apart with the bone ends no longer in their usual position. The main sign of a dislocation is deformity—there is often a bizarre appearance compared to the uninjured side. In addition to deformity, dislocations have other signs and symptoms similar to those of a fracture, including severe pain and the inability of the victim to move the injured joint. The shoulders, elbows, fingers, hips, kneecaps, and ankles are the joints most frequently affected.

What to Do

Evaluation and management of dislocations are similar to those of fractures. If medical care will be delayed or there is compromised circulation, attempt to reduce (put back in place) the dislocation.

▶ Sprains

A sprain is an injury to a joint in which the ligaments and other tissues are damaged by stretching or twisting. The ankles, knees, and thumbs are the joints most often sprained. It may be difficult to distinguish between a severe sprain and a fracture. Some sprains involve small fractures, but this does not change their management in the field.

What to Look For

- Pain
- Tenderness that may be more over the soft tissues than the bone
- Swelling
- Stiffness and decreased function of the joint
- Bruising occurs within hours or days
- The joint may be unstable (moves in abnormal directions) if the ligaments are completely torn

What to Do

1. Evaluate as for a fracture. If in doubt, treat as a fracture.
2. Apply the RICE procedures.
3. Splint or tape for support.

Muscle Injuries

▶ Strains and Tendon Injuries

A muscle strain occurs when a muscle is stretched beyond its normal range of motion; a muscle strain can also occur from overuse. Tendons can be strained or develop tendinitis. If a muscle or tendon completely ruptures, there is often marked swelling and bruising, and a gap may be present in the muscle or tendon.

What to Look For

- Limited movement due to pain and stiffness.
- Variable tenderness.
- Variable swelling and bruising depending on the extent of damage.
- Tendonitis may have a grating or crackling sensation when the affected tendon is moved.
- A gap may be present in the tendon or muscle.
- Delayed symptoms, possibly for 1 to 2 days depending on the severity of the injury.

What to Do

1. Apply the RICE procedures.
2. Stretch the affected muscle gently.
3. Give anti-inflammatory medication, such as ibuprofen or naproxyn, especially for tendinitis.
4. Splint if pain is severe.

▶ Muscle Cramps

A cramp is an uncontrolled spasm and contraction resulting in sudden pain and restriction of movement. Cramps can result from a sudden injury, overuse, poor conditioning, lack of stretching or warm-up before exercise, and heat exposure with dehydration.

What to Look For

- Sudden onset of severe pain in the muscle
- Spasm that prevents movement
- Firm area in the muscle that may be tender
- Often occurs during or after strenuous activity

What to Do

Try one or more of the following:

1. Have the victim gently stretch the affected muscle.
2. Apply steady pressure over the muscle.
3. Apply ice to the cramped muscle.
4. If the cramping has followed hard exertion in the heat, give mildly salted water (0.25 to 1 teaspoon of salt in 1 quart of water) or a sports drink.
   To prevent nocturnal cramps, try taking diphenhydramine (eg, Benadryl) at bedtime.
5. Do not give salt tablets alone. Water needs to be replaced as well. One to two salt tablets can be dissolved in a quart of water.

▶ Emergency Care Wrap-up

What to Look For	What to Do
Bone Injuries	
Fractures	1. Control bleeding.
• Deformity	2. Expose the injury.
• Open wounds	3. Check damage to blood vessels and nerves.
• Swelling	4. Realign deformities.
• Tenderness	5. Splint the fracture to stabilize it.
• Abnormal movement	6. Limit swelling and pain with RICE procedures.
Open Fractures	1. Clean off dirt and debris and irrigate the bone end.
• Bleeding	2. Do not push the bone end back under the skin.
• Protruding bone end	3. Cover all open fracture wounds with a dry, sterile dressing before applying a splint.
	4. Make a written note about the injury.
	5. Splint and wrap the extremity.
Joint Injuries	
Dislocations	1. Evaluate and manage as for a fracture.
• Deformity	
• Severe pain	
• Limited movement	
Sprains	1. Evaluate as for a fracture.
• Pain	2. Apply the RICE procedures.
• Tenderness	3. Splint or tape for support.
• Swelling	
• Decreased movement	
• Bruising	
• Limited use of the joint	

What to Look For	What to Do
Muscle Injuries	
Strains • Limited movement • Variable tenderness • Variable swelling and bruising • Grating or crackling sensation • Gap in the tendon or muscle • Delayed symptoms	1. Apply the RICE procedures. 2. Stretch the affected muscle gently. 3. Give anti-inflammatory medication. 4. Splint if pain is severe.
Muscle Cramps • Sudden pain • Uncontrolled spasm • Tenderness • Occurs during or after strenuous activity	1. Gently stretch the affected muscle. 2. Apply steady pressure over the muscle. 3. Apply ice to the cramped muscle. 4. Give victim mildly salted water or a sports drink. 5. Do not give salt tablets alone.

Specific Bone and Joint Injuries

8

© Josh Schutz/ShutterStock/Thinkstock

Managing specific bone and joint injuries in remote environments requires common sense, some diagnostic skills, and sensitivity to the needs of the victim and the group. For example, with a painful ankle injury, consider the desire and ability of the injured person to walk; whether people are available for transportation; and the terrain, weather, and distance involved. Try to encourage self-rescue without calling for outside help. Support the ankle with a splint or tape and use an ice axe, ski pole, or wooden stick for balance. Although causing more pain, the decision to walk out may be safer than waiting for help.

The skeletal system is shown in **Figure 8-1**.

chapter
at a glance

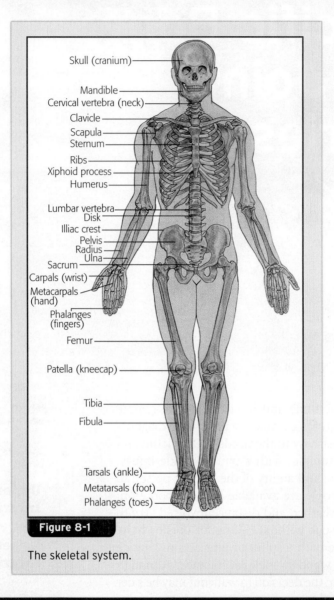

Skull (cranium)

Mandible
Cervical vertebra (neck)
Clavicle
Scapula
Sternum

Ribs
Xiphoid process
Humerus

Lumbar vertebra
Disk
Illiac crest
Pelvis
Radius
Ulna
Sacrum
Carpals (wrist)
Metacarpals (hand)

Phalanges (fingers)

Femur

Patella (kneecap)

Tibia
Fibula

Tarsals (ankle)
Metatarsals (foot)
Phalanges (toes)

Figure 8-1

The skeletal system.

Upper Extremity Injuries

▶ Shoulder Injury

The collarbone (clavicle) is easily seen and felt along its entire length. It could be injured by a direct blow or by a fall onto the shoulder. The shoulder is made up of the clavicle (collarbone), scapula (shoulder blade), and the upper end of the humerus (upper arm bone). The joint between the collarbone and shoulder blade is frequently injured, and is referred to as a shoulder separation. Fractures of the upper end of the humerus (the arm bone) are treated as shoulder injuries.

What to Look For

- Local tenderness, swelling, or deformity, indicating a fracture.
- Tenderness and a bump at the junction of the collarbone and shoulder, usually due to a sprain.
- Level of pain. Clavicle fractures are extremely painful, but sprains are not too painful except when the victim tries to lift the arm on the side of the sprain. In either case, the victim is able to use the hand.
- Severe pain with swelling. Fractures of the humerus at the shoulder cause severe pain and marked swelling. These fractures are often not significantly displaced, and the fractured bone ends may not move very much.
- Position of the affected arm. Generally, a victim with a fractured arm holds it against the chest wall, whereas with a dislocation, the victim holds the arm away from the body wall.
- Local pain, tenderness, and muscle spasm. These can be caused if the scapula has been fractured, which can be caused by a direct blow.

What to Do

1. Treat all of these injuries with a sling.
2. If bandages are not available, a sling can be fashioned from any available cloth or improvised by using safety pins to pin the arm of a long-sleeved shirt to the upper part of the victim's shirt **Figure 8-2A**. The forearm can be tucked into the space between the buttons of a button-down shirt. If the victim is wearing a jacket or shirt, fold the lower edge up over the arm and pin it to the shirt **Figure 8-2B**. A piece of webbing or rope looped around the arm can also make an improvised sling.

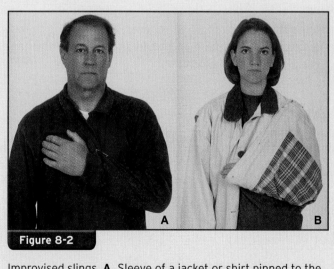

Figure 8-2

Improvised slings. **A.** Sleeve of a jacket or shirt pinned to the clothing. **B.** Lower edge of a jacket or shirt pinned up over the injured arm.

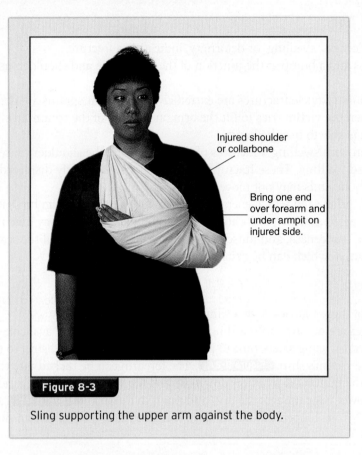

Injured shoulder
or collarbone

Bring one end
over forearm and
under armpit on
injured side.

Figure 8-3

Sling supporting the upper arm against the body.

3. For the best immobilization of shoulder injuries, apply a sling as shown **Figure 8-3**.
4. Allow some freedom of the forearm and hand and access to the hand to check circulation, sensation, and movement.

▶ Shoulder Dislocation

Nearly all dislocations of the shoulder joint occur with the arm in the cocked, throwing, or kayak high-brace position with the hand above and behind the shoulder. The head of the humerus is forced out of the socket and lodged in front of the shoulder **Figure 8-4**. A person who has had a dislocated shoulder before will recognize the injury if it happens again.

What to Look For

As you look for the following, document what you find:

- The upper arm is usually held away from the body, and it is more painful to lay the forearm against the abdomen.

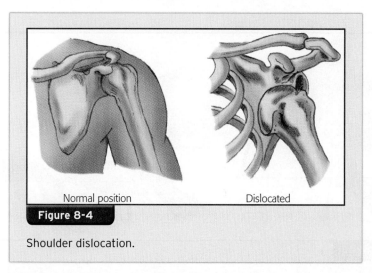

Normal position   Dislocated

Figure 8-4

Shoulder dislocation.

- Compare the injured shoulder with the uninjured one. In a dislocated shoulder, the shoulder looks squared off rather than rounded as in an uninjured shoulder **Figure 8-5**.
- Check circulation, sensation, and movement of the hand.

What to Do

1. Pull the arm, bent to a right angle at the elbow, steadily out to the side **Figure 8-6**. Have an assistant pull in the opposite direction, using straps, a sleeping bag, or

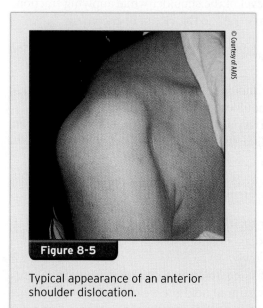

© Courtesy of AAOS

Figure 8-5

Typical appearance of an anterior shoulder dislocation.

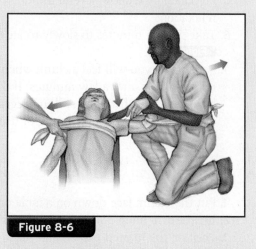

Figure 8-6

Applying traction on the arm to relocate a dislocated shoulder.

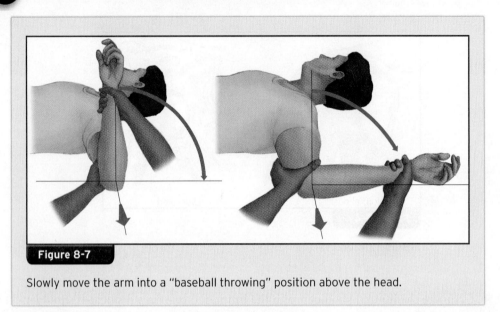

Figure 8-7

Slowly move the arm into a "baseball throwing" position above the head.

clothing around the chest, just below the armpit. You can use muscle relaxation through massage or guided imagery to keep the victim relaxed and enhance attempts at relocation.

2. Pad the armpit, chest wall, and front of the elbow, where pressure will be applied during traction.
3. Lean back, using your body weight for traction.
4. Gradually elevate the victim's arm to the level of the shoulder while applying traction.
5. Be patient and allow several minutes to pass. Talk to the victim to encourage relaxation.
6. Take 5 to 15 minutes to slowly rotate the arm into a baseball-throwing position **Figure 8-7**.
7. Sometimes you will feel a clunk when the shoulder pops back into its socket; if not, relax traction after a few minutes. If the shoulder moves freely without pain, it has been reduced. If you are still unsuccessful, try again but rotate the arm outward, then inward while applying traction, or use a different method, such as the method described next.

Alternate Method of Shoulder Dislocation Reduction

1. Put the victim face down on a table or flat rock **Figure 8-8**.
2. Let the arm hang down toward the ground.
3. Position the injured person and the arm slowly.
4. Tie a 10- to 15-lb weight to the arm or wrist (eg, rocks in a day pack, water in a bucket, or sand in a bag). Do not ask the victim to hold the weight, which would prevent the arm from relaxing. This method is time consuming (it could take up to

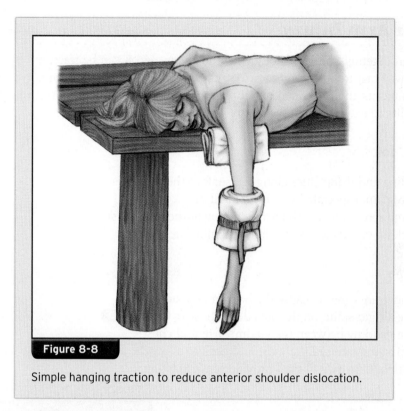

Figure 8-8

Simple hanging traction to reduce anterior shoulder dislocation.

an hour) and relaxation is critical, but the muscle will eventually fatigue and allow the shoulder to be replaced.

5. Once the muscles are relaxed, gently but firmly grasp the upper arm below the shoulder and pull outward. Then remove the weight. The shoulder will slide back into position as the victim's muscles contract.

6. Stabilize the shoulder with a sling and swathe. Place padding (pillows, towels) between the upper arm and chest to support the arm.

7. Check circulation, sensation, and movement in the arm and fingers.

8. For paddlers or climbers who need some motion of the shoulder to travel out of the wilderness, fashion a tether to limit motion of the upper arm **Figure 8-9**.

9. If reduction attempts are not successful, use a sling and swathe with clothing wadded beneath the arm to support it in a comfortable position.

10. If you are unable to reduce the dislocation, evacuate the victim.

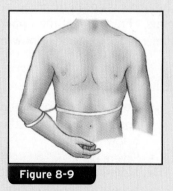

Figure 8-9

Wrap straps around the waist and mid-forearm to avoid redislocation.

▶ Upper Arm Injury

The humerus extends from the shoulder to the elbow, and it can be fractured by a fall, twist, or direct blow. Fractures of the humerus are usually obvious. An important nerve runs directly along the humerus and is frequently injured with humerus fractures. Nerve injury will result in the inability to extend (cock) the wrist.

What to Look For

- Swelling and deformities along the shaft of the humerus
- Severe pain, especially with movement
- Grating sensation and abnormal motion at the fracture site
- Check for circulation, sensation, and movement

What to Do

1. Remove any rings because the hand might swell.
2. Place a rigid splint on the outside of the arm **Figure 8-10**.
3. Place padding between the victim's arm and chest.
4. Loop a strap around the wrist and neck to allow the arm to hang in the sling position. Gravity will then provide gentle traction.

▶ Elbow Injury

The elbow joint is made up of the lower end of the humerus and the upper ends of the forearm bones. The elbow can be injured by a direct blow or indirectly by a fall on an outstretched hand. The elbow is one of the more frequently dislocated joints. Fractures of the upper forearm or lower humerus are treated as elbow injuries.

What to Look For

- Deformity indicates an elbow dislocation or serious fracture of the bones above or below the joint.
- Severe pain.
- Swelling, tenderness.
- Inability to move the elbow without severe pain.
- Impaired circulation, sensation, or movement below the injury.

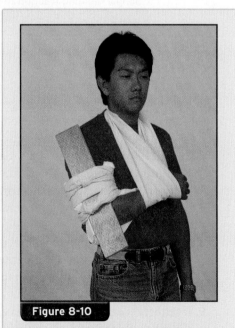

Figure 8-10

Splinted upper arm with sling, swathe, and padding between the arm and the chest.

What to Do

1. Remove any rings because the hand might swell.
2. Immobilize the affected arm with a sling, with the elbow bent as comfort allows.
3. Keep the elbow in the position found to prevent blood vessel and nerve damage.
4. If there is significant deformity, and medical care will be delayed more than a few hours, attempt to realign the fracture or relocate a dislocated elbow.
   - If circulation is impaired, and medical care is not immediately available, the injury should be realigned.

ADVANCED PROCEDURE

Traction for a Dislocated Elbow

If circulation is obstructed (the victim would have a cool, bluish hand, no pulse at the wrist, a numb hand, and would be unable to move his or her fingers) or help is many hours away, attempt to improve the alignment. Otherwise, splint the elbow in the position in which it is found.

- Apply slow, steady traction to the wrist and forearm with the elbow partially bent (this is usually how it is found). Have an assistant apply countertraction to the upper arm **Figure 8-11** .
- If no one else is available to help, put one hand on the upper arm and grasp the wrist with the other hand.
- A dislocation can usually be reduced without a strong pull, but deformed fractures might be only slightly improved at best.

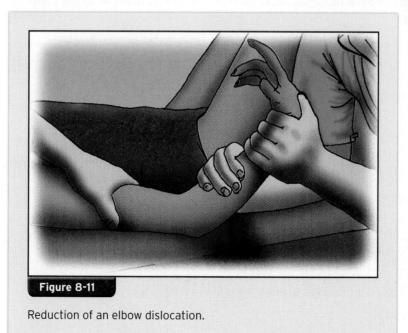

Figure 8-11

Reduction of an elbow dislocation.

▶ **Lower Arm Injury**

What to Look For

The forearm or wrist can be fractured by a direct blow or a fall in which the victim lands on the outstretched hand, resulting in a deformity.

What to Do

1. Remove any rings the victim is wearing.
2. Attempt to straighten severe angulation of the forearm. While one person holds the arm just above or below the elbow, a second first aid provider grasps the hand and pulls firmly. If you are the only rescuer available, grasp above the elbow and push up above the elbow while pulling down below the injury.
3. Apply a splint from the middle of the palm to just below the elbow. A splint on the palm side of the hand and forearm allows the elbow to bend and the arm to rotate. A second splint goes from the back of the elbow and extends to the back of the hand. This allows some bending at the elbow, but it prevents rotation of the hand and forearm **Figure 8-12** . Simple splints can also be made by folding and rolling a foam pad around the forearm or padding the forearm with clothing or a foam pad and sandwiching it with any straight, firm materials (stays from backpacks, pieces of wood, and so forth). If the thumb hurts when it is moved, include it in the splint.
4. Leave the fingers free or wrapped in the functional position (as if holding a ball, glass, or can) with a rolled-up sock, glove, or other soft material in the palm.

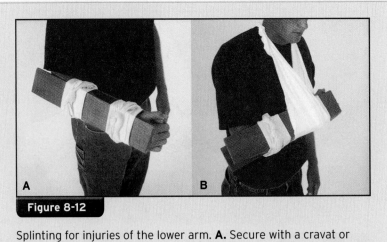

Figure 8-12

Splinting for injuries of the lower arm. **A.** Secure with a cravat or roller bandage. **B.** Place the arm in a sling.

5. For maximal immobilization and comfort, include the elbow bent to a right angle (90° of flexion) in the splint.
6. Have the victim exercise the fingers to help circulation and reduce swelling.
7. The victim should seek medical care.

▶ Hand Injury

What to Look For

- Deformities, tenderness, and swelling.
- Fingers may be moved out of alignment by injuries in the hand.
- Check circulation, sensation, and movement.

What to Do

1. Place the injured hand in the position of function (the hand will look like it is holding a baseball) by placing a rolled pair of socks or similar item in the palm.
2. Gently realign any displaced fingers. Buddy tape as described in the "Finger Dislocation and Fractures" section in this chapter.
3. Attach a rigid splint along the forearm and under the hand **Figure 8-13** .

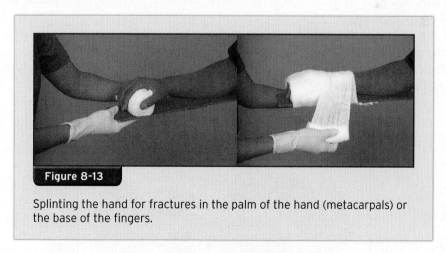

Figure 8-13

Splinting the hand for fractures in the palm of the hand (metacarpals) or the base of the fingers.

▶ Finger Dislocation and Fractures

The fingers are easily injured, and even a minor injury may cause a dislocation. Finger injuries include fractures, sprains, dislocations, and tendon injuries.

What to Look For

- Deformity and inability to use or bend the finger
- Pain and swelling
- Restricted movement
- Bruising
- An abnormal position of two adjoining bones; looks like a lump at the joint
  Figure 8-14

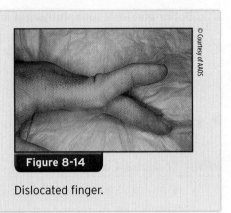

Figure 8-14

Dislocated finger.

What to Do

Immediately after injury, dislocations of the fingers can be reduced with only minimal discomfort, using the following steps:

1. Grasp the end of the finger in one hand, using gauze or cloth to avoid slipping.
2. Pull steadily and firmly on the finger, then push the base of the dislocated segment back in place **Figure 8-15**. Remove any rings.
3. If unsuccessful, try hyperextending the joint before pushing the base back into place.
4. Splint the finger in a functional position.
5. For unstable and painful fractures at the base of the finger or the bones in the palm of the hand, tape the injured finger to its neighbor, place a soft roll of material in the palm, and then wrap the whole hand with an elastic bandage, roller gauze, or torn strips of clothing.
6. For fractures of the middle segment of the finger or dislocations on either side, realign any deformity and splint to an adjacent finger (buddy taping).
7. Place gauze between the fingers to absorb moisture and tape the fingers together in the position of function.

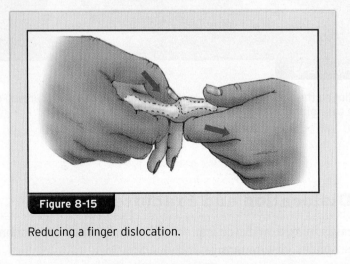

Figure 8-15

Reducing a finger dislocation.

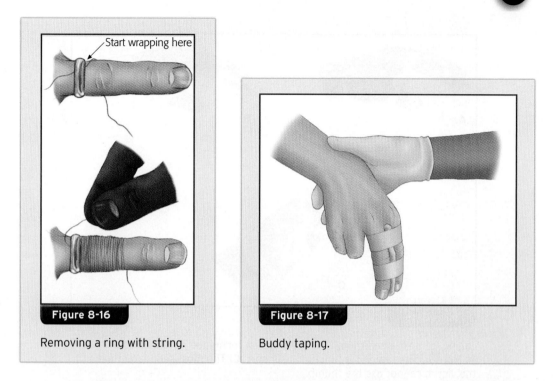

Figure 8-16

Removing a ring with string.

Figure 8-17

Buddy taping.

8. If the injured person cannot tolerate any movement, add a rigid splint or bulky wrap. After any significant injury to the arm or hand, especially if immobilization is needed, the hand can swell. Remove rings to ensure that circulation to the finger is not impaired by swelling. If fingers are already swollen or a ring cannot be removed, try elevating the arm, applying a cold pack to the finger and soap for lubrication. If you are still unsuccessful in your attempts to remove a ring, wrap the finger with string, dental floss, or fishing line as illustrated in **Figure 8-16** to remove the ring. If you are still unsuccessful and the ring is becoming painfully tight, use the file on a pocket knife to cut the ring.

9. Two types of hand dislocation are difficult to reduce in the field: the base of the index finger and the thumb. Make only one attempt, and then immobilize the joint in a position of function.

10. Tape a finger to its neighbor to allow functional support of the finger after reducing a dislocation or for a sprained finger **Figure 8-17**. For less movement, pad between the fingers and wrap or tape them together without space between. Alternatively, splint the middle joint for comfortable function.

11. Mallet finger is an injury to the last joint of a finger that results from the sudden bending ("jamming") of the joint and results in tearing of the tendon that extends the joint. The tip of the finger will droop and the victim will be unable to fully extend the joint. Fashion a short splint to hold the joint fully extended.

12. For thumb comfort, fashion a splint that includes the thumb and wrist; for best function, try taping **Figure 8-18A-C**. A small chip of bone might be broken off, but urgent evacuation is not necessary.

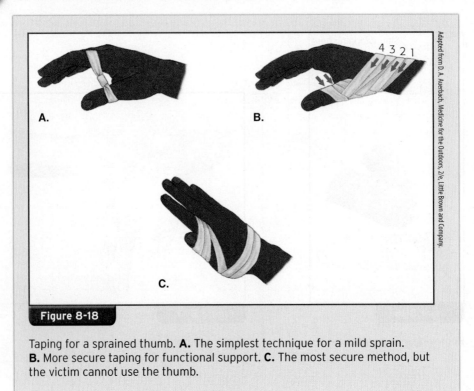

Figure 8-18

Taping for a sprained thumb. **A.** The simplest technique for a mild sprain. **B.** More secure taping for functional support. **C.** The most secure method, but the victim cannot use the thumb.

Lower Extremity Injuries

▶ Hip Injury

The hip is a ball-and-socket joint. The socket is in the pelvic bone. The ball is on the top of the femur, or thighbone. The hip can be dislocated or fractured. These injuries are usually the result of high-energy accidents such as falls from height or motor vehicle accidents, but they can also result from simple falls.

What to Look For

- Pain around the hip that is made more severe with any movement
- Inability to bear weight
- The foot may be rotated outward or inward to an abnormal degree
- The injured limb may appear shorter than the uninjured limb
- With a hip dislocation, the hip and knee are both held bent, with the knee turned inward

What to Do

1. Plan to carry the victim out of the wilderness on a litter or sled.
2. Gently realign the limb and rotate the foot into a normal position. If there is significant resistance to movement, suspect a possible hip dislocation.
3. Splint the affected leg to the uninjured leg.
4. For greater stabilization, secure a splint using a long board, oar, or ski along the side of the body and leg from the armpit to the heel.
5. Put padding between the legs and around the injured leg.
6. Evacuate.
7. With a hip dislocation, there is severe pain, and the hip and knee are held bent with the knee turned inward. Because realigning the joint is very difficult, do not attempt it. Stabilize a hip injury in the position in which it was found **Figure 8-19** and **Figure 8-20** .

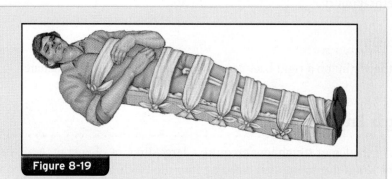

Figure 8-19

Splint for hip or femur fracture. Note the padding under the splint and between the legs. The splint extends to the armpit to prevent hip movement. Possible splint materials include a board, ski, or oar. Tie the injured person's legs together with padding between the legs.

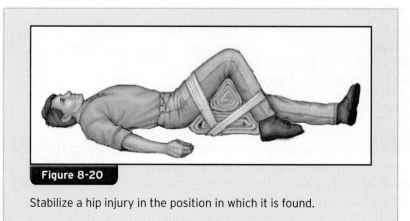

Figure 8-20

Stabilize a hip injury in the position in which it is found.

▶ Pelvic Injury

Major falls can fracture the pelvis.

What to Look For

- The injured person indicates pain when the affected area is pressed or the pelvis is squeezed side to side or front to back.
- The victim can tolerate walking, but with pain; this indicates minor fractures around the pelvic bone.
- The victim is unable to bear walking and even sitting; this indicates a major pelvic fracture.
- There are signs of shock due to internal bleeding.
- The injured person has blood in the urine or is unable to urinate due to bladder or urethral injury.

What to Do

Stabilize the victim on a rigid backboard, litter, or sled, and then evacuate.

▶ Thigh Injury

Fractures of the femur (thighbone) require a large amount of energy. A victim can lose up to 2 quarts of blood due to internal bleeding into the thigh. A victim of an open femur fracture can actually bleed to death. Stabilization of a femur fracture can reduce bleeding and be life-saving. Femur fractures are usually obvious, due to abnormal motion and pain. Femur and hip fractures may have a similar appearance.

What to Look For

- Severe pain, unable to bear weight.
- Motion at the fracture site, possibly with a grating sensation.
- Swelling and deformity.
- Thigh or leg may appear to be shortened.
- Foot may be rotated abnormally.

What to Do

1. Begin applying manual traction to the extremity by grasping the ankle and maintaining a straight pull on the leg. Traction decreases blood loss, relieves pain, stabilizes fracture fragments, prevents converting a closed fracture into an open fracture, and reduces further soft-tissue damage.

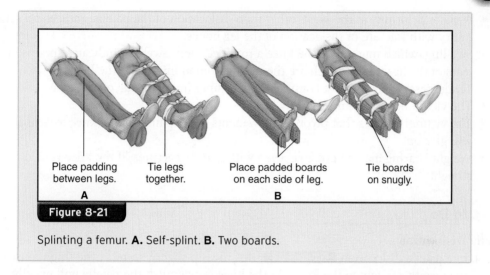

Place padding between legs.   Tie legs together.   Place padded boards on each side of leg.   Tie boards on snugly.

A   B

Figure 8-21

Splinting a femur. **A.** Self-splint. **B.** Two boards.

2. If the victim needs to be moved without traction, stabilize in the position of maximum comfort by splinting the injured leg to the uninjured leg **Figure 8-21A**. Another method is shown in **Figure 8-21B**.
   - Pad between the legs and under the knees to produce a slight bend.
   - For greater support, add a rigid splint from the armpit to below the heel, as for a hip fracture.
3. Monitor circulation beyond the injury. Loosen the laces, but do not remove the boot and sock in cold weather. The toe of the boot may be cut away to help monitor circulation.

▶ Knee Injury

The knee consists of the lower end of the femur, the upper end of the leg (tibia), and the patella (kneecap). Knee injuries include fractures, dislocations, and sprains. Knee sprains are often severe and, unlike many other joint injuries, often require surgery. Knee injuries often make it difficult for the victim to walk. A good rule of thumb is that if a victim of a knee injury can walk without severe pain, can actively straighten the knee, and the knee does not buckle or give way, the injury probably is not severe.

What to Look For

- The victim indicates pain when attempting to bend or straighten the knee without help lifting the lower leg.
- A gap or marked tenderness along the edges of the kneecap suggests a fracture.
- A patella that is displaced to the outside (laterally) with the knee held bent (in flexion) indicates a dislocation of the kneecap, which is caused by a pivoting injury with a partially bent knee.

- A major deformity at the knee, other than dislocation of the patella, indicates a serious injury with fracture or dislocation of the leg bones.
- Swelling, which might give the knee a rounded look. Swelling indicates sprains or tears of the ligaments, which are the most common injuries to the knee.
- Tenderness, which is most common on the inner (medial) side of the knee.
- The victim holds the knee slightly bent.
- The victim indicates that pivoting movements cause pain and the knee feels as if it will give out.
- Weight bearing may be possible, even with patella fractures, if the knee is held straight.

What to Do

Patella Dislocation

1. In a patella dislocation **Figure 8-22**, flex the hip slightly to relax the thigh muscle, then gently straighten the knee. As the knee is extended, the patella will usually realign itself. If not, with the knee straight, push the patella back into place with pressure on the outside edge.
2. Wrap the leg in a cylinder splint made from a foam sleeping pad **Figure 8-23**, or sandwich on both sides with two rigid splints. This will stabilize the knee, and the injured person might be able to walk unaided.
3. Improvise a cane or crutch if needed.

Sprains

1. Wrap the knee firmly with an elastic bandage or cylinder splint.
2. If the sprain is mild to moderate, the victim may walk. However, walking will be difficult in steep or rugged terrain.
3. Improvise a walking stick, if needed.

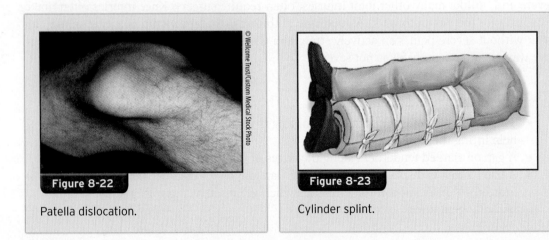

Figure 8-22

Patella dislocation.

© Wellcome Trust/Custom Medical Stock Photo

Figure 8-23

Cylinder splint.

Severe Pain, Major Deformity, and Moderate to Severe Swelling

1. Check for diminished blood flow (cool, bluish foot, no pulse at the ankle, a numb foot, and pain on movement of the toes).
2. If circulation in the foot appears to be poor, attempt to improve alignment with direct traction along the normal long axis of the leg.
3. Splint securely but without compromising circulation to the foot.
4. If the leg is bent at the knee at a strange angle, realign the leg. This is easier than splinting at odd angles.
5. Do not ask the victim to stand or walk.
6. Evacuate the victim.

▶ Lower Leg Injury

The shinbone (tibia) can easily be felt under the skin along the front and inner side of the lower leg.

What to Look For

- Fractures are generally obvious with severe pain, early swelling, instability, some deformity, and an inability to bear weight.
- Tibia fractures often puncture the skin, creating an open fracture.
- Isolated tenderness and pain on the outer part of the leg with no tenderness of the shinbone indicates a possible fibula fracture (the fibula is the smaller bone on the outer side of the leg).

What to Do

1. Correct angular deformities with gentle traction by pulling at the ankle. Splint lower leg fractures to immobilize the knee and ankle. Use any padded materials to secure the leg and prevent movement of the ankle and knee **Figure 8-24**. Provide support with a small pad under the knee. Wrap the leg first in a sleeping pad. Hold the foot and provide traction on the leg while another person applies the splint.

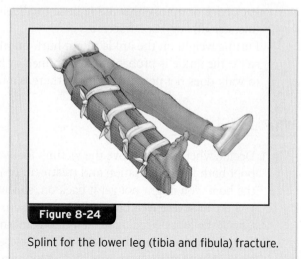

Figure 8-24

Splint for the lower leg (tibia and fibula) fracture.

2. Traction splinting is not generally done for lower leg fractures. However, manual traction can be used to further reduce pain, muscle spasm, and bleeding while applying a splint.
3. Evacuate the victim.
4. If the fibula alone is fractured with the tibia intact, the victim can walk with a cane or crutch and ankle support.

▶ Ankle Injury

Most ankle injuries are sprains of the outside (lateral) ligaments, caused by the foot turning inward. It is difficult to tell the difference between a severe sprain and a fracture **Figure 8-25**. Ligament injuries and fractures often occur together, and dislocations are nearly always associated with multiple fractures. Treat an injury as a fracture whenever there is diffuse, marked swelling, inability to bear weight, or obvious signs of fracture, such as a deformity or crepitus (crunching with movement).

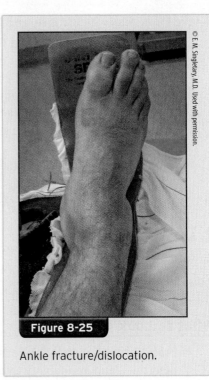

Figure 8-25

Ankle fracture/dislocation.

© E. M. Singletary, M.D. Used with permission.

What to Look For

- The typical sprained ankle is swollen, tender, and bruised just in front of the knob of bone on the outer side of the ankle (lateral malleolus).
- Pain and marked tenderness over the bones (press gently along the bones) at either the back edge or tip of either ankle bone (malleolus) or the outside bone of the foot (metatarsal) suggest a fracture.
- Putting weight on the ankle might hurt, but if the victim is able to take four or more steps, the ankle is probably only sprained or has a minor fracture. However, inability to walk does not necessarily mean there is a fracture.

What to Do

1. Decide whether to remove the victim's footwear or leave it on. Remove the shoe or boot both for examination and treatment or if the foot is wet. However, if you take off the boot, you might not get it back on, so leave it on if the person needs to walk or you are in severe weather or difficult terrain.
2. Check the foot's circulation, sensation, and movement.
3. Straighten any deformity of the ankle. Hold the toes and back of the heel, lift the leg, and apply traction. Improved alignment results without much effort.

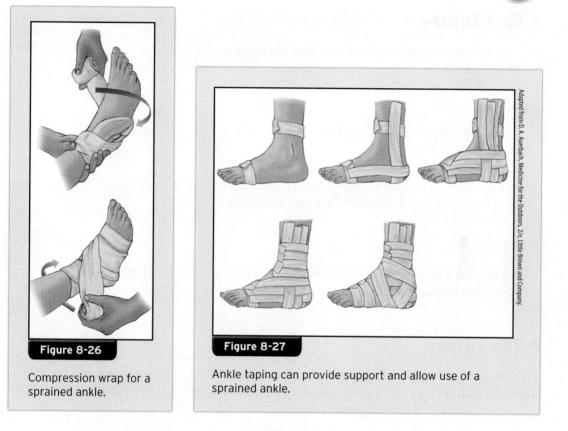

Figure 8-26

Compression wrap for a sprained ankle.

Figure 8-27

Ankle taping can provide support and allow use of a sprained ankle.

Adapted from D. A. Auerbach, Medicine for the Outdoors, 2/e, Little Brown and Company.

4. Use the RICE procedures. The goal of RICE is to limit swelling.

5. After applying an ice pack for 20 minutes, wrap with an elastic bandage in a figure-8 pattern or simple overlapping from the toes upward **Figure 8-26**. For extra compression, add a U-shaped pad (made of a rolled bandanna, a piece of ground foam, or other material) around the outer knob of the ankle. For a mild sprain, taping the ankle will provide enough support to reduce swelling but will still allow the victim to walk **Figure 8-27**.

6. Splint ankle fractures with a parka, foam sleeping pad, folded or rolled blanket, SAM splint, or pillow arranged in a U shape around the foot and lower leg **Figure 8-28**. With less severe ankle injuries, if the ankle is supported by a splint or tape and the pain is bearable, the victim might be able to walk.

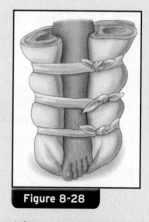

Figure 8-28

A foam sleeping pad or rolled or folded blanket in a U shape will immobilize the foot and ankle.

▶ Foot Injury

Fractures of the long bones of the foot (metatarsals) can occur from a direct blow, a sudden twisting injury, or the stress of repetitive activity such as hiking.

What to Look For

- Local tenderness and pain with walking.
- Swelling and bruising.
- Tenderness over bone prominences.
- Pain that occurs after repetitive stress. Pain may not occur initially, and often reoccurs after a reproducible distance or length of activity.

What to Do

1. Provide a stiff-sole boot and cane or crutch to allow the victim to walk.
2. If pain increases with walking, the victim should not continue. Evacuate the victim.

▶ Toe Injury

Toes are usually fractured by a direct blow, such as stubbing or by dropping a heavy object. Although painful, they are usually not serious injuries, unless they involve the big toe. Most toe fractures do well with realignment and buddy taping.

What to Look For

Compare injured and uninjured sides, looking for swelling and deformities in the injured toe or toes.

What to Do

1. If a toe has a different bend or angle compared with the same toe on the other foot, pull traction in line with its normal position to realign it.
2. Immobilize an injured toe by buddy taping it to its neighbor with padding in between, similar to an injured finger.
3. The victim should not have any trouble walking. A stiff-sole boot might be more comfortable than a soft shoe.

Spinal Injuries

The spine is a column of vertebrae extending from the base of the skull to the tailbone Figure 8-29 . Each vertebra is a bony ring through which the spinal cord passes. The vertebrae are separated by flexible pads called disks. The spinal cord is made up of long tracts of nerves that join the brain with the rest of the body. If a broken vertebra pinches the spinal cord, paralysis can result. A ruptured disk can cause severe pain radiating down the arm or leg and may cause partial or complete paralysis and numbness. Fractures most often occur from severe incidents in which the victim strikes the head or lands on the upper back or buttocks, compressing the spine. Falls, collisions such as in skiing, and vehicle crashes are examples of high-energy incidents that can cause spine fractures. Ruptured or "herniated" disks can also result from these types of injuries, or from less severe injuries such as sports or heavy lifting. Urban first aid advises not to move victims with potential spinal injury; in the wilderness, however, it might be necessary to move these people for a more thorough evaluation or to a safer place.

In addition to deciding whether to move a victim with a possible spinal injury, you also need to decide when to allow a conscious person to get up and move. Full spine immobilization involves a potentially hazardous, long, and costly rescue.

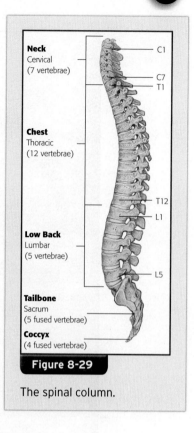

Neck
Cervical
(7 vertebrae)

C1

C7
T1

Chest
Thoracic
(12 vertebrae)

T12
L1

Low Back
Lumbar
(5 vertebrae)

L5

Tailbone
Sacrum
(5 fused vertebrae)

Coccyx
(4 fused vertebrae)

Figure 8-29

The spinal column.

▶ Assessing and Treating Spinal Injuries

What to Look For

- Numbness, tingling, weakness, or burning sensation in the arms or legs
- Loss of bowel or bladder control
- Paralysis of the arms and/or legs
- Tenderness along the midline prominence of the spine

Ask a responsive victim the following questions (related to **Figure 8-30A-F**):

- *Is there pain?* Often a victim will describe nerve pain as an electric shock or shooting pain down the arm or leg. The pain from nerve injuries in the neck radiates to the arms; from upper back injuries, around the ribs; and from lower back injuries, down the legs.
- *Can you move your feet?* Ask the victim to move each foot, pushing downward and upward against your hand despite pain in the back or other areas. If a good effort produces no movement or very weak movement, the victim might have injured the spinal cord.

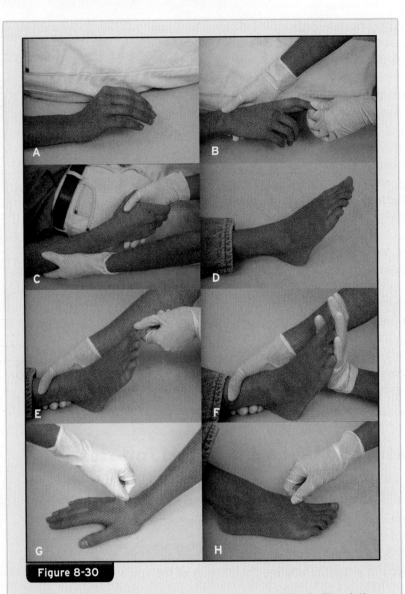

Figure 8-30

Assessment of a spinal injury. For a responsive victim: **A.** The victim wiggles his or her fingers. **B.** The rescuer pinches or squeezes the victim's fingers. **C.** The victim squeezes the rescuer's hand. **D.** The victim wiggles his or her toes. **E.** The rescuer pinches or squeezes the victim's toes. **F.** The victim pushes his or her foot against the rescuer's hand. For an unresponsive victim: **G.** The rescuer pinches the victim's hand. **H.** The rescuer pinches the victim's foot.

- *Can you move your fingers?* Ask the victim to grip your hand. A strong grip, equal on both sides, indicates that a spinal cord injury is unlikely, but a weak or absent grip on one or both sides indicates a possible spinal cord injury in the neck.

For an unresponsive victim:

- Ask bystanders what happened. If there was a significant fall, blow to the head, or diving injury, assume that the victim has a spine injury until a good evaluation shows otherwise.
- Look for injuries around the head and spine (cuts, bruises, and deformities).
- A lack of reaction to painful stimuli could mean spinal cord damage. Pinch the victim's hands (either the palm or the back of the hand) and feet (either the sole or the top of the bare foot) **Figure 8-30G-H**.

What to Do

1. Check the injured person's breathing.
2. Tell the injured person to remain still. If the victim has spine pain, is unresponsive, or is confused following a head injury, stabilize the spine, especially the neck, to avoid further damage. To some degree, the ribs stabilize the thoracic spine and the large muscles of the lumbar area stabilize the lower spine.
3. Tell a responsive and cooperative victim not to move. To stabilize the neck initially, grasp the victim's shoulders and cradle the head between the insides of your forearms **Figure 8-31A**. If the victim is sitting upright, support the head with your hands. Hold the head and neck still and lower the victim slowly onto the back **Figure 8-31B**. There should be no need to manipulate the neck into an uncomfortable position. A responsive, sober person will try to protect a painful neck from damaging movements.
4. Hold the victim's head still (support using rocks padded with clothing or similar objects) while improvising better immobilization.
5. Improvise a short backboard from a backpack, lifejacket, paddles, snowboard, snowshoe, or snow shovel.
6. Place the board behind the head, neck, and chest with rolled clothing on either side of the head (to prevent rotation) and padding beneath the back of the head.
7. Be sure that the head and neck are in the neutral position, with the eyes looking straight forward and the nose in line with the navel.
8. Secure the trunk firmly to the board around the chest, below the arms, and around the forehead. A similar partial backboard can be used for the lumbar or thoracic spine.
9. Fashion a simple neck collar from an aluminum foam splint (SAM splint), a rolled jacket or towel, or a padded hip belt from a backpack **Figure 8-32**. A neck collar alone is not adequate for immobilizing someone with a high suspicion of serious neck injury, but it can be used for comfort after a strain or after waking up with a painful neck.

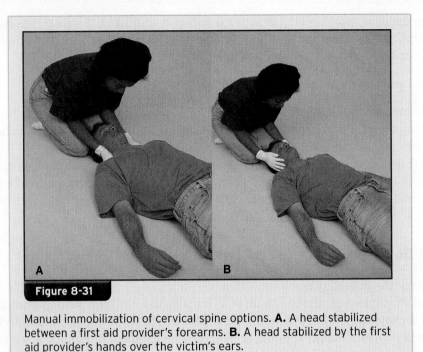

Figure 8-31

Manual immobilization of cervical spine options. **A.** A head stabilized between a first aid provider's forearms. **B.** A head stabilized by the first aid provider's hands over the victim's ears.

▶ Moving a Victim With a Spinal Injury

A victim in an awkward position after a fall, wedged between trees or rocks, or lying face down should be extricated and placed on the back with the spine straight. Straighten the head and neck of an unresponsive victim to maintain an open airway. Injured persons might need to be moved to a secure place where you can provide further first aid. If you are alone, correctly moving a victim with suspected spine injury without a litter or backboard is impossible. Be especially cautious if you note any of the signs of spinal injury mentioned previously. To place a backboard under a victim, assign one person to control the head and neck and to give the commands for any movement to other rescuers. This person cradles the head between the insides of the forearms while holding the top of the shoulder or simply holds the head and jaw firmly with a hand on either side. Gently straighten the injured person's head and neck, if necessary. To examine the back and spine, to turn the victim onto his or her back, or to place someone on an improvised

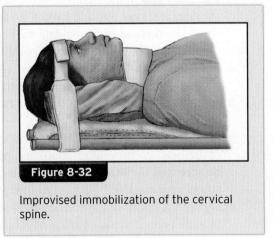

Figure 8-32

Improvised immobilization of the cervical spine.

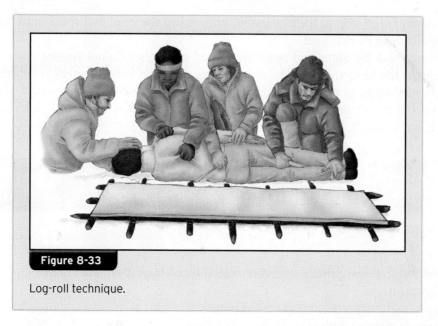

Figure 8-33

Log-roll technique.

backboard, roll the victim like a log, with no twisting or bending **Figure 8-33**. Lifting requires one or more rescuers on each side to support the chest, pelvis, and legs, and one at the head.

▶ When to Remove Spine Immobilization

In the wilderness, seek a balance between the difficulties and dangers of evacuating an immobilized victim and the risks of not immobilizing a spine injury. Fortunately, spine injuries are rare.

To exclude the possibility of a spine injury in a victim with a suspicious mechanism of injury (fall, blow to the head, or diving injury) and to rule out the necessity of spine immobilization, use the following criteria:

- The victim has calmed down from the initial reaction to injury and is fully alert, cooperative, and not intoxicated.
- There are no signs or symptoms of spinal cord injury (numbness, tingling, or burning sensation in arms or legs or paralysis or weakness of fingers, toes, hands, or feet, unless explained by injury to that part).
- There is no marked tenderness when pressing on the spine (not including muscles on either side of the spine).
- There is no marked muscle spasm (this can develop hours later or the next day if there has been a sprain/strain).
- There is no severe midline spine pain with movement (exclude muscle tightness to the side of the spine and extending along the top and inside of the shoulder blade).
- There are no other painful injuries that could make the spine difficult to evaluate (such as multiple broken ribs, fractures of the arms or legs, or major injury close to the spine).

If the victim fails a step in the evaluation, immobilize the head and spine until help and better equipment can be obtained.

In the event that the signs and symptoms listed previously do not suggest spine injury, you can support the head and have the victim rotate and then bend the neck slowly through his or her normal range of motion. You can then support the victim in an attempt to sit and stand, then slowly try rotation and side and forward bending. Mild soreness only, with minimal limitation of motion, indicates no serious spine injury.

Guidelines for Evacuation of Musculoskeletal Injuries

Evacuate as rapidly as possible for the following injuries:

- Open fractures.
- Injuries with nerve damage or compromised blood supply not alleviated by realignment.
- Injuries with suspected spinal-cord damage.
- Injuries associated with serious blood loss.
- Major fractures (hip, femur, pelvis, injury with deformity at the knee, ankle, or elbow).
- Major dislocations or those that cannot be relocated.

Provide nonurgent or assisted evacuation for injuries that cause sufficient pain or disability such that the injured person cannot safely or effectively continue travel.

Evacuation is unnecessary for the following injuries:

- Digit (finger or toe) injuries.
- Minimal injuries to other joints.
- Suspected fractures with no deformity or dislocations after reduction when splinting provides comfort and adequate function, and function is adequate to continue safely.

▶ Emergency Care Wrap-up

What to Look For	What to Do
Upper Extremity Injuries	**Note:** For all of these injuries, check circulation, sensation, and movement.
Shoulder Injury • Local tenderness, swelling, or deformity • Bump at the junction of the collarbone and shoulder • Level of pain • Severe pain with swelling • Position of the affected arm • Muscle spasm	1. Put the arm in a sling with one end over forearm and under armpit on the injured side and the other around neck.
Shoulder Dislocation • The upper arm is usually held away from the body • Deformity • Painful movement	1. Consider attempting relocation if medical care is delayed. 2. Pad and splint the affected limb.
Upper Arm Injury • Swelling and deformities • Impaired motor nerve function • Severe pain	1. Remove any rings. 2. Splint the arm. 3. Place padding between the arm and chest. 4. Use a strap or cravat bandage for a sling.
Elbow Injury • Major deformities • Severe pain • Swelling, tenderness • Painful movement • Impaired motor nerve function	1. Remove any rings. 2. Immobilize with a sling. 3. Keep elbow in the position found. 4. Consider attempting relocation if medical care is delayed.
Lower Arm Injury • Deformity of the wrist or forearm	1. Remove any rings. 2. Attempt to straighten severe angulation of the forearm. 3. Apply a splint to immobilize the hand, wrist, and forearm. 4. Exercise the fingers to help circulation and reduce swelling.

What to Look For	What to Do
Hand Injury • Deformities and swelling • Fingers moved out of alignment	1. Place a pad in the palm. 2. Realign any displaced fingers. 3. Attach a rigid splint along the forearm and under the hand.
Finger Dislocation and Fractures • Bent fingertip that cannot be straightened • Inability to grasp or pinch • Pain and swelling • Restricted movement • Bruising • Abnormal position of two adjoining bones	1. Pull steadily on the finger with the joint straight or hyperextended. 2. Push the base of the dislocated segment back in place. 3. Splint the finger in the position of function. 4. Tape a finger to its neighbor to restrict movement.

Lower Extremity Injuries

What to Look For	What to Do
Hip Injury • Serious injury with pain around the hip • Inability to bear weight • Leg lengths often unequal • Limb locked in an unusual position	1. Realign the limb. 2. Splint the affected leg to the uninjured leg. 3. Put padding between the legs and around the injured leg. 4. Evacuate.
Pelvic Injury • Pain upon compression • Walking or sitting may be unbearable • Signs of shock • Blood in the urine or inability to breathe	1. Stabilize the victim on a rigid backboard, litter, or sled. 2. Evacuate.
Thigh Injury • Severe pain • Swelling, deformity • Abnormal motion • Grating • Leg lengths unequal	1. Manual traction. 2. Stabilize the victim in a position of comfort. 3. Evacuate.

What to Look For	What to Do
Knee Injury • Pain on bending or straightening the knee • Marked tenderness along the edges of the kneecap • Major deformity • Swelling	1. Relocate the kneecap if it is dislocated. 2. Wrap the leg or knee. 3. Improvise a cane or crutch if needed. 4. Evacuate if necessary.
Lower Leg Injury • Severe pain • Swelling • Abnormal motion with grating • Deformity • Inability to bear weight • Open fractures	1. Correct angular deformities with gentle traction. 2. Splint lower leg fractures to immobilize the knee and ankle. 3. Evacuate.
Ankle Injury • Swelling • Tenderness • Bruises • Pain	1. Determine whether to remove the victim's footwear or leave it on. 2. Realign deformity of the ankle. 3. Use the RICE procedures. 4. For a sprain, use an elastic bandage. 5. For a fracture, splint the ankle.
Foot Injury • Local tenderness and pain • Swelling and bruising	1. Provide a stiff-sole boot and crutch. 2. If pain increases with walking, do not continue. 3. Evacuate.
Toe Injury • Swelling • Deformity	1. Apply traction if needed. 2. Immobilize an injured toe with buddy taping. 3. Walking is allowed with a stiff-sole boot.
Spinal Injuries • Numbness, tingling, weakness, or burning sensation in arms or legs • Loss of bowel or bladder control • Paralysis of arms and/or legs • Tenderness along the midline prominence of the spine	1. Check breathing. 2. Tell the person to remain still. 3. Hold the head still. 4. Immobilize the spine with a backboard. 5. Evacuate immediately.

9 Circulatory Emergencies

▶ Anatomy and Physiology

There are three components to the circulatory system: the heart **Figure 9-1**, the blood vessels, and the blood.

The heart is a four-chambered muscular pump that receives oxygen-deficient blood from the body, pumps it through the lungs (where it gets rid of carbon dioxide and is refilled with oxygen), then pumps the oxygen-rich blood back to the body. Heart function is variable, with the capacity to slow down during periods of rest and accelerate during exercise or stress to meet the demands of the body.

Blood vessels are reactive tubes that can expand or contract based on the dynamic need for blood flow to the various parts of the body. Arteries carry blood away from the heart to the tissues, and veins carry blood back to the heart. As arteries get farther away from the heart, they decrease in size and eventually become a network of microscopically small capillaries. It is through the capillaries that the exchange of oxygen and carbon dioxide takes place, with oxygen passing into the tissues and carbon dioxide passing back into the blood. The blood then travels through veins, which become larger as they approach the heart. The smaller blood vessels have the ability to dilate or contract in response to numerous stimuli, such as heat, cold, exercise, and meals.

Blood is a suspension of cells in a protein-rich fluid called plasma. Red cells, which carry oxygen, make up most of the cells; white cells defend the body against infections; and platelets are essential for clotting.

The circulatory system works at its best only when all of the parts are functioning well. It requires a healthy heart, normal blood volume, enough red cells to carry oxygen, and blood vessels that are neither overly dilated nor excessively contracted.

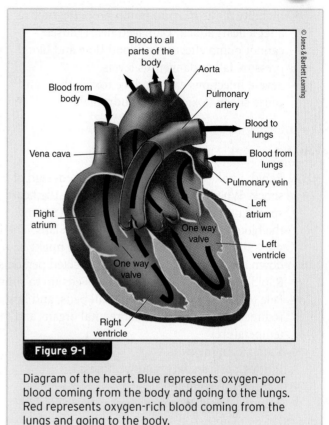

© Jones & Bartlett Learning

Figure 9-1

Diagram of the heart. Blue represents oxygen-poor blood coming from the body and going to the lungs. Red represents oxygen-rich blood coming from the lungs and going to the body.

▶ Shock

Shock occurs when blood flow is inadequate to maintain the supply of oxygen. Oxygen, the fuel of life, is carried by the red blood cells from the lungs to all living tissues in the body. The two most important causes of shock are low blood volume and low blood pressure. Loss of 1 to 1.5 pints of blood from an adult can cause the first stages of shock.

Low blood volume can result from the following:

- Internal or external blood loss (internal blood loss usually occurs in the abdomen)
- Severe dehydration due to diarrhea, vomiting, or sweating, especially if combined with a lack of fluid intake

Low blood pressure can be due to the following:

- Dilation of the blood vessels, as in anaphylaxis (severe allergic reaction) or with spinal cord damage. Small blood vessels dilate and the blood volume is insufficient to fill the enlarged space, causing blood pressure to fall.

- Inability of the heart to pump properly, such as after a heart attack. Damaged heart muscle cannot pump effectively; blood flow and blood pressure fall to dangerous levels.
- Severe infections can produce toxins that can cause shock (toxic shock syndrome).

CAUTION

DO NOT confuse true shock with emotional shock. True shock can be fatal; emotional shock is not usually dangerous. Fainting results from a brief drop in blood pressure and is preceded by some of the signs of shock, but it is usually harmless and temporary.

What to Look For

- Rapid, weak pulse—the most consistent sign of shock. When blood volume is reduced, the heart speeds up, trying to compensate by circulating the blood more rapidly. Blood pressure falls. The faint pulse is due to low blood pressure. In early shock the pulse rate might be normal when the victim is lying down, but it speeds up when the affected person sits or stands.
- Rapid breathing. Breathing also speeds up to supply more oxygen to the blood.
- Pale or bluish (cyanotic) skin, nail beds, and lips. Blood vessels in the skin constrict, redirecting blood flow to more vital organs and producing changes in skin color and temperature.
- Damp, clammy skin.
- Restlessness, anxiety, and weakness.
- Nausea and vomiting.
- Altered level of responsiveness.

Shock requires hospital treatment. Do not expect true shock to improve spontaneously. Your treatment will reduce the effects, at best.

What to Do

1. Check breathing and examine the victim, both in front and in back, for bleeding. If external bleeding seems insufficient to cause shock, consider internal bleeding into the abdomen, chest, stomach, or intestines.
2. Control all bleeding and treat any major injuries.
3. Lay the victim on his or her back.
4. Keep the victim sheltered and warm. Use spare clothes, coats, blankets, or sleeping bags over and under the victim to prevent heat loss.
5. Do not give food to a victim in traumatic shock. If the victim is alert enough to swallow, give only clear liquids.
6. If shock is due to dehydration and the victim is alert enough to swallow safely, give the victim lightly salted water or sports drinks orally. Water replacement is most important.
7. Treat a severely injured person as if shock is inevitable.
8. Evacuate the victim as quickly as possible.

PEDIATRIC NOTE

Children's bodies respond to shock by increasing the heart rate. The normal maximum heart rate for infants is 160 beats/min; for preschool children, 140 beats/min; and for school-age children, 120 beats/min. The pulse can also be elevated due to pain or fear. The blood pressure in a child who is bleeding will be maintained until approximately 40% of the blood volume has been lost. The unwary first aid provider can get false comfort from an apparently normal, strong pulse. After 40% of the blood volume has been lost, a child's condition deteriorates rapidly. An increasing pulse rate, prolonged capillary refill time, and diminishing consciousness, with lethargy or restlessness, are signs of impending shock. Monitor the vital signs and alertness to detect impending shock before the situation turns critical.

▶ Internal Bleeding

Internal bleeding comes from disorders such as stomach ulcers, miscarriages, and injuries that do not break the skin (such as injuries to the lung that bleed into the chest or injuries to the spleen or liver that bleed into the abdominal cavity). Fractures of the pelvis, hip, or thigh also can result in serious hidden bleeding. Because no blood is seen, internal bleeding can be difficult to detect, can seldom be controlled in the field, and can be life threatening.

What to Look For

- A painful, tender, rigid abdomen (this indicates possible bleeding into the abdomen).
- Fractured ribs or bruises on the chest; shortness of breath.
- Unexplained signs of shock (weakness, dizziness, or fainting; a rapid pulse; cold, moist skin).
- Vomiting or coughing up blood.
- Stools that are black or contain large amounts of blood (the black color results from digested blood).
- In a pregnant woman, vaginal bleeding or abdominal pain are signs of serious problems.

What to Do

1. Check breathing repeatedly to evaluate the severity of bleeding.
2. Be prepared for vomiting. If the victim is not alert, place in the recovery position to prevent inhalation of vomit.
3. If the victim is alert, treat shock, and keep the victim warm.
4. Evacuate to medical care immediately.

▶ Heart Disease and Chest Pain

Causes of chest pain include heart disease, lung problems, infections such as pneumonia and bronchitis, muscle strain, contusions, and abdominal problems such as stomach ulcers and gallstones. Consider serious disease when chest pain is associated with shortness of breath, weakness, cyanosis (bluish tinge to skin and lips), and cold, clammy skin; when it is a heavy, crushing, burning, or squeezing pain beneath the breastbone; when it radiates to the neck, jaw, throat, arms, or shoulders; or when it occurs in a person with a history of heart or lung disease with previous attacks of similar pain. Someone who complains of indigestion brought on by exercise might have heart disease.

The cause of most heart pain is coronary artery disease. Cholesterol deposits narrow the coronary arteries and block the supply of blood to the heart muscle (myocardium). If the narrowing is minor, the victim might be able to perform everyday activities without difficulty. During exercise or strong emotion, however, more blood is needed by the heart muscle than can pass through the narrowed arteries, and the relative lack of blood to the heart muscle causes pain.

A characteristic story is that the victim walks uphill after a heavy meal and develops crushing central chest pain that brings the person to a halt. After a minute or two of rest, the pain goes away but returns after the victim continues to walk.

Pain relieved by rest or nitroglycerin (a medication that improves blood flow) or lasting less than 15 minutes is called angina. More severe, longer-lasting pain not relieved by rest or nitroglycerin can signal that the victim is having a heart attack, which is an emergency. The victim is typically anxious, is short of breath, has cold, clammy, and/or cyanotic skin, might feel light headed, and might prefer to sit rather than lie down. Occasionally, however, the victim will experience little discomfort and might deny that a heart attack is occurring.

What to Look For

Perform a primary assessment. Signs that the person is obviously in distress include the following:

- The victim's SAMPLE history indicates previous similar pain, a history of heart or lung disease, recent chest injury, unusual physical activity involving the chest muscles (lifting, climbing, paddling, carrying a heavy pack), or a recent respiratory infection. Ask about previous digestive system disease such as an ulcer or gallbladder disease, nervous stomach, hiatus hernia, and irritable bowel disease. Ask about medicines being taken and why they are needed.

> **NOTE**
>
> After an angina attack, the victim might look and feel normal. During a heart attack the victim may be nervous, may be obviously in pain, and will look sick.

- Abnormal pulse, abnormal respirations, and altered responsiveness.
- Location, type, severity, and duration of pain; change in pain; possible relation to breathing, coughing, or physical activity; shortness of breath. Ask the victim to describe the pain.
- Symptoms of infection (chills, fever, cough, shortness of breath, sore throat, earache, or stuffy head that might suggest a chest infection).

- Indigestion.
- Changes in the vital signs, especially temperature, pulse, breathing rate, and skin characteristics (color and moisture).

What to Do

For angina, do the following:

1. Suspect angina if typical pain occurs in a middle-aged or elderly person, especially one with a history of known heart disease or angina.
2. If the victim has had previous attacks, he or she will usually be carrying nitroglycerin (a spray or small, white pills about half the size of an aspirin), and will know how to use it. Assist the victim in using the medicine according to the directions on the container. Nitroglycerin enlarges the blood vessels and increases blood flow to the heart muscle. Be sure the victim is sitting or lying down when taking nitroglycerin, because it occasionally causes a drop in blood pressure and often causes a pounding headache.
3. If the pain stops within 15 minutes, it was likely angina. If it continues, suspect a heart attack (see the next list of steps).
4. Evacuate anyone you suspect has angina. The person may walk out of the wilderness if he or she is able to do so without pain.

If you suspect a heart attack, do the following:

1. Keep the victim sheltered and warm.
2. If the victim is not allergic to aspirin, give one aspirin. Aspirin, given early during a heart attack, reduces mortality.
3. Give the victim nothing but water or clear, bland liquids to drink.
4. Arrange immediate evacuation.

Changes in Cardiac Rhythm

The normal heartbeat is regular in rhythm—sometimes slow and sometimes fast, but always regular. As you feel a pulse you might occasionally feel a skipped beat—a break in the regularity of the beat—or total irregularity. Most rhythm irregularities are harmless. Total irregularity (atrial fibrillation, not to be confused with fatal ventricular fibrillation) is sometimes found at high altitude and in victims of hypothermia. In both instances, the condition reverts to normal when the person is removed from the contributing environment.

Evacuate the victim if the heart rate is greater than 120 beats per minute at rest and if the afflicted person is unable to function normally.

▶ Emergency Care Wrap-up

What to Look For	What to Do
Shock	
Shock • Rapid, weak pulse • Rapid breathing • Pale or bluish (cyanotic) skin, nail beds, and lips • Damp, clammy skin • Restlessness, anxiety, weakness • Nausea and vomiting • Altered level of responsiveness	1. Check breathing and examine the victim. 2. Control all bleeding and treat any major injuries. 3. Lay the victim on his or her back. 4. Keep the victim sheltered and warm. 5. Do not give food to a victim in traumatic shock. 6. If shock is due to dehydration, give water and electrolyte replacement solutions orally. 7. Treat a severely injured person as if shock is inevitable. 8. Evacuate as quickly as possible.
Internal Bleeding	
• A painful, tender, rigid abdomen • Fractured ribs or bruises on the chest • Unexplained signs of shock • Vomiting or coughing up blood • Stools that are black or contain large amounts of blood • Vaginal bleeding and/or abdominal pain in a pregnant woman	1. Check breathing. 2. Place the victim in the recovery position. 3. Treat shock and keep the victim warm. 4. Evacuate to medical care immediately.
Heart Disease and Chest Pain	
Angina and Heart Attack • Victim's SAMPLE history • Abnormal pulse; abnormal respirations; altered responsiveness • Location, type, severity, and duration of pain • Symptoms of infection • "Indigestion" • Changes in the vital signs	1. If available, give the victim nitroglycerin spray or tablets. 2. Give one aspirin if the victim is not allergic to aspirin. 3. Evacuate.

Respiratory Emergencies

10

Our bodies require a constant supply of oxygen from the air we breathe. Bodily functions create carbon dioxide, a waste gas that must be exhaled. The respiratory system is the collection of organs that function to exchange oxygen and carbon dioxide. Ventilation is the process of moving air in and out of the lungs. Respiration includes the exchange of gases in the lungs. Respiratory problems may be severe or mild. Severe problems can be rapidly progressive and life threatening.

Anatomy and Physiology

The respiratory system includes the air passages, lungs, chest wall, and diaphragm. The diaphragm is the muscular sheet that separates the chest from the abdomen. The ribs, chest muscles, and diaphragm provide the pumping mechanism for ventilation.

PEDIATRIC NOTE

The normal respiratory rate is higher in children than in adults and is age dependent. The rate is 30 breaths/min for preschool children; 20 breaths/min for school-age children; and 12 breaths/min for adolescents. Difficult, labored breathing and grunting, with a rapid respiratory rate, indicate a problem. The ribs are very resilient in children. A severe direct blow to the chest might fail to fracture ribs, but it can produce serious bruising of the lungs and other structures.

The chest is bounded by the collarbones above and the lower margin of the rib cage below. There are 12 ribs on each side, which are attached to the vertebral column posteriorly. The top 10 ribs join the sternum in front, but the eleventh and twelfth ribs are short and do not extend around to the front.

Air enters the chest through the mouth and nose, passes between the vocal cords, and travels down the trachea (windpipe), which divides behind the middle of the breastbone into left and right bronchi, one to each lung. The bronchi subdivide into smaller and smaller tubes until they end in the alveoli, or air sacs, which are smaller than can be seen with the naked eye. The alveoli are where oxygen and carbon dioxide move across a thin membrane, into and out of the blood.

The main structures within the chest are the lungs, the heart, and large arteries and veins attached to the heart. The lungs are each surrounded by a membrane, the pleura, which also lines the inside of the chest wall. The potential space between each lung and the chest wall, the pleural space, can fill with blood or air after injuries to the lungs or the chest wall. It is possible to have blood or air in one pleural space and not in the other. The lungs are kept expanded by a negative pressure in each pleural space. If the pleural space is opened, the partial vacuum is broken and the lungs collapse.

Respiratory emergencies are either illnesses or injuries. Injuries are classified as either open or closed. Open injuries have a wound that penetrates the chest wall. Closed injuries include fractured ribs, flail chest, and lung or heart contusions. Illnesses can affect the air passages (colds, bronchitis, and asthma), the lungs (pneumonia), the chest wall (pleurisy), or all three areas. Heart disease can cause secondary breathing problems such as shortness of breath and pulmonary edema ("water on the lungs").

Chest Injury

Serious chest injuries usually result from high-energy incidents such as motor vehicle crashes and falls from a height. High-energy trauma to the chest is often associated with other severe injuries such as head and spine injuries. Less severe injuries such as muscle strains and contusions can occur from lower-energy incidents such as simple falls or direct blows, or from overuse of the chest and arm muscles. Consider the mechanism of injury as a clue to the nature and severity of injury.

▶ Assessment and Treatment of Chest Injuries

Preliminary assessment and treatment for all chest injuries are the same. First, evaluate the airway and breathing. Is the victim in respiratory distress or breathing easily? Be sure to examine the bare chest in adequate light. Examine both the injured and uninjured sides and compare. Remember DOTS from the chapter *Victim Assessment and Urgent Care*.

What to Look For

- Abnormal breathing or obstruction. Look for rapid, shallow breaths.
- Painful breathing and coughing.
- Noisy breathing.
- Bluish lips or fingernails (cyanosis) indicating poor oxygenation.
- Coughing up blood or pink froth.
- Wounds.
- A sucking noise from air moving in and out of a wound.
- Decreased movement of one or both sides of the chest **Figure 10-1**.
- Grating or clicking from broken ribs.
- Increased pulse rate.
- Signs of internal bleeding and shock.
- Shoulder pain may result from irritation of the diaphragm.
- Air under the skin leaking from a punctured lung. Look for puffiness (sometimes extreme) with a spongy, cracking feeling.
- Assess for other injuries (spine, head, abdomen injuries, and extremity fractures).

What to Do

1. Keep the airway open.
2. Help the victim into a comfortable position.
3. If laying down, lay the victim on the injured side if possible.
4. Encourage deep breathing.
5. If breathing or coughing are painful, splint the affected area by having the victim hold a pad or pillow firmly against the painful area while taking deep breaths and coughing.
6. Evacuate if the victim is so short of breath that he or she cannot speak in complete sentences, if there is cyanosis, or if the condition worsens at all.

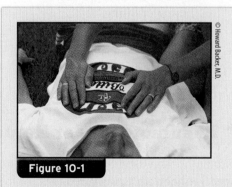

© Howard Backer, M.D.

Figure 10-1

Look and feel for differences in movement between the two sides of the chest.

▶ Rib Fractures

Ribs can be fractured in one or more places. Rib fractures can be isolated or can be associated with internal organ damage. In higher-energy injuries, internal damage, such as a punctured lung, is more common. Lower-rib fractures can be associated with abdominal injuries.

Multiple adjacent ribs may be broken; if each is broken in more than one place, this can result in flail chest, where the chest wall loses support for breathing. A flail chest results in abnormal movement, where the flail segment moves inward during inhalation and outward during exhalation. This opposite movement is called paradoxical motion.

What to Look For

- Assess for chest injury as discussed previously.
- Severe, localized chest pain, especially with deep breathing and coughing.
- Tenderness directly over one or more ribs.
- Deformity, such as a step-off at a rib, or flail chest.
- Grating or clicking sound caused by the movement of broken ribs.
- Shortness of breath.
- Coughing up blood or pink froth.
- Abdominal pain, distention, and tenderness.

What to Do

1. Give the victim painkillers.
2. Hold a pad or pillow against the painful area.
3. Do not splint the chest with a tight wrap unless the pain with movement is very bad.
4. A single, simple rib fracture is not an urgent problem and does not require the victim to be evacuated, although it may limit the ability to do strenuous activity such as hiking or lifting.
5. Have the victim lie on the affected side to splint it.
6. For flail chest, splint the area by taping or strapping a bulky pad over the area.
7. Evacuate all severe injuries, such as flail chest, or if there is cyanosis or significant shortness of breath.

▶ Pneumothorax or Hemothorax

Normally, there is only a thin film of lubricating fluid in the pleural space. If air enters this space, either from a punctured lung, or from a penetrating wound, a pneumothorax occurs. Air can also enter the pleural space spontaneously, without an injury, by rupture of a small bleb (blister) on the surface of the lung. The vacuum normally present in the chest cavity is broken and the lung collapses.

A hemothorax occurs when bleeding occurs into the pleural space **Figure 10-2**. If there is a serious injury, the chest can fill with blood, causing collapse of the lung. Bleeding can be

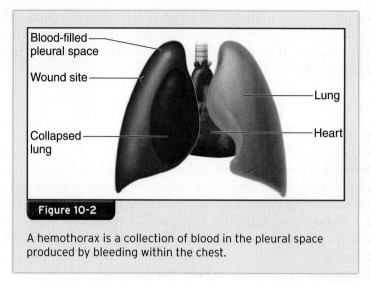

Figure 10-2

A hemothorax is a collection of blood in the pleural space produced by bleeding within the chest.

severe, and it can lead to shock. A small hemothorax often occurs with a rib fracture, and may cause referred pain to the shoulder. In most cases, a pneumothorax will also have some degree of associated bleeding, and is then properly called a hemopneumothorax.

What to Look For

- Signs of serious chest injury.
- Progressively worse shortness of breath.
- Penetrating wound may or may not be present.
- One side of the chest may be moving less well than the other.
- The trachea (windpipe) may be shifted toward the affected side.

What to Do

1. Allow the person to adopt the most comfortable position that does not hinder breathing.
2. Evacuate the victim immediately.

▶ Tension Pneumothorax

In a tension pneumothorax, a flaplike tear on the surface of the lung can act as a one-way valve. Air is sucked into the pleural space with each breath, but the flap-valve closes on expiration. More and more air is trapped in the pleural space. The pressure within the chest increases rapidly, with serious and immediate effects on the functions of the lung and heart. As the pressure in the chest increases, it can become impossible for the victim to breathe, and suffocation ensues. The increased pressure can also reduce blood flow to and from the heart, causing circulatory collapse (shock). If the affected person appears to be dying, act urgently—tension pneumothorax kills quickly.

What to Look For

- Gasping, labored breathing, with heaving chest and neck muscles.
- Increased blueness of the lips and fingernails.
- Less movement of the affected side of the chest than of the normal side.
- Shortness of breath progressing to the inability to move any significant air.
- Bulging of the affected chest, especially noticeable above the collarbone.
- Affected side of the chest may seem larger, and moves less than the unaffected side.
- Trachea (windpipe) is shifted away from the affected side (in contrast to a regular pneumothorax).
- Bulging veins may be visible in the neck and face.
- Signs of shock.
- Victim appears near death.

ADVANCED PROCEDURE

Tension Pneumothorax

In the event of tension pneumothorax, the following medical procedure is the only hope of saving the victim's life and is beyond the scope of standard first aid:

1. Push a large medical needle or catheter into the affected chest cavity to allow air to escape and to relieve pressure within the chest.
2. Evacuate the victim immediately.

▶ Open Injury

An open injury has a wound large enough for air to enter the chest from outside, causing a pneumothorax. The lung collapses and cannot be expanded until the wound is sealed. If air flows in and out of the chest cavity through the wound, a sucking sound may be made, hence the term "sucking chest wound."

What to Look For

- Injury after a severe blow or fall
- Broken skin, with an obvious hole in the chest wall through which air may move noisily during both inhalation and exhalation
- Signs of a pneumothorax

What to Do

1. Seal an open, sucking wound with a thick, impermeable dressing (petroleum jelly on gauze and a bulky dressing, or an improvised dressing of a plastic bag or kitchen wrap padded with bulky cloth) taped closely to the skin to prevent escape or entry of air.
2. Sometimes sealing the wound is harmful. If there is a tear in the lung in addition to the wound in the chest wall, air can continue to escape into the pleural space and build up pressure. If the victim's condition becomes worse, release a corner of the dressing to allow escape of air with expiration.

Respiratory Illness

Illnesses of the respiratory system are common. They can be either mild or severe. Some illnesses, such as asthma, are chronic or recurring but can be treated to allow participation in wilderness activities. Other illnesses are acute, such as pneumonia, and cause the victim to become very ill.

Respiratory illnesses are generally divided into upper and lower respiratory infections, noninfectious problems such as asthma, and chest wall problems such as muscle strains. Upper respiratory infections are problems such as the common cold, sore throat, and sinus infections. Lower respiratory infections include bronchitis (infection of the lower air passages) and pneumonia (infection of the lung itself). Infections can be either viral or bacterial. Viral infections are usually less severe and self-limited, but bacterial infections usually require medical treatment. It is often difficult to tell the difference between viral and bacterial illness, and the first aid is the same. Shortness of breath and cough can also be due to heart problems. Smoking predisposes people to respiratory illnesses and should be strongly discouraged. Victims of respiratory illness should absolutely not smoke or be exposed to secondhand smoke.

What to Look For

- Shortness of breath, cough, and possibly pain.
- SAMPLE history. Is there a history of asthma, smoking, or other respiratory or heart problems? Is the victim using medication for respiratory illness?
- Pain with movement of the arms and tenderness of the chest suggest irritation of the chest wall, ribs, or muscles.
- Fever and generalized muscle aches suggest infection.
- Exertional chest pain, not associated with movement of the arms, suggests heart problems.
- Coughing up sputum (thick green or yellow material) is associated with lower respiratory infection. Blood streaks may be present.
- Signs of upper respiratory infection such as runny nose, sore throat, and stuffy nose.
- Headache around the eyes, nose, or forehead can be associated with sinus infection.
- Signs of severe breathing problems such as rapid breathing, shortness of breath, cyanosis, or increased heart rate.

- Swollen lymph nodes ("glands") around the neck or jaw are associated with infection.
- Asymmetric expansion of the chest may be present with pneumonia.

Consider a respiratory problem to be serious when the following is present:

- There is shortness of breath, weakness, cyanosis, or cold, clammy skin.
- It occurs in a person with a history of lung disease with previous attacks of similar pain.
- There is difficulty either in taking air in or blowing it out, accompanied by wheezing, grunting, or snoring.
- There is blood in the sputum.
- The victim has difficulty with inspiration accompanied by a crowing sound—stridor.
- There is known heart disease, pain suggesting a heart attack, an abnormal heart rate or rhythm, and/or marked ankle swelling.
- There is persistent cyanosis of the skin, lips, and nail beds.
- The victim has shortness of breath of uncertain cause that does not respond to rest or other simple measures.

What to Do

If you suspect a serious respiratory problem, do the following:

1. Keep the victim sheltered and warm.
2. Have the victim adopt a position that allows the most comfortable breathing.
3. Give the victim nonprescription pain medication if pain is prominent.
4. Assist the victim with use of his or her own medication.
5. Arrange immediate evacuation.

For a nonurgent problem, do the following:

1. Help the victim to a comfortable position.
2. Encourage rest and fluids.
3. Most respiratory illnesses will benefit from moist, warm air. Have the victim breathe the vapors from a boiling kettle or pan of water.
4. Acetaminophen or anti-inflammatory drugs such as ibuprofen are usually very helpful for aches and pains. Do not give aspirin to children; a serious, even fatal complication called Reye syndrome can result.
5. Use decongestants for upper respiratory symptoms.

▶ Chest Pain

Chest pain is common and is usually not due to serious disease, but it should never be ignored, because it can occasionally signal life-threatening illness. The cause can be obscure and difficult to discover, even in a hospital. Chest pain causes anxiety because of its association with heart trouble. If chest pain is due to exertion or is associated with shortness of breath, seek medical attention immediately. Most chest pain is caused by one of the following:

- Irritation of ribs, muscles, or joints in the chest wall
- Heart disease
- Respiratory disease
- Gastrointestinal disease

▶ Chest Wall Pain

Exercise or a minor injury can sprain or bruise ribs, chest muscles, or the joints between the ribs and the breastbone. The afflicted person can point to the site of the pain, which is tender on examination. The pain is aching or sharp and aggravated by deep breathing, coughing, twisting the trunk, or moving the arms and shoulders. It is usually only necessary to treat the symptoms with activity modification, stretching, and painkillers.

▶ Asthma

Asthma is a lung condition with recurring spells of shortness of breath, wheezing, and cough due to spasm and swelling of the small air passages. Attacks result from allergies (to pollen, dust, and animal dander); irritants such as smoke, air pollution, and cold air; or exercise. Asthmatics might be perfectly healthy otherwise and able to participate in strenuous, outdoor activities, especially if the asthma is controlled by medication.

What to Look For

The victim may have a history of asthma. Symptoms range from mild to severe and life threatening, including the following:

- Shortness of breath with difficulty in breathing out
- Audible wheezing
- Exposure to environmental triggers (animal dander, smoke, or pollen)

What to Do

1. Place the victim in a comfortable, upright position to help breathing.
2. Assist the victim in using medicines as directed on the labels or by the victim. Most asthmatics carry prescribed medicines (an inhaler and/or pills) and know how to use them **Figure 10-3**.
3. Give the victim clear fluids.
4. Evacuate the victim if:
   - There is no improvement after using medications. Inhaled medications usually work within a few minutes. Pills make take several hours to help.

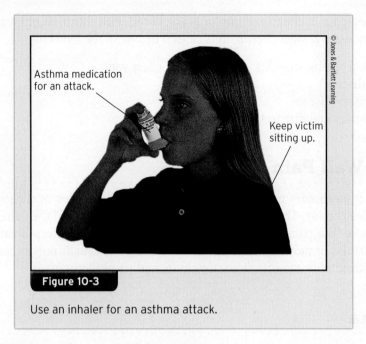

Asthma medication
for an attack.

Keep victim
sitting up.

©Jones & Bartlett Learning

Figure 10-3

Use an inhaler for an asthma attack.

- There are repeated attacks.
- There is a severe and prolonged attack.
- There is no history of asthma and/or no asthma medicines are available.

▶ Colds

A cold is an upper respiratory infection, usually caused by a virus, that is self-limited. Treatment is usually directed toward symptom relief. Antibiotics are not helpful for the common cold.

What to Look For

- Victim complains of a runny nose, headache, or feeling poorly (malaise).
- Fever and chills.
- Cough, usually dry or with clear sputum.

What to Do

1. Encourage rest.
2. Encourage fluids.
3. Use decongestants and painkillers as needed.
4. Breathing warm water vapor may help.

▶ Bronchitis

Bronchitis is an infection of the lower airways, usually due to a virus. Bronchitis can trigger asthma. Most bronchitis is mild and self-limited, but sometimes severe complications such as shortness of breath and pneumonia can result. Bronchitis is common in smokers.

What to Look For

- Productive cough, usually with green or yellow sputum, sometimes blood-streaked
- Symptoms of a cold: fever, malaise, congestion

What to Do

1. Treat as for a cold.
2. Have the victim immediately quit smoking and eliminate exposure to secondhand smoke.
3. Evacuate if there is shortness of breath or signs of pneumonia.

▶ Pneumonia

Pneumonia is an infection of the lungs and can be either viral or bacterial. Viral pneumonias are usually self-limited and can be treated like a cold or bronchitis. Bacterial pneumonias are often very severe and require antibiotics.

What to Look For

- Very ill victim, often with productive cough, high fever.
- Localized chest pain, often worse with breathing or coughing (pleuritic pain).
- Shortness of breath may be present.
- One side of the chest may not expand fully.

What to Do

1. Treat as for bronchitis or a cold.
2. Evacuate the victim if not improving.

▶ Benign Hyperventilation

Many people react to anxiety by overbreathing, or hyperventilating. Although the victims feel like they are not getting enough air, they are actually getting too much. Hyperventilation causes

> **CAUTION**
>
> **DO NOT** have the affected person breathe into a bag because it can dangerously stress the heart and respiratory system.

the victim to blow off too much carbon dioxide, which results in abnormal chemical balance in the blood and causes the following:

- Dizziness or light-headedness
- Increasing shortness of breath
- Numbness, coldness, and/or tingling of the mouth, hands, and feet
- Chest tightness or discomfort

The victim—who believes that these are signs of a heart attack, stroke, or other serious problem—becomes more anxious, causing more overbreathing, which eventually leads to spasmodic contractures of the hands and feet, as well as fainting. Fainting allows return of normal breathing with recovery.

In the injured, the elderly, and those with diabetes, heart disease, or lung disease, always consider serious causes of hyperventilation.

What to Do

If you believe that the hyperventilation is not due to a serious condition, do the following:

1. Reassure the person who is suffering, removing him or her from the cause of anxiety (for example, a cliff).
2. Encourage slow, regular breathing.
3. If the hyperventilation persists without a precipitating cause, consider other respiratory problems and plan to evacuate the victim.

▶ Emergency Care Wrap-up

What to Look For	What to Do
Chest Injuries	
• Abnormal breathing or obstruction • Painful breathing and coughing • Noisy breathing • Bluish lips or fingernails • Coughing up blood or pink froth • Wounds • A sucking noise from air moving in and out of a wound • Decreased movement of one or both sides of the chest • Grating or clicking from broken ribs • Increased pulse rate • Signs of internal bleeding and shock • Shoulder pain may result from irritation of the diaphragm • Air under the skin leaking from a punctured lung • Assess for other injuries	1. Keep the airway open. 2. Help the victim into a comfortable position. 3. If laying down, lay on the injured side if possible. 4. Encourage deep breathing. 5. If breathing or coughing are painful, splint the affected area by having the victim hold a pad or pillow firmly against the painful area. 6. Evacuate if the victim is so short of breath that he or she cannot speak in complete sentences, if there is cyanosis, or if the condition worsens at all.
Rib Fractures • Assess for chest injury as above • Severe, localized chest pain, especially with deep breathing and coughing • Tenderness directly over one or more ribs • Deformity, such as a step-off at a rib, or flail chest • Grating or clicking due to movement of broken ribs • Shortness of breath • Coughing up blood or pink froth • Abdominal pain, distension, and tenderness	1. Give the victim painkillers. 2. Hold a pad or pillow against the painful area. 3. Do not splint the chest with a tight wrap unless the pain with movement is very bad. 4. A single, simple rib fracture is not an urgent problem and does not require the victim to be evacuated, although it may limit the ability to do strenuous activity such as hiking or lifting. 5. Have the victim lay on the affected side to splint it. 6. For flail chest, splint the area by taping or strapping a bulky pad over the area. 7. Evacuate all severe injuries, such as flail chest, or if there is cyanosis or significant shortness of breath.

What to Look For	What to Do
Pneumothorax or Hemothorax • Signs of serious chest injury • Progressively worse shortness of breath • Penetrating wound may or may not be present • One side of the chest may be moving less well than the other • The trachea (windpipe) may be shifted toward the affected side	1. Allow the person to adopt the most comfortable position that does not hinder breathing. 2. Evacuate immediately.
Tension Pneumothorax • Gasping, labored breathing • Increased blueness of lips and fingernails • Less movement of the affected side of the chest • Shortness of breath progressing to the inability to move any significant air • Bulging of the affected chest, especially noticeable above the collarbone • Affected side of the chest may seem larger, and moves less than the unaffected side • Trachea (windpipe) is shifted away from the affected side (in contrast to a regular pneumothorax) • Bulging veins may be visible in the neck and face • Signs of shock • Victim appears near death	1. Advanced-trained medical providers would perform the following procedure; it is beyond the scope of first aid. Push a large medical needle or catheter into the affected chest cavity to allow air to escape and to relieve pressure within the chest. 2. Evacuate immediately.
Open Injury • Injury after a severe blow or fall • Broken skin, with an obvious hole in the chest wall • Signs of a pneumothorax	1. Seal an open, sucking wound with a thick, impermeable dressing. 2. If the victim's condition becomes worse, release a corner of the dressing to allow escape of air with expiration.

What to Look For

What to Do

Respiratory Illnesses

What to Look For	What to Do
• Shortness of breath, cough, and possibly pain • SAMPLE history. Is there a history of asthma, smoking, or other respiratory or heart problems? Is the victim using medication for respiratory illness? • Pain with movement of the arms and tenderness of the chest suggest irritation of the chest wall, ribs, or muscles • Fever and generalized muscle aches suggest infection • Exertional chest pain, not associated with movement of the arms, suggests heart problems • Coughing up sputum (thick green or yellow material) is associated with lower-respiratory infection. Blood streaks may be present • Signs of upper-respiratory infection such as runny nose, sore throat, and stuffy nose • Headache around the eyes, nose, or forehead can be associated with sinus infection • Signs of severe breathing problems such as rapid breathing, shortness of breath, cyanosis, or increased heart rate • Swollen lymph nodes ("glands") around the neck or jaw are associated with infection • Asymmetric expansion of the chest may be present with pneumonia	1. Keep the victim sheltered and warm. 2. Have the victim adopt a position that allows the most comfortable breathing. 3. If pain is prominent, give the victim nonprescription pain medication. 4. Assist the victim with use of his or her own medication. 5. Arrange immediate evacuation.
Asthma • Shortness of breath with difficulty in breathing out • Audible wheezing • Exposure to environmental triggers (animal dander, smoke, or pollen)	1. Place the victim in a position of comfort. 2. Assist the person in using medications. 3. Give clear fluids. 4. Evacuate if necessary.
Colds • Runny nose, headache, or feels poorly • Fever and chills • Cough, usually dry or with clear sputum	1. Encourage rest. 2. Encourage fluids. 3. Use decongestants and painkillers as needed. 4. Breathing warm water vapor may help.

What to Look For	What to Do
Bronchitis • Productive cough, usually with green or yellow sputum, sometimes blood-streaked • Symptoms of a cold: fever, malaise, congestion	1. Treat as for a cold. 2. Have the victim immediately quit smoking and eliminate exposure to secondhand smoke. 3. Evacuate if there is shortness of breath or signs of pneumonia.
Pneumonia • Very ill victim, often with productive cough, high fever • Localized chest pain, often worse with breathing or coughing (pleuritic pain) • Shortness of breath may be present • One side of the chest may not expand fully	1. Treat as for bronchitis or a cold. 2. Evacuate if not improving.
Benign Hyperventilation • Dizziness or light-headedness • Increasing shortness of breath • Numbness, coldness, and/or tingling of the mouth, hands, and feet • Chest tightness or discomfort	1. Calm the person down. 2. Encourage slow, regular breathing. 3. If hyperventilation persists, evacuate.

Neurologic Emergencies

11

Anatomy and Physiology

The nervous system consists of three interconnected parts: the brain, the spinal cord, and the peripheral nerves **Figure 11-1**.

The brain is composed of soft nerve tissue suspended in cerebrospinal fluid, which cushions movement within the rigid, protective skull. The blood supply comes from arteries that run up both sides of the neck and enter the skull from below, and then form a delicate network over the surface of the brain. Swelling or bleeding into or around the brain increases pressure within the skull and compresses the brain, compromising cerebral function.

The brain is the command and control center of the nervous system, controlling thought and emotion as well as vital bodily functions. The rest of the nervous system is a collection of message lines, conveying signals to and from the brain.

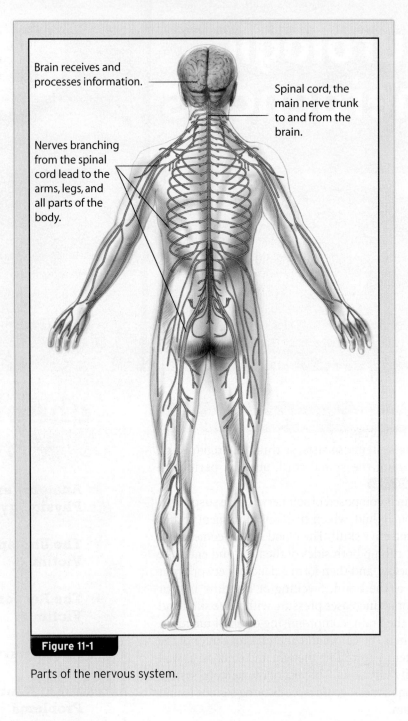

Brain receives and processes information.

Spinal cord, the main nerve trunk to and from the brain.

Nerves branching from the spinal cord lead to the arms, legs, and all parts of the body.

Figure 11-1

Parts of the nervous system.

The spinal cord, composed of nerve fibers from the brain, extends from the base of the skull to the lower back. It lies in the spinal canal, protected by the bones of the vertebral column. The peripheral nerves, which arise from the cord and leave the spinal canal between each vertebral bone, carry motor and sensory signals to and from the muscles, skin, and organs of the body. An injury to the spinal cord affects all functions below the level of the damage.

The Unresponsive Victim

▶ Causes and Treatment for Unresponsive Conditions

An unresponsive victim presents one of the most difficult problems in the wilderness. Regardless of the cause of unresponsiveness ▭ Table 11-1 ▭, the first-aid management is much the same.

If the victim was observed falling, a traumatic head injury is the likely cause of the unresponsiveness. If there are no witnesses and the victim is unresponsive, determining the cause could be impossible. Remember that the victim of an unwitnessed head injury may have become unresponsive from another cause, and then sustained the head injury.

If the victim is with another person or group, find out what you can about that person's history. Has the affected person had a head injury, such as from a fall? Has he or she had seizures in the past? Has he or she suffered any known neurologic or other disease? Has he or she taken any medications or drugs—medicinal or illegal? Has he or she eaten anything unusual? Has he or she suffered allergies to food, an insect bite, or other possible causes of an allergic reaction?

Table 11-1 Some Causes of Altered Responsiveness	
Head injury	Neurologic illness:
Shock:	• Stroke
• Heart failure	• Meningitis
• Severe injury	• Seizure
• Bleeding	Asphyxia:
• Spinal injury	• Avalanche burial
Drugs or poisoning:	• Near drowning
• Alcohol	Metabolic and environmental:
• Legal or illegal drugs	• Low blood glucose (sugar)
• Wild plants or mushrooms	• Diabetic coma
	• Hypothermia
	• Heatstroke

Survey the scene to look for clues to the cause if the victim's history is unobtainable. Consider the time of year and environment (for example, in winter, consider hypothermia; in summer, consider heatstroke). Look for evidence of a fall, boating incident, or other causative event.

PEDIATRIC NOTE

Closed head injuries are common in children. Direct injury with brain swelling can result in permanent damage. Failure to recognize an inadequate airway can produce a secondary brain injury in children due to lack of oxygen. A child's alertness is a sensitive gauge of adequate oxygenation.

What to Look For

- Try to determine if there has been an injury or if the unresponsiveness is due to illness.
- Assess responsiveness with the AVPU scale. Look for changes in level of responsiveness. Decreases are worrisome.
- If there has been a head injury, look for other injuries, and assume there is a spinal injury as well.
- If there does not appear to be an injury, look for signs of illness (discussed later in this chapter).
- Signs of seizures (bitten tongue, incontinence of urine, ongoing seizures).
- Abnormalities of the eyes (deviated to one side, unequal pupils).
- Paralysis. Look at the victim's face as well as the limbs. Do both sides move equally?
- Medical identification tags.

What to Do

Unresponsiveness has many causes, but all unresponsive or poorly responsive victims need an open airway, protection from aspiration (inhaling into the lungs) of saliva and vomit, and a steady, normal body temperature. The general care of all unresponsive victims is similar, regardless of the cause.

With evidence of a head injury:

1. Protect the spine in case of fracture or spinal-cord injury.
2. Roll the victim carefully onto the back for better examination.
3. Check breathing; open and maintain an airway.
4. Stop bleeding from any scalp wounds.
5. Monitor vital signs. One member of the party should stay with the victim at all times to do so.
6. Move the victim to safety, comfort, and shelter.

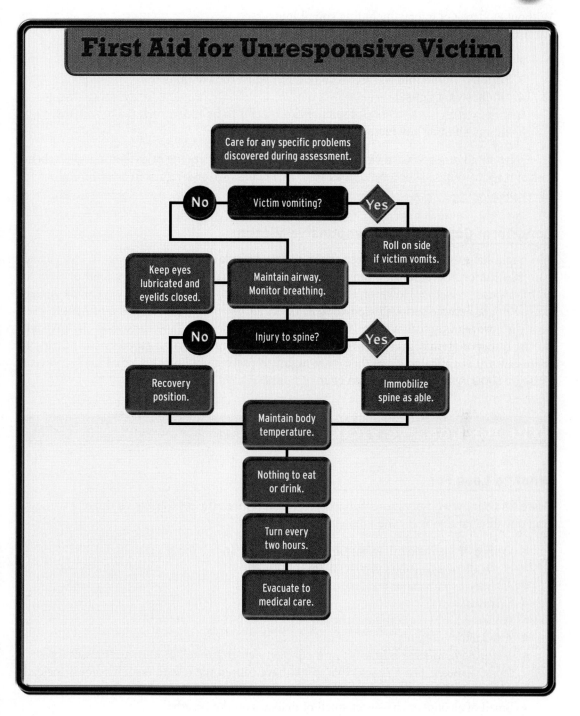

First Aid for Unresponsive Victim

Care for any specific problems discovered during assessment.

No — Victim vomiting? — Yes

Roll on side if victim vomits.

Keep eyes lubricated and eyelids closed.

Maintain airway. Monitor breathing.

No — Injury to spine? — Yes

Recovery position.

Immobilize spine as able.

Maintain body temperature.

Nothing to eat or drink.

Turn every two hours.

Evacuate to medical care.

Without evidence of injury (including spinal injury):

1. Roll the victim carefully onto the back.
2. Check breathing; open and maintain an airway.
3. Turn the victim into the recovery position when the victim is stable.
4. Monitor vital signs.
5. If the victim has a history of seizures and seems to be recovering, make sure the victim is taking any medications properly.

Evacuate all unresponsive victims other than those experiencing brief fainting spells, brief loss of responsiveness after a mild head injury (concussion), or seizures in a victim known to have epilepsy.

Long-Term Care of the Unresponsive Victim

You might have to care for an unresponsive victim for a day or more. If this is the case, avoid pain medications because they can conceal neurologic changes. Do not give food or fluid to an unresponsive victim. However, if the victim is unable to take fluids over several days, that person might become seriously dehydrated. Lubricate the eyes with any eye ointment to prevent the corneas from developing ulcers from dry-air exposure. Tape the eyelids lightly shut during transportation. Unresponsive victims may be incontinent of urine or feces. If they soil themselves, it is critical to clean them thoroughly to prevent skin breakdown. Finally, prevent pressure sores by turning the victim every 2 hours.

The Responsive Victim

What to Look For

Based on your own observations and a careful history from the responsive victim or a witness, find out about and look for the following:

- Details of the incident: exact time, length of fall, and so forth.
- Duration of unresponsiveness, if any.
- Alterations in behavior or level of responsiveness.
- Seizures.
- Potential for hypothermia at the site.
- Any known diseases.
- Medical identification bracelet or medallion, which can tell of known illnesses (epilepsy, diabetes, heart attack) that might have caused the loss of responsiveness instead of a head injury.
- Smell of alcohol or the sweet smell of diabetes on the breath.
- Level of responsiveness; use the AVPU scale to measure. Restlessness may be due to brain injury or pain.

- Unequal pupil size, indicating possible damage to one side of the brain.
- Spinal injury, which can occur with a head injury.
- Blood or clear fluid oozing or dripping from the nose or ears, without a local injury to account for it, which can suggest bleeding or leaking of cerebrospinal fluid from a fracture at the base of the skull.
- Examine the face and limbs for paralysis.

Head Injury

People with serious head injuries tend to get worse and die; those with less severe head injuries tend to get better. Very few head injuries need surgery; those that do need it at once.

▶ Concussion

A concussion is the brief disruption of brain function due to a blow to the head. Even a mild blow to the head can jar the brain against the skull and momentarily disrupt mental function. Anyone who has been unresponsive from a head injury, however briefly, must not walk or be left unattended because intracranial bleeding (bleeding within the skull) can occur during the next few hours, resulting in disorientation or even coma.

What to Look For

- No loss or brief loss (less than 30 seconds) of responsiveness.
- Victim may see "stars" (visual changes).
- Nausea, dizziness, headache.
- After a severe concussion the victim may not remember events that occurred immediately before the injury, or may not remember facts such as the date.

What to Do

1. Following a concussion, allow the victim to sleep, but wake the affected person every 2 to 3 hours to check the level of responsiveness.
2. If no symptoms appear 8 hours after injury, wake the victim once during the first night.
3. Seek medical care if any of the following are present:
   - Vomiting.
   - Persistent ringing in the ears.
   - Impaired balance.
   - Loss of taste or smell.
   - Loss of responsiveness occurs after regaining responsiveness or lasts longer than 30 seconds.

▶ Head Injury With Delayed Deterioration

More severe injury can bruise the brain or rupture blood vessels. The resulting swelling or bleeding causes increased pressure inside the skull, which interferes with brain function. The victim will die unless the blood under pressure is released by surgery. Brain damage from compression can be permanent, because brain cells cannot regenerate (unlike cells in other parts of the body).

Often there is a brief loss of responsiveness followed by a period of near-normal responsiveness lasting minutes or hours. As pressure from bleeding builds up, there is deterioration of mental function and eventual unresponsiveness.

What to Look For

- After a head injury, the victim may regain responsiveness, appear quite normal for a time (lucid interval), and continue the expedition. However, continued bleeding or swelling of the brain causes pressure inside the skull to rise. Decreased level of responsiveness occurs, followed by coma and death.
- Victim complaints of severe, progressive headache not relieved by common medications.
- Repeated vomiting.
- Altered behavior including confusion, combativeness, irrationality, or apparent intoxication, then drowsiness and progressive unresponsiveness.

What to Do

1. Protect and maintain the airway.
2. Maintain a stable body temperature.
3. Treat the victim as though he or she were unresponsive.
4. Evacuate the victim immediately.

▶ Severe Diffuse Brain Injury

Severe, diffuse injury to the brain can be caused either by the initial severe head injury and subsequent swelling or by lack of oxygen (hypoxia) secondary to inadequate breathing. This type of brain injury generally causes complete unresponsiveness immediately. There may be some recovery of responsiveness but with an altered level that may persist permanently.

What to Look For

- The victim is deeply unresponsive from the time of injury.
- The airway can be obstructed and breathing can be impaired.
- Changes in responsiveness on the AVPU scale. Over time, these changes are extremely important. Improvement is a good sign; deterioration is ominous.

- The speed at which the victim regains normal responsiveness. This indicates roughly the severity of the injury and forecasts the final outcome.

Good Signs

- The victim starts to awaken, responds verbally, and knows his or her name, whereabouts, the month, and the year.
- The victim's body movements become normal and are equal on both sides.
- The victim blinks in response to a hand waved closely in front of the eyes.

Bad Signs

- The victim's pupils fail to respond to light and become dilated (enlarged).
- One of the victim's pupils becomes larger than the other.
- The pulse slows.
- Breathing becomes irregular.
- The victim's body temperature rises.
- The victim awakens, but there is evidence of brain or spinal damage with loss of feeling, one-sided weakness, or paralysis.

What to Do

1. Clear and maintain the airway; if there is no breathing, start CPR.
2. Assume the victim has spinal cord injuries.
3. Apply a neck collar or otherwise restrain the head from moving.
4. Repeat your examination periodically to determine the victim's progress; record your observations.
5. Prevent additional injury. Move the victim to shelter and safety.
6. Evacuate the victim quickly.

▶ Skull Fractures

Fractures can be closed or open. A closed fracture occurs without a break in the scalp. A fracture is open when the scalp over the fracture is lacerated and the brain or its coverings are exposed. Skull fractures can occur without displacement of bone or with a depressed segment of bone that could press on the brain.

What to Look For

- Broken bone edges in the wound. A smooth, exposed white bone surface might not be serious if there is no associated skull fracture.
- Clear or blood-tinged fluid dripping from the nose or ear without an apparent injury to those areas. This indicates a possible fracture at the base of the skull.

What to Do

1. If a depressed skull fracture is present, protect the area with a doughnut dressing slightly larger than the depressed area.
2. If there is an open fracture, cover the wound with a sterile dressing.
3. Control any bleeding by applying a sterile or clean dressing and applying pressure around the edges of the wound, not directly on it.
4. Evacuate the victim.

Other Neurologic Problems

▶ Stroke

Stroke is caused by blockage of a blood vessel or bleeding in the brain. If an artery is partially blocked, the stroke symptoms might be temporary. These little strokes, known as transient ischemic attacks (TIAs), last from a few minutes to several hours, after which the victim recovers.

Stroke is most common in those with hardening of the arteries (arteriosclerosis), the elderly, and people with high blood pressure or diabetes. In the wilderness, symptoms of stroke occasionally occur in young, healthy persons due to a head injury, decompression sickness, or cerebral edema (thickening of the blood due to altitude).

What to Look For

The signs and symptoms of stroke depend on the part of the brain involved.

- Altered responsiveness: assess as for unresponsive victim
- Numbness, weakness, or paralysis of the face, arm, or leg, usually on one side of the body
- Turning of the head and eyes to one side
- Noisy breathing, drooling
- Visual changes, including double vision, sudden blurring, or loss of vision in one or both eyes
- Loss of balance or coordination
- Difficulty speaking or inability to understand simple statements
- Sudden, very severe, unexplained, long-lasting headache
- Convulsions
- A history of diabetes, hypertension, heart disease, or previous stroke

What to Do

1. Keep the victim in the recovery position, with the head and upper body slightly raised to lessen brain swelling.
2. If awake, allow the victim to find a comfortable position.
3. Offer the victim clear liquids with caution.
4. Evacuate the victim.

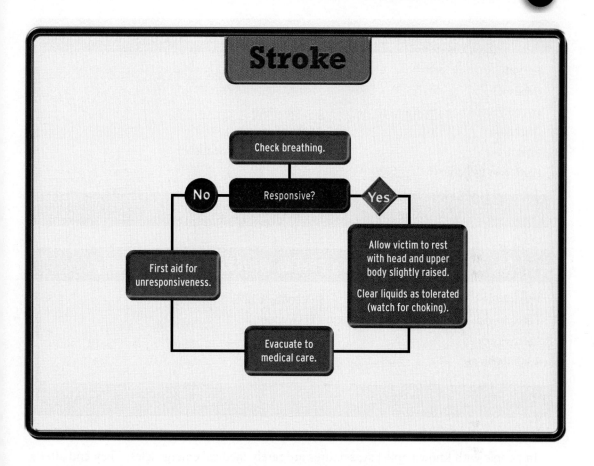

► Seizures

Seizures are due to sudden, temporary, abnormal electrical discharges in the brain Table 11-2 . Recurrent seizures occur in epilepsy.

There are two types of seizures. Partial seizures may be experienced as a momentary lack of awareness, an involuntary movement of an arm, leg, and/or the face, a sensation of numbness or tingling, or abnormal vision or smell. Responsiveness might or might not be affected. Generalized seizures are frequently preceded by an aura—a momentary vision, smell, or other sensation that forewarns the victim of the seizure—then start with a sudden spasm of body muscles, causing the victim to cry out hoarsely and fall to the ground with a rigid back and limbs. A few seconds later, violent, rhythmic contractions of the neck, back, and extremities occur. During this phase, which usually lasts only a few minutes, the victim might bite his or her tongue or be incontinent. After a seizure, the victim is unresponsive for minutes to an hour or longer, then gradually awakens. Immediately after a seizure, the victim breathes deeply, might look blue, and might foam at the mouth.

Table 11-2 Causes of Seizures in People Without Known Epilepsy

Epilepsy	Stroke
Head injury	Lightning injury
Hypoglycemia (low blood sugar)	Illegal drugs
Poisoning	Lack of oxygen
Heatstroke	Pregnancy (complications)
High fever (children)	

Table 11-3 Medications That a Person With Epilepsy May Carry

Phenytoin	Phenobarbital
Carbamazepine	Primidone
Valproic acid	Ethosuximide
Trimethadione	

In people with known epilepsy, seizures are rarely medical emergencies. They end after a few minutes and aren't associated with harm unless the victim is in a dangerous or exposed location or is injured during the seizure. The victim usually does not require medical attention. Epilepsy typically begins in childhood. Seizures that begin later in life often are due to serious medical conditions. New onset of seizures requires evacuation and immediate medical care. Seizures in individuals with diabetes should be treated as hypoglycemia.

Most people with epilepsy can control their seizures with medication and live normal lives, including participating in wilderness activities Table 11-3 . However, they should avoid higher risk activities (climbing, alpine skiing, riding chair lifts, unsupervised swimming, boating, scuba diving, and caving) unless they have a history of reliably taking medicine on schedule, have been seizure free for at least 2 years, and have approval from their neurologist.

What to Do

1. Concentrate on preventing injury; an oncoming seizure cannot be prevented. Help the victim to lie down in a safe area.
2. Don't restrain the victim. If possible, remove nearby objects that the victim might strike. Don't open or insert anything into the victim's mouth.

3. After the seizure, make sure the airway is open. Breathing might stop temporarily, but it will restart without help unless there is an airway obstruction.

4. Discourage onlookers and arrange for privacy. The victim might have been incontinent and might be embarrassed.

5. Afterward, assess as you would for an unresponsive victim; the victim will have an altered mental status or be sleepy. In particular, take the body temperature (to assess for heatstroke) if you have a thermometer, feel the skin temperature, and look for lacerations of the tongue or injuries caused by muscle spasms or a fall. Look for a medical identification tag. Keep the victim in the recovery position until he or she is awake and alert.

6. Check for a history of seizures. If there is a history of seizures, determine whether medicine is being taken to prevent seizures. Ask whether any doses have been missed.

7. If there is no history of epilepsy, ask about diabetes, a recent head injury, eating wild plants, and medicines or illegal drugs that have been taken. If the victim is a child, ask the parents whether he or she has had a high fever.

8. Evacuate if:
   - There is no history of epilepsy with similar episodes.
   - The seizure lasts more than 5 minutes or seizures are repetitive.
   - Responsiveness does not return within 20 to 30 minutes.
   - The victim is in the second half of pregnancy.

▶ Simple Fainting

Simple fainting is a common, benign, and usually brief form of rapid drop in blood pressure that results in inadequate blood flow to the brain and loss of normal responsiveness. It might have either a physical or an emotional cause, such as pain, the sight of blood, excitement, fear, or standing for a long time, especially in the heat. Someone who is dehydrated or has lost blood might faint when trying to stand.

What to Look For

In a previously healthy person:

- Reports of seeing spots, feeling dizzy, hot or cold, and nauseated
- Paleness, with cold, clammy skin
- Passing out, slumping, or falling down

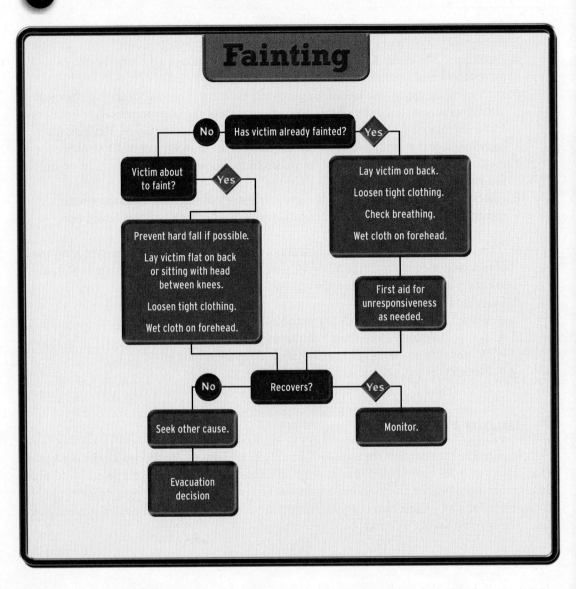

Fainting

Has victim already fainted?

No → Victim about to faint?

Yes →

Yes →
Prevent hard fall if possible.

Lay victim flat on back or sitting with head between knees.

Loosen tight clothing.

Wet cloth on forehead.

Yes →
Lay victim on back.

Loosen tight clothing.

Check breathing.

Wet cloth on forehead.

First aid for unresponsiveness as needed.

Recovers?

No → Seek other cause. → Evacuation decision

Yes → Monitor.

What to Do

For a person who is about to faint:

1. Prevent a hard, injury-causing fall.
2. Lay the person flat. If there is no place for the victim to lie down, the afflicted person should sit with the head between the knees. When a person who has fainted is flat on the ground, blood flow to the brain increases, blood pressure returns rapidly to normal, and the victim wakes up.
3. Loosen tight clothing, especially around the neck.
4. Place a cool, wet cloth on the victim's forehead.

If someone has fainted:

1. Check the victim's breathing.
2. Lay the victim flat.
3. Loosen tight clothing.
4. Check for injuries caused by the fall.
5. Place a cool, wet cloth on the victim's forehead.
6. Provide care for unresponsiveness.
7. Keep persons who have fainted lying down until they have recovered, and then have them stand up slowly.
8. Evacuate the victim if he or she:
   - Appears to have a serious illness or injury.
   - Has fainted repeatedly.
   - Does not awaken within 30 seconds.
   - Was lying down when the episode occurred.
   - Continues to be light-headed when attempting to get up.

Unresponsiveness due to a sudden serious illness (heart attack, stroke, internal bleeding with shock) can be mistaken at first for a simple faint. A middle-aged or elderly victim or one who doesn't recover rapidly after lying flat should be assessed and cared for as for any unresponsive victim. If fainting occurs each time the victim stands, suspect dehydration or shock.

▶ Headache

Most headaches are harmless and can be controlled by resting, avoiding eye fatigue, and by taking mild, nonprescription medications (aspirin, acetaminophen, or ibuprofen). In the wilderness, headaches also can be caused by dehydration, altitude, glare off of snow or water, and traction on the neck muscles from carrying a heavy pack. Rarely, a headache can be the first sign of a serious condition, such as high-altitude cerebral edema, stroke, meningitis (infection of the brain or spinal cord), or severe high blood pressure.

What to Look For

- Head trauma.
- Tenderness over the scalp, neck, and shoulders due to chronic muscle contraction.
- Pupils unequal in size.
- Complaints of double vision (stroke).
- Fever.
- Severe neck stiffness (a sign of meningitis).
- Impaired sensation or movement of the extremities (stroke).
- Impaired balance. Have the victim stand with the eyes closed or walk a straight line (test for high-altitude cerebral edema).
- Ask the victim if he or she is drinking adequate water and passing pale yellow urine (a sign of adequate hydration).

Suspect serious illness or injury if a headache:

- Causes vomiting, inability to sleep, or inability to eat or drink for more than a day in someone without previous recurrent headaches (even if infrequent).
- Lasts more than a day, is unresponsive to nonprescription medication, and is steadily getting worse.
- Is sudden and severe, unlike any previous headaches, and does not improve with rest and mild pain medicine.
- Is associated with drowsiness, stiff neck, altered mental status, high fever, personality changes, visual changes, weakness or loss of sensation on one side of the body, and/or loss of balance.

What to Do

1. If the headache is mild to moderate, give the victim nonprescription pain medication.
2. Encourage adequate hydration.
3. If acute mountain sickness is a possibility, descend to an altitude below that at which the headache started (at least 2,000 feet lower). Do not go higher!
4. If the cause appears serious, evacuate.

▶ Migraine

Migraine headaches are usually periodic, one-sided, and throbbing, and they frequently are accompanied by nausea and vomiting. They tend to run in families and affect men less frequently than women, in whom they might occur around the time of the menstrual period. The headaches are frequently accompanied by visual changes such as spots and flashing lights. Migraine sufferers usually carry medication to be taken at the onset of a headache; if not, sometimes mild nonprescription pain medications help. During the headache, allow the victim to rest in a dark area.

▶ Diabetes

People with diabetes are subject to alterations in blood sugar that affect their responsiveness.

Low blood sugar (hypoglycemia) can be caused by taking too much insulin or by taking insulin without taking enough food. Exercise lowers blood sugar and people with diabetes who are not used to strenuous hiking or other exercise might not eat enough extra food to prevent a significant drop in blood sugar. Hypoglycemic fainting comes on quickly, with dizziness, sweating, and alteration of responsiveness. Treat by giving the victim sugar immediately. Recovery usually is rapid.

High blood sugar levels (hyperglycemia) result from too little insulin. Blood sugar levels climb slowly, sometimes over a day or two. The condition is recognized by excessive thirst, large urine output, exhaustion, or a fruity smell to the breath. As the condition worsens, the person with diabetes might lapse into a coma. This is very dangerous and requires evacuation.

▶ Emergency Care Wrap-up

What to Look For	What to Do
Head Injuries	
Concussion • No loss or brief loss of responsiveness • May briefly "see stars" • Nausea, dizziness, headache	1. Following a concussion, allow the victim to sleep, but wake the person every 2 to 3 hours to check level of responsiveness. 2. If no symptoms appear 8 hours after injury, wake once during the first night.
Bruising or Hemorrhage • Lucid interval • Severe, progressive headache • Repeated vomiting • Altered behavior or loss of responsiveness	1. Protect and maintain the airway. 2. Maintain a stable body temperature. 3. Treat as though unresponsive. 4. Evacuate immediately.
Severe Diffuse Brain Injury • Deeply unconscious from the time of injury • Obstructed airway or impaired breathing	1. Clear and maintain the airway. 2. Assume spinal cord injuries. 3. Apply a neck collar. 4. Repeat examination periodically to determine progress. 5. Move the victim to shelter and safety. 6. Evacuate quickly.
Skull Fractures • Depressed area in skull • Broken bone edges in a scalp wound • Clear or blood-tinged fluid dripping from the nose or ear	1. Control bleeding with pressure around the wound edge on undamaged skull using a doughnut dressing so there is no pressure on the fracture. 2. Cover open wounds with sterile dressings. 3. Evacuate.

What to Look For

What to Do

Other Neurologic Problems

What to Look For	What to Do
Stroke • Altered responsiveness • Numbness, weakness, or paralysis of face, arm, or leg • Turning of the head and eyes to one side • Noisy breathing, drooling • Visual changes • Loss of balance or coordination • Difficulty speaking or inability to understand simple statements • Sudden, very severe, unexplained, long-lasting headache • Seizures • A history of diabetes, hypertension, heart disease, or previous strokes	1. Keep victim in the recovery position. 2. If victim is awake, allow the person to find a comfortable position. 3. Offer clear liquids with caution. 4. Evacuate.
Seizures • Momentary lack of awareness • Involuntary movement of a limb • Sensation of numbness or tingling • Abnormal vision • Sudden spasm of body muscles	1. Concentrate on preventing injury. 2. Don't restrain the victim. 3. After the seizure, make sure the airway is open. 4. Evacuate if necessary.
Simple Fainting • Reports of "seeing spots," feeling dizzy, hot or cold, and nauseated • Paleness, with cold, clammy skin • Passing out, and slumping or falling down	1. Check breathing. 2. Lay the victim flat. 3. Loosen tight clothing. 4. Check for injuries caused by the fall. 5. Place a cool, wet cloth on forehead. 6. Keep the person lying down. 7. Evacuate if necessary.

What to Look For	What to Do
Headache • Head trauma • Tenderness over the scalp, neck, and shoulders • Pupils unequal in size • Complaints of double vision • Fever • Severe neck stiffness • Impaired sensation or movement of the extremities • Impaired balance	1. If headache is mild to moderate, give nonprescription pain medication. 2. Encourage adequate hydration. 3. If acute mountain sickness is a possibility, descend to an altitude below that at which the headache started (at least 2,000 feet lower). Do not go higher! 4. If the cause appears serious, evacuate.

12 Abdominal Emergencies

Abdominal problems are difficult to diagnose even in a hospital, and a first aid provider should not be expected to distinguish among the many causes of abdominal pain; usually, first aid will be similar regardless of the cause. For wilderness first aid, it is most useful to consider abdominal problems according to the few common symptoms they cause rather than offer a diagnosis. A few common specific problems are discussed. The major decision in the wilderness is when to evacuate the victim.

Anatomy of the Abdomen

The abdomen is bordered by the diaphragm above and the bony pelvis below. The diaphragm is the sheet of muscle that separates the chest from the abdomen. Within the cavity of the abdomen are the liver, the kidneys, the spleen, the stomach, and the small and large intestines. The intestines are enclosed in a membrane, the peritoneum, and are surrounded by the peritoneal space or cavity in which blood or other fluids can collect. The aorta and inferior vena cava, the two largest blood vessels in the body, run along the back wall of the abdomen against the vertebral column.

When communicating to potential rescuers or considering certain problems, divide the abdomen into four quadrants. Pain localized in one of these areas might indicate a particular problem. For example, pain or soreness with pressure in the right upper quadrant might be caused by a liver injury or infection (hepatitis) or the gallbladder blocked by a stone. Pain in the right lower quadrant might be from appendicitis, an ovarian or pregnancy problem, kidney stone, or hernia on that side; left lower quadrant pain might be from a problem in the bowel, ovary, kidney stone, or hernia on that side. Left upper quadrant pain might be from an injury to the spleen, stomach, or pancreas **Figure 12-1A-B** .

Pain in both front and back often points to one of the organs in the posterior abdomen. When it is on one side, the problem might be in the kidney (infection or stone), gallbladder (on the right), or a major blood vessel. When in the midline, it might be from the pancreas, stomach, aorta, or uterus. Injuries to intra-abdominal organs can be categorized as closed (resulting from falls and blows) or open (resulting from penetration by items such as a knife, stick, rock, or bullet). Illnesses include diarrhea diseases (such as gastroenteritis), bleeding, and appendicitis.

Abdominal Injuries

Serious injury to the abdomen, whether blunt, without a break in the skin (closed), or with penetration of the peritoneal cavity (open), can cause internal bleeding or leakage of intestinal contents that result in irritation and infection (peritonitis) within the peritoneal cavity. Surgery is the treatment for most serious internal abdominal injuries. Look for an associated abdominal injury with injuries of the lower chest.

▶ Closed Injuries

Any abdominal organ can be injured by a direct blow. Higher-energy injuries are more likely to damage organs, but some organs can be damaged by lower-energy injuries such as a punch or sports collision. Solid-organ injuries usually result in significant bleeding. Hollow-organ injuries are more likely to cause peritonitis.

A blow to the left upper abdomen or fractured lower left ribs can rupture the spleen. Consider splenic rupture after a lower left chest injury. Shock, due to progressive severe bleeding, develops after rupture. Silent, symptomless bleeding can continue within the spleen for up to 3 weeks after an injury. The spleen can then suddenly burst. This delayed rupture of the spleen can cause severe bleeding and shock.

Injuries to the kidneys can be caused by a direct blow to the back or flank, possibly with a fracture of the lowest rib.

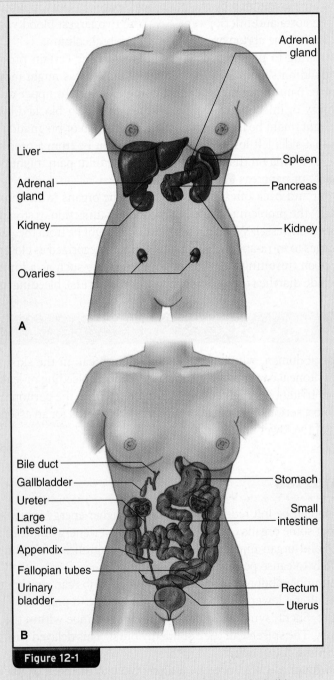

Figure 12-1

The solid and hollow organs of the abdomen. **A.** Solid organs include the liver, spleen, pancreas, kidneys, and (in women) ovaries. **B.** Hollow organs include the gallbladder, stomach, small intestine, large intestine, and bladder.

What to Look For

- Mechanism of injury.
- Bruising or abrasions of the abdominal wall or lower chest.
- Abdominal pain and tenderness of varying severity. If the pain and tenderness are severe, the injured person lies quite still. Pain usually starts around the navel, and then spreads to the region of the injured organ. If blood or intestinal contents are in the abdominal cavity, pain might be felt in one or both shoulders.

Possible Spleen Injury

- Signs of shock.
- Pain in the left upper abdomen.

Possible Kidney Injury

- Pain in the flank, sometimes radiating into the groin.
- Blood in the urine.
- Signs of shock.

> **PEDIATRIC NOTE**
>
> The abdominal contents are less well protected in a child than in an adult. The rib cage does not cover the liver or spleen, and the pelvis is relatively shallow, allowing greater exposure to injury.

- A combination of an enlarged tight abdomen, increasing pain and tenderness, fever, and nausea and vomiting. These are highly suspicious signs of peritonitis, caused either by injury or by illness. The abdomen becomes more rigid as peritonitis spreads; movement, coughing, and tapping or pressing on the abdomen causes pain.

What to Do

1. Have the victim rest completely and allow only sips of water by mouth.
2. Record written observations frequently, especially the pulse rate and changes in general condition.
3. Evacuate if any signs of shock or peritonitis appear.

▶ Open Injuries

An abdominal injury is open if there is more than a superficial injury to the skin, with or without obvious penetration of the peritoneal cavity. A small puncture wound can be as dangerous as an obvious gash. A long, sharp object that punctures the skin can be withdrawn, but the bowel may have been punctured, allowing leakage of intestinal contents and causing peritonitis.

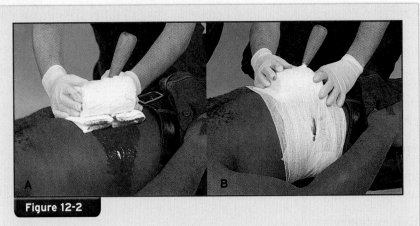

Figure 12-2

Stabilizing a penetrating wound. **A.** Stabilize a penetrating object with bulky padding. **B.** Secure padding and object.

What to Look For

- Protruding bowel or fat.
- External bleeding from a laceration of the abdominal wall.
- Signs similar to a closed injury, as listed above.

What to Do

If the object that caused the injury is still in the wound, and if medical help is close by, leave the object there—as taught in urban first aid **Figure 12-2A-B**. If the object has penetrated one of the large blood vessels but is blocking the escape of blood, severe bleeding might occur with removal. If it is not possible to evacuate the victim without removing a penetrating object, and medical care is not available, it may be necessary to remove the object. The rescuer must realize that removal may lead to severe, rapid bleeding and death. Whenever possible, stabilize the object in place. Consider shortening a large object that is preventing evacuation, but carefully stabilize it prior to cutting, to prevent further damage.

1. Treat as for closed injuries.
2. If bowel is protruding **Figure 12-3** and has not been torn, two options are available. If help is far away, try to return the bowel gently to the abdominal cavity; then dress the wound. If help is close at hand, cover the bowel with a moist (preferably sterile) cloth. Keep the wound moist during transportation.
3. If the bowel has been torn, it must not be returned to the abdominal cavity. Cover it and keep it moist.

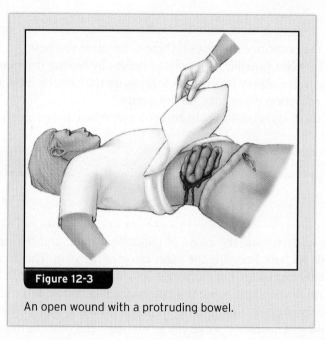

Figure 12-3

An open wound with a protruding bowel.

▶ Hernia

Hernias occur when loops of intestines protrude through a weak spot in the abdominal wall, but not through the skin. This condition is more common in men than in women, and the most common site is the groin. Other possible sites are the navel and old surgical scars. Hernias may appear suddenly or enlarge gradually. They rarely require urgent surgery, and most hernias will easily slide back inside with relaxation and gentle pressure. Occasionally a hernia is trapped and the blood supply to the protruding loop of intestine is cut off (strangulated hernia). This requires emergency medical care.

What to Look For

Unstrangulated Hernia

- Bulging in the groin, sometimes extending into the scrotum; easier to see when the victim is straining or coughing; and disappears (reduces) if the victim lies on his or her back and relaxes the abdomen.
- Swelling, usually soft and painless.
- Soreness, burning, or feeling of pressure (variable).

Strangulated Hernia

- Hernia that will not reduce.
- Firm bulge with rapidly increasing pain, tenderness.
- Pain spreading to the abdomen; possible vomiting.

What to Do

1. The victim may continue activities if there is minimal soreness.
2. Attempt to reduce a possible strangulated hernia by having the victim lie on his or her back and relax. Apply steady, gentle pressure to push the hernia back through its opening. If reduction is not easy, do not persist.
3. Evacuate if there is increasing pain and you are unable to reduce the hernia.

Abdominal Illnesses

▶ Pain

It often is difficult to determine the cause of abdominal pain, and the decision to evacuate usually can be made without knowing the exact cause of the pain. The decision to evacuate is sometimes immediately apparent, but you might have to observe the victim for several hours to determine the course of the illness. (See the criteria for evacuation at the end of this chapter.) The difficulty in obtaining help, the number of people in the group (and whether the injured person can be left alone, if necessary, while you go for help), and other factors affect this decision.

What to Look For (All Causes)

- Signs of shock, which could be caused by internal bleeding or infection.
- A SAMPLE history.
- The location of the pain. The cause of the pain can be in the organ underlying the site.
- Pain that is decreasing, increasing, or staying the same.
- Associated diarrhea or vomiting.
- Signs of dehydration—dry tongue, rapid pulse, and dizziness on standing, especially if there has been repeated vomiting and/or diarrhea.
- Others in the party who have the same problem.
- Ingestion of potentially poisonous wild plants or unpurified water.
- Associated conditions such as diabetes or pregnancy.
- A painful, rigid, or abnormally swollen abdomen.

What to Do

1. Make an initial check and assess vital signs.
2. Allow slow sipping of clear fluids, including water, diluted juice, sports drinks, soup broth, and herbal tea. Avoid alcohol- or caffeine-containing drinks. (See the appendix *Fluid and Electrolyte Replacement* for fluid and electrolyte replacement guidelines.)
3. Give the victim an antacid.

4. Apply heat, such as a canteen filled with warm water, to the abdomen.
5. Be prepared for vomiting.
6. Allow the victim to assume the most comfortable position, which is often lying with bent knees.

▶ Appendicitis

The appendix is a small tube attached to the large intestine. It can become infected and can rupture, causing peritonitis.

> **CAUTION**
>
> **DO NOT**
> - Give the victim an enema or laxative. These can worsen the condition or cause complications.
> - Give the victim nonclear fluids to drink as long as the pain continues.
> - Give the victim solid foods.
> - Give the victim milk products.

What to Look For

- Intermittent pain that begins in the midabdomen, then moves to the lower right abdomen. The pain increases over 6 to 24 hours, becomes constant, and is accentuated by movement or cough, causing the victim to lie still with the knees drawn up.
- Tenderness to pressure or touch over the lower right abdomen.
- Intermittent vomiting.
- Loss of appetite.
- Low-grade fever.
- Later, pain and tenderness are felt throughout the abdomen, indicating a ruptured appendix, which will spread infection throughout the abdominal cavity (peritonitis). Victims with peritonitis are usually very ill and in severe pain.

What to Do

1. Place the victim in the most comfortable reclining position.
2. Give the victim sips of fluid to avoid dehydration, but do not give food.
3. Evacuate the victim.

▶ Nausea and Vomiting

Nausea and vomiting can occur with many conditions, such as mild altitude sickness, motion sickness, head injury, intestinal viruses, food poisoning, excessive eating or drinking, carbon monoxide poisoning, or emotional stress. In minor illnesses, this should improve within a couple of days. Persistent or increasing nausea and vomiting can signal more serious illnesses, such as appendicitis or bowel obstruction. If the condition lasts longer than 1 or 2 days, serious dehydration can develop, especially in young children and the elderly.

What to Look For

- Abdominal pain.
- Blood or brown, grainy material (which looks like coffee grounds) in the vomit; this could be blood from the stomach.
- Diarrhea. Vomiting and diarrhea together are often a self-limited viral infection.
- Chills and fever.
- Signs of dehydration (dizziness when standing, dry mouth and tongue, cracked lips, concentrated urine, thirst, and rapid pulse).
- Others in the group with similar symptoms (this suggests food poisoning or an infectious cause).
- A recent head injury.
- Ingestion of wild plants/mushrooms or unpurified water.

What to Do

1. Give the victim small amounts of clear fluids, such as sports drinks, clear soups, flat soda, apple juice, or cranberry juice.
2. If the victim is able to keep fluids down, offer carbohydrates (starches, bread, cereal, and pasta); these are the easiest foods to digest. Avoid any milk products or meat for 48 hours.
3. Have the victim rest; avoid exertion until he or she is able to eat solid foods easily.
4. Evacuate if vomiting persists beyond 48 hours or is bloody.

▶ Diarrhea

Diarrhea is the frequent passage of loose, watery, or unformed stools. Common causes are intestinal infections (bacterial, viral, or parasitic), food poisoning, food sensitivity/allergy, and stress. A common wilderness source of infection is unpurified drinking water. Even small amounts of crystal clear water may have severe contamination. Dehydration occurs if the victim cannot drink enough fluid to replace the losses from diarrhea. The elderly and the very young are especially prone to dehydration. Replacement of fluids and electrolytes (sodium and potassium) is of primary importance in any diarrhea victim.

What to Look For

- Bloody mucus or pus in the stool
- Signs of dehydration
- Cramping abdominal pain, usually in the lower abdomen
- Lack of bowel control
- Fever
- Others in the group with similar symptoms

What to Do

1. Have the victim drink enough clear fluids to replace losses plus the usual intake. Watch urine output to gauge adequacy of fluid intake. Scant, dark urine indicates dehydration.
2. When clear fluids are tolerated, have the victim return gradually to a normal diet. Initially, try crackers, soup, toast, rice, pasta, and applesauce.
3. If it is available, give the victim pink bismuth (adult dose: 2 tablets 4 times per day for 1 or 2 days or 2 tablespoons every half hour for 8 doses).
4. Give the victim loperamide HCL (capsule or liquid, 2–4 mg initially, then 1–2 mg 4 times a day if diarrhea persists) or diphenoxylate atropine (which is a prescription drug). Do not use if there is fever and diarrhea with blood or pus in the stools.

Avoid

- Milk products or meat for 48 hours after diarrhea stops, because there might be intolerance to fat or lactose after infections.
- Caffeine, because it stimulates the intestine and increases urination and dehydration.

▶ Constipation

Minor changes in diet, fluid intake, activity, and emotional state can cause constipation. Changing these will relieve constipation in most cases.

What to Look For

- Painful, hard bowel movements.
- Bowel movements less often than every 1–2 days.

What to Do

1. Increase intake of high-fiber foods, such as whole grains and fruits.
2. Maintain adequate fluid intake (urine should be pale yellow if enough water is being consumed).
3. Try to have a bowel movement each day.
4. Use a stool softener such as mineral oil or Colace.
5. Avoid:
   - Strong laxatives
   - Alcohol
   - Foods that cause constipation, such as bananas, cheese, meat, and sugary foods.

▶ Bloody Stools and Hemorrhoids

Small amounts of bright-red blood on the stool and toilet paper or in the toilet water is alarming but is usually not serious. More serious bleeding from growths farther inside the rectum is usually darker in color. There are two common causes of bloody stools: hemorrhoids (piles) and fissures. Hemorrhoids are inflamed, swollen veins, and fissures are cracks in the skin around the anus. Both may be caused by constipation with hard, dry stools that require straining to evacuate. Constipation and these resulting problems are common at high altitudes or in other environments where it might be impossible to drink enough fluids and eat enough fruit, vegetables, and fiber. Hemorrhoids also can occur with frequent diarrhea. Hemorrhoids and fissures can resolve by themselves, but they commonly recur.

What to Look For

External Hemorrhoid

- A firm, painful, pink or bluish lump next to the anus present for several days.
- Bleeding with passage of stool.
- Bright red blood and small dark clots possibly extruding from the swelling. With bleeding, the pain and swelling decrease. The discomfort of external hemorrhoids resolves naturally in about 1 week, with or without bleeding.

Internal Hemorrhoid

- Soft swelling, often painless, that is frequently protruding from the rectum during or after a bowel movement; might be invisible.
- Bleeding with passage of stool.

Fissure

- A fissure is a painful crack in the skin at the margin of the anus.

Signs of Serious Bowel Bleeding

- Painless bowel movements with large quantities of red, maroon, or brownish blood (there might be some abdominal cramping).
- Signs of shock from blood loss.

What to Do

For minor hemorrhoids and fissures with bleeding:

1. Adjust the victim's diet to soften stool by increasing fluids, fruits, vegetables, and whole grains.
2. Give the victim warm baths to soothe and cleanse.
3. Have the victim wear cotton underwear and loose clothing.

4. Apply cold compresses, zinc oxide, or petroleum jelly to control irritation.
5. Apply hemorrhoid suppositories to help relieve pain.
6. If a grapelike cluster or large swelling protrudes from the rectum, have the victim get on the knees and elbows with the buttocks higher than the head, and apply gentle steady manual pressure to the protruding tissue until it slips back inside. The person should remain in this position or lie on the side for about 30 to 60 minutes.

For major bleeding:

1. Have the victim walk if he or she is not dizzy or weak.
2. Evacuate the victim.

Evacuation Guidelines for Abdominal Problems

Evacuate the victim to medical care if:

- The victim has sustained a serious injury.
- There is persistent abdominal pain for more than 8 hours.
- The victim is unable to drink or retain fluids for more than 24 hours.
- The victim is a pregnant woman with abdominal pain.
- The abdomen is rigid or swollen and painful.
- The abdominal pain increases with cough or movement.
- The victim has persistent pain that begins around the navel and later moves to the lower right abdomen (appendicitis).
- The victim has abdominal pain with high fever.
- There is vomiting or diarrhea with severe pain.
- There is vomiting with severe headache (and no history of migraine or a recent head injury).
- There are signs of internal bleeding, such as the stool or vomit is bloody; the stool appears black and tarry (pink bismuth may harmlessly turn stools black); or vomitus appears brown and grainy, like coffee grounds.
- The victim has diarrhea with fever and stools containing bloody mucus.
- There are signs of severe dehydration or shock, including fainting or extreme light-headedness when trying to stand, rapid pulse, or altered mental status.

▶ Emergency Care Wrap-up

What to Look For	What to Do
Abdominal Injuries	
Closed Injury • Mechanism of injury • Bruising or abrasions of the abdominal wall or lower chest • Abdominal pain and tenderness • Signs of shock • Nausea and vomiting • External bleeding	1. Have the victim rest. 2. Evacuate if any signs of shock or peritonitis appear.
Open Injury • A small puncture wound • Obvious gash • A long, sharp object that punctures the skin • Protruding bowel or fat	1. If the object is still in the wound, leave it there. 2. Treat as for closed injuries. 3. If bowel is protruding and has not been torn, try to return the bowel gently to the abdominal cavity, or cover the bowel with a moist cloth. 4. If the bowel has been torn, cover it and keep it moist.
Unstrangulated Hernia • Bulging in the groin • Swelling • Soreness	1. The victim may continue activities if there is minimal soreness. 2. Evacuate if there is increasing pain and you are unable to reduce the hernia.
Strangulated Hernia • Hernia that will not reduce • Firm bulge with rapidly increasing pain • Tenderness • Vomiting is possible	1. Have the victim lie on the back and relax. 2. Apply steady, gentle pressure to push the hernia back through its opening. 3. Evacuate if there is increasing pain and you are unable to reduce the hernia.

What to Look For	What to Do
Abdominal Illnesses	
Pain • Signs of shock • A SAMPLE history • Diarrhea or vomiting • Diabetes or pregnancy • Rigid or swollen abdomen	1. Make an initial check and assess vital signs. 2. Allow slow sipping of clear fluids. 3. Give an antacid. 4. Apply heat to the abdomen. 5. Be prepared for vomiting. 6. Allow victim to assume the most comfortable position.
Appendicitis • Intermittent pain • Tenderness • Intermittent vomiting • Diarrhea • Loss of appetite • Low-grade fever	1. Place the victim in the most comfortable reclining position. 2. Give sips of fluid to avoid dehydration. 3. Evacuate.
Nausea and Vomiting • Abdominal pain • Blood or brown, grainy material in the vomit • Chills and fever • Signs of dehydration • Others in the group with similar symptoms • Recent head injury • Ingestion of wild plants/mushrooms or unpurified water	1. Give small amounts of clear fluids. 2. If victim is able to keep fluids down, offer carbohydrates. 3. Have the victim rest.
Diarrhea • Bloody mucus or pus in the stool • Signs of dehydration • Cramping abdominal pain • Lack of bowel control • Fever • Others in the group with similar symptoms	1. Have the victim drink clear fluids. 2. When clear fluids are tolerated, have the victim return gradually to a normal diet. 3. If available, give pink bismuth. 4. Give loperamide hydrochloride.

What to Look For	What to Do
Constipation	1. Increase intake of high-fiber foods. 2. Maintain adequate fluid intake. 3. Use a stool softener such as mineral oil or Colace. 4. Avoid strong laxatives, alcohol, and binding foods.
Bloody Stools and Hemorrhoids • A firm, painful lump next to the anus • Bleeding with the passage of stool	1. Adjust diet to soften stool. 2. Give the victim warm baths. 3. Have the victim wear cotton underwear and loose clothing. 4. Apply hemorrhoid medications.
Serious Bowel Bleeding • Painless bowel movements with large quantities of blood • Signs of shock	1. Have victim walk if he or she is not dizzy or weak. 2. Evacuate the victim.

Diabetic Emergencies and Allergic Reactions

Diabetic Emergencies

Normally, the body can effectively maintain a constant and proper supply of glucose in the blood. When the body can no longer regulate the blood-sugar level effectively and too much glucose is present in the blood, the person is said to have diabetes mellitus, or simply "diabetes."

Diabetes occurs when either: (1) insulin is not produced, (2) not enough insulin is produced, or (3) the body has become resistant to insulin. When a person eats a meal, glucose is absorbed from the small intestine into the bloodstream. The pancreas secretes insulin, which transports glucose molecules out of the bloodstream and into the cells. This provides the cells with the energy they need to function properly. If not enough insulin is present, glucose cannot enter cells, so it accumulates in the bloodstream and raises blood sugar levels.

▶ Diabetes

There are two types of diabetes:

1. *Type 1:* This formerly was known as insulin-dependent diabetes. With this condition, the person with diabetes does not have enough insulin to transfer glucose into the cells. It usually affects children and young adults and is treated with insulin that is usually self-administered via injection.

2. *Type 2:* This was formerly known as non-insulin dependent diabetes and it is the most common form of diabetes. Once thought to affect only older individuals, it is increasingly being diagnosed in children, especially those who are obese. With type 2 diabetes, the body's cells resist insulin, which prevents glucose from entering the cells. Initially, most individuals with type 2 diabetes do not require insulin injections and treatment includes through exercise, weight loss programs, and medications to lower blood-glucose levels. Later, low doses of insulin may be needed to regulate blood glucose.

Managing Diabetes in the Wilderness

All people with diabetes need to eat on a regular schedule and plan the timing and amount of exercise, because physical exertion acts like insulin. An individual with diabetes who plans to exercise vigorously needs to take less diabetic-control medicine or eat more in order to avoid serious drops in blood sugar. If a person's blood sugar level remains abnormal for long, a wilderness emergency will occur. Good diabetes management requires frequent measurement of blood-glucose levels with a chemically treated paper strip or a blood-glucose meter (an electronic device that analyzes blood sugar).

Before starting on a wilderness trip, individuals should inform the wilderness group leader that they have diabetes, discuss the planned trip with their physician, and carry adequate supplies of necessary medicines and other equipment (ie, insulin, syringes, needles, pills, etc.), including extra supplies for emergencies **Table 13-1**. An injectable medication called glucagon can raise blood sugar in an emergency. Another group member might agree to help carry these extra supplies. Individuals with diabetes should also carry extra food and snacks, so that they do not have to rely on others in the group if food is needed quickly.

Table 13-1 **Diabetic Supplies**
• Insulin or diabetes control pills
• Syringes, needles, alcohol wipes
• Equipment to measure blood sugar
• Oral glucose tablets, candy bars, and/or plastic bottles of thick oral glucose solution
• Injectable medicine to raise low blood sugar (glucagon)

If you are a trip leader and a member of your group has diabetes, refresh your memory regarding diabetes identification and first aid, see that at least one other group member is also familiar with these, and, ideally, if the person takes insulin, ensure that at least one additional group member knows how to give injections.

Insulin and glucagon should be protected from the cold (in an inside pocket in cold weather) or heat (in a closed vacuum bottle or buried in the pack). Also, remember that insulin will not work in hypothermic victims if the body temperature is below 30°C (88°F).

▶ Acute Complications of Diabetes

Hypoglycemia (Blood Sugar Too Low)

The condition of low blood glucose is called hypoglycemia. Hypoglycemia is the most dangerous of the acute complications of diabetes. Low blood sugar can rapidly result in unconsciousness brain damage and death. Hypoglycemia is caused when the person with diabetes does any one of the following:

- Takes too much insulin (rapidly depletes sugar)
- Does not eat (reduces sugar intake)
- Over-exerts or exercises (uses sugar faster)
- Vomits (empties stomach of sugar)

Most people with diabetes monitor their blood-glucose levels as often as four times a day to maintain the proper levels and to prevent a diabetic emergency **Figure 13-1** .

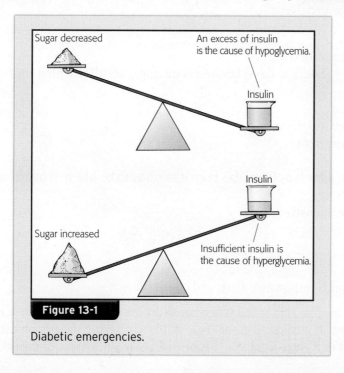

Figure 13-1

Diabetic emergencies.

Hyperglycemia (Blood Sugar Too High)

The opposite reaction of hypoglycemia is hyperglycemia. This condition occurs when a person with diabetes has too much glucose in his or her blood. Several scenarios can cause this medical condition (ie, insufficient insulin, overeating, illness, inactivity, stress, or a combination of these factors). Hyperglycemia can also cause loss of consciousness but it is a slower process than with hypoglycemia, and is not as immediately dangerous. However, untreated, hyperglycemia can eventually lead to death.

Hyperglycemia in remote locations is rarely encountered unless a person is stranded and has either lost or run out of diabetes medication. Those who do not know they have diabetes commonly show the signs of hyperglycemia.

What to Look For

Hypoglycemia

- Medical identification tag
- Sudden onset (minutes to an hour) because no sugar is reaching the brain
- Staggering, poor coordination, clumsiness
- Anger, bad temper
- Cold, pale, moist, or "clammy" skin
- Confusion, disorientation
- Sudden hunger
- Excessive sweating
- Trembling, shakiness
- Seizure (no sugar reaching the brain)
- Eventual unresponsiveness

Hyperglycemia

- Medical identification tag
- Gradual onset (hours to days) because some sugar is still reaching the brain
- Drowsiness
- Extreme thirst
- Very frequent urination
- Warm, red, dry skin
- Vomiting
- Fruity breath odor (has been also been described to be like nail polish remover)
- Heavy breathing
- Eventual unresponsiveness

What to Do

Hypoglycemia

If the affected person is responsive, alert, and can swallow:

1. The person may be able to tell you what to do. He or she should check his or her blood glucose. If it is low, use the "rule of 15s" by having the person eat 15 grams of sugar (i.e., 3 to 5 glucose tablets, 1 tube of glucose gel, 2 tbsp. of raisins, or 4 oz. of

orange or apple juice). If the person is not able to test his or her blood glucose, and you strongly suspect that the person has low blood glucose, give him or her 15 grams of fast-acting sugar.

2. Wait 15 minutes for the sugar to get into the blood.
3. If the affected person is able, check the blood glucose level again. If it is still low, the person should consume 15 more grams of sugar. If testing is not available, and there is no improvement in 15 minutes after the first eating of 15 grams of sugar, give the person 15 more grams of sugar.
4. If there is no improvement, seek immediate medical care. Hypoglycemia can be a life-threatening emergency.

If the individual is unresponsive:

1. Place the person onto his or her side.
2. If it is available, give glucagon. When in remote locations, a person with diabetes should be carrying glucagon, which raises blood glucose quickly. Glucagon requires a physician's prescription and comes in a kit containing powdered glucagon that is mixed with a solution and drawn up into a syringe. It is injected into the buttocks or thigh. Glucagon works the opposite of insulin. It mobilizes glucose stored in the muscles and liver as glycogen. Be aware that many people vomit after receiving glucagon. Family members, a friend, and group leaders should learn when and how to inject glucagon in a hypoglycemic emergency.
3. Place glucose gel or a paste made of water and sugar between a cheek and the gum, where it may be swallowed reflexively, or rub sugar into the victim's gums where some may be absorbed into the blood. These procedures may take some time so do not give up too quickly.
4. If there is no improvement, seek immediate medical care. Hypoglycemia can be a life-threatening emergency.

All diabetic emergencies should seek medical care following the emergency.

Hyperglycemia

Most persons with diabetes can recognize what is happening and will adjust their insulin dose or seek medical care before serious problems develop.

1. Give frequent, small sips of water if the person can swallow.
2. If uncertain whether the individual has a high or low blood glucose level, and the person is responsive and able to swallow, use the "rule of 15s" for giving sugar described above. "Sugar (glucose) for everyone" is the rule of thumb for all diabetic emergencies—hyper- or hypoglycemia—so you don't really need to distinguish between them. The extra sugar will not cause any significant harm in an individual experiencing hyperglycemia if the person can be evacuated for immediate medical care.
3. Do not give insulin unless the person can self-administer.
4. Seek immediate medical care.

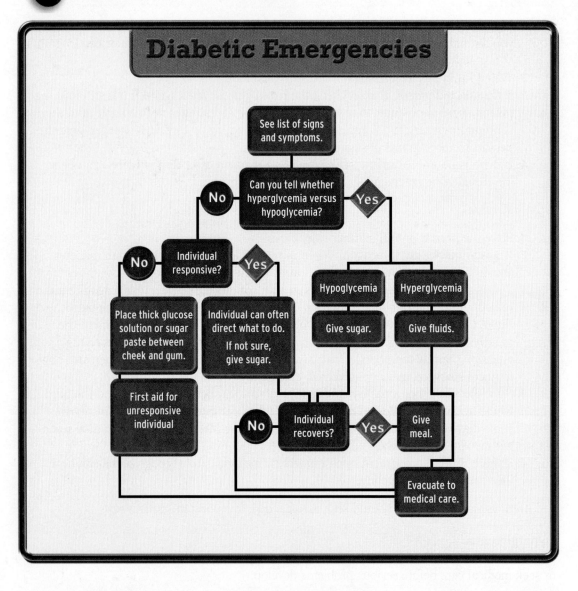

Diabetic Emergencies

See list of signs and symptoms.

Can you tell whether hyperglycemia versus hypoglycemia?
- No
- Yes

No path:

Individual responsive?
- No
- Yes

No: Place thick glucose solution or sugar paste between cheek and gum. → First aid for unresponsive individual

Yes: Individual can often direct what to do. If not sure, give sugar.

Yes path:

Hypoglycemia → Give sugar.

Hyperglycemia → Give fluids.

Individual recovers?
- No
- Yes

Yes: Give meal.

No: Evacuate to medical care.

Allergic Reactions

Allergic reactions can be mild and recurrent (for example, hay fever, hives, and mild asthma) or sudden and severe (such as allergic swelling and severe asthmatic attacks). The most serious type is anaphylactic shock, an immediate and overwhelming allergic reaction seen in people who are extremely sensitive to insect stings, drugs, or foods.

Unlike milder allergic reactions such as hay fever, anaphylactic shock is a massive allergic reaction that overwhelms the body's systems with potentially fatal results. The majority of anaphylactic deaths result from the inability to breathe because of swollen air passages. The next most common cause of death is from shock resulting from the collapse of the circulatory system. Wilderness first aid providers must attend to these crises as quickly as possible.

▶ Severe Allergic Reactions (Anaphylactic Shock)

What to Look For

While eating, after taking medicine, or after being stung by an insect, the victim suddenly (or, rarely, within hours) develops some or all of the following symptoms or signs:

- Severe itching or hives
- Sneezing, coughing, or wheezing
- Shortness of breath
- Tightness and swelling of the throat
- Tightness in the chest
- Dramatic swelling of the face, tongue, and/or mouth
- Vomiting, cramps, or diarrhea
- Convulsions or loss of responsiveness

What to Do

1. Act quickly. Every second counts.
2. Immediately check breathing and give the victim CPR if needed.
3. Injected epinephrine can be a life-saving procedure **Figure 13-2**. It opens the airway, raises blood pressure, and relieves swelling. If the victim has physician-prescribed epinephrine, ask if you can help the victim self-administer it. If the victim is unable to do so and state law permits it, inject the epinephrine by following the directions on the epinephrine kit.
4. If you don't have epinephrine:
   - Use an asthma inhaler.
   - If the victim can swallow, give a dose of an antihistamine or nasal decongestant medication.
5. Give the victim first aid for unresponsiveness and/or seizures as necessary.
6. Allow a conscious victim to assume a comfortable position. Sitting up usually makes breathing easier; place an unresponsive victim in the recovery position.
7. After the victim improves, give 25–50 mg of antihistamine (diphenhydramine [Benedryl]; one to two of the over-the-counter capsules) every 3 hours for 24 hours (or longer if hives or other symptoms recur after stopping the antihistamine).
8. If there is no improvement, evacuate the victim rapidly.

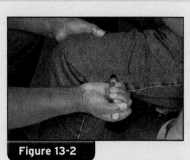

Figure 13-2

The only lifesaving treatment for anaphylactic shock is epinephrine.

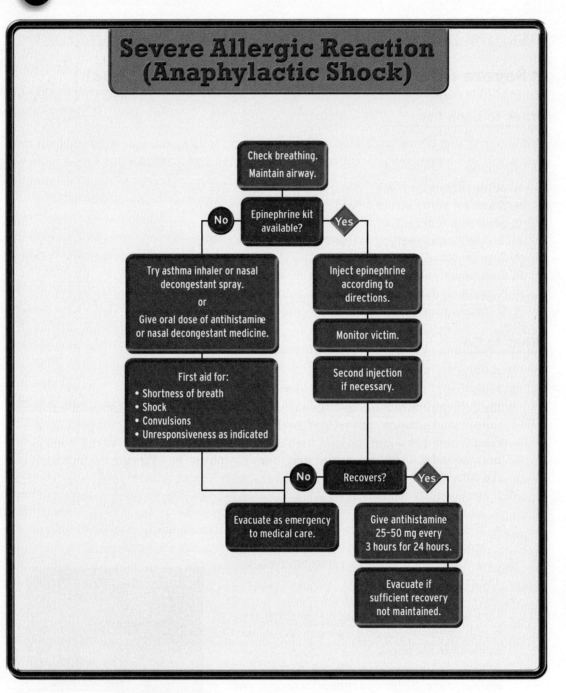

Severe Allergic Reaction (Anaphylactic Shock)

Check breathing. Maintain airway.

Epinephrine kit available?

No →

Try asthma inhaler or nasal decongestant spray.
or
Give oral dose of antihistamine or nasal decongestant medicine.

First aid for:
• Shortness of breath
• Shock
• Convulsions
• Unresponsiveness as indicated

Yes →

Inject epinephrine according to directions.

Monitor victim.

Second injection if necessary.

Recovers?

No → Evacuate as emergency to medical care.

Yes → Give antihistamine 25–50 mg every 3 hours for 24 hours.

Evacuate if sufficient recovery not maintained.

▶ Allergic Rhinitis

Allergic rhinitis affects the nose, sinuses, and eyes. There are two main types: hay fever, due to windborne pollen and occurring only at certain seasons of the year; and perennial rhinitis, due to substances present year round, such as house dust, mites, feathers, animal dander, or molds.

What to Look For

- Itching of the nose, the roof of the mouth, the throat, and the eyes
- Stuffy, runny nose; runny eyes
- Sneezing

What to Do

1. Avoid the cause, if known and if possible.
2. Give the victim oral antihistamines or antihistamine/decongestant combinations (nonprescription or prescription). The main drawbacks are drowsiness and a tendency to raise the blood pressure.

▶ Hives

Hives can result from an allergy to a drug, insect sting or bite, or food (particularly eggs, nuts, fruit, or shellfish). They occasionally occur during a viral infection.

What to Look For

- Pink, blotchy, itchy bumps on the skin (wheals) that range in size from less than ½" to several inches in diameter and that might be localized or cover the entire body.
- Occasional massive, itchy swelling of a lip, eyelid, hand, or foot.

What to Do

1. Be prepared for anaphylactic shock; hives can precede anaphylactic shock (discussed previously). Treat accordingly.
2. Give the victim nonprescription antihistamines such as diphenhydramine as necessary. Most cases are self-limited and last only a few days to a week.

▶ Emergency Care Wrap-up

What to Look For　　　　　　　　　　**What to Do**

Diabetic Emergencies

What to Look For	What to Do
Hypoglycemia (low blood sugar) • Sudden onset • Pale, cold, clammy skin • Rapid pulse • Headache, hunger, dizziness, nervousness, weakness • Staggering, poor coordination, trembling • Personality changes: anger, bad temper • Altered mental status (confusion, disorientation, eventual coma)	1. Immediately check persons with diabetes whose behavior is unusual. 2. Look for a medical alert tag. 3. Do an initial check and care for immediate problems. 4. Determine what has happened, history of diabetes or other medical conditions, and whether the individual has been taking any medicines or shots. 5. Immediately give sugar. 6. If the person is unable to swallow, place a thick glucose solution or a paste made of water and sugar between the cheek and the gum. 7. Consider glucagon injection. 8. Evacuate those who become worse or do not recover.
Hyperglycemia (high blood sugar) • Gradual onset • Flushed, dry, warm skin • Rapid pulse • Rapid, deep respirations • Extreme thirst • Fruity odor of breath • Vomiting • Frequent urination • Altered mental status (drowsiness, confusion, eventual coma)	1. Immediately check persons with diabetes whose behavior is unusual. 2. Look for a medical alert tag. 3. Do an initial check and care for immediate problems. 4. Determine what has happened, history of diabetes or other medical conditions, and whether the individual has been taking any medicines or shots. 5. Assist the responsive person with any medications necessary. 6. Evacuate those who don't recover or who become worse.

What to Look For	What to Do
Allergic Reactions	
Anaphylactic Shock • Severe itching or hives • Sneezing, coughing, wheezing • Shortness of breath • Tightness and swelling of the throat • Tightness in the chest • Dramatic swelling of the face, tongue, and/or mouth • Vomiting, cramps, diarrhea • Convulsions, loss of responsiveness	1. Act quickly. Every second counts. 2. Immediately check breathing and give CPR if needed. 3. If epinephrine kit is available, administer it immediately according to directions.
Allergic Rhinitis • Itching of the nose, roof of mouth, throat, and eyes • Stuffy, runny nose; runny eyes • Sneezing	1. Avoid the cause, if known. 2. Give nonprescription or prescription oral antihistamines or antihistamine/decongestant combinations.
Hives • Pink, blotchy, itchy bumps on the skin that range in size • Occasional massive, itchy swelling of a lip, eyelid, hand, or foot	1. Give nonprescription antihistamines.

14 Genitourinary Problems

The term genitourinary refers to the reproductive and urinary systems. The urinary system includes the kidneys, ureters, bladder, and urethra **Figure 14-1**. The female reproductive system includes the ovaries, fallopian tubes, uterus, and vagina. The male reproductive system includes the testicles, prostate spermatic cords, and penis.

Problems of the genitourinary system are often mild but irritating; however, they can be severe and life threatening. Mild problems such as bladder infections are common in healthy, active adults, and often cause significant discomfort, especially in the wilderness, where medical care may not be available.

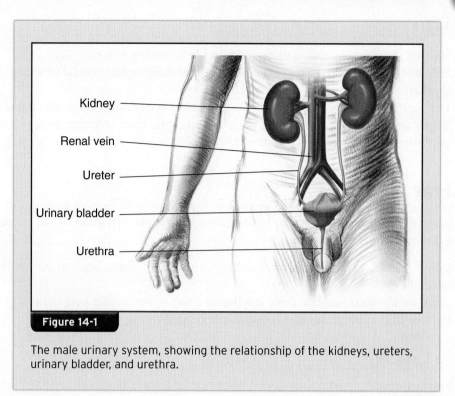

Figure 14-1

The male urinary system, showing the relationship of the kidneys, ureters, urinary bladder, and urethra.

(labels on figure: Kidney, Renal vein, Ureter, Urinary bladder, Urethra)

Problems Specific to Women

▶ Vaginitis

Vaginitis occurs when the normal balance of microbes in the vagina is altered, resulting in an irritating vaginal discharge. Common causes are infections by yeasts, bacteria, or protozoa (trichomonas). Although uncomfortable, vaginal infections are not dangerous and do not require evacuation from the wilderness.

What to Look For

- Vaginal soreness, burning, and/or itching
- Increased vaginal discharge
- Pain with urination

What to Do

1. Women should wear cotton underwear and loose-fitting pants.
2. Irrigate the vulva with clean water several times daily to remove the irritating discharge, and then dry with a towel.
3. Use vaginal antifungal medication (nonprescription clotrimazole or miconazole), which are highly effective against yeast vaginitis (the most common variety) and partially effective against trichomonas.

▶ Vulvar Irritation

The vulva is the area of external skin folds around the vagina. Irritation of the vulva, called vulvitis, has many causes, including:

- Allergic reaction or irritation from soaps, perfumes, or plants (such as poison ivy).
- Infection.
- Constant moisture, such as from leaving on a wet swim suit for long periods of time.
- Mechanical irritation, such as horseback or bicycle riding.

What to Look For

- Vulvar soreness, burning, or itching not associated with increased vaginal discharge
- Vulvar redness
- Pain with urination

What to Do

1. Avoid further contact with the irritating substance (if known).
2. Wash the vulva with clean water and mild soap; rinse generously.
3. Apply hydrocortisone cream (nonprescription) externally three times daily.

▶ Problems With Urination

Pain with urination, in the absence of vaginitis, vulvitis, and genital sores, often is caused by a urinary tract infection.

What to Look For

- Frequent, burning urination (strong urge with only small amounts of urine)
- Low abdominal pain and cramping
- Cloudy or bloody urine
- Foul-smelling urine

What to Do

1. Have the victim drink a lot of water. The victim's urine should be pale yellow.
2. Have the victim drink acidic fluids or juices (such as cranberry juice).
3. Have the victim take vitamin C to acidify the urine.
4. Have the victim avoid sexual intercourse.

Most antibiotics become concentrated in the urine and will treat these infections. Have the victim begin a 3-day course of antibiotics. If pain while urinating is accompanied by fever, flank pain, pus or blood in the urine, nausea, or vomiting, seek medical care immediately.

▶ Missed Menses

The normal menstrual cycle usually occurs about once per month. Each month, an egg is released from the ovary. If the egg is not fertilized, the lining of the uterus is shed, resulting in vaginal bleeding, called menstruation. Temporary absence of menstrual periods is not necessarily abnormal, and is more common in teenagers and women older than 40. Irregularity or absence of menstrual periods can result from stress, illness, starvation, and eating disorders such as anorexia. Heavy, regular exercise also can suppress ovulation and menstruation.

What to Look For

- A history of unprotected intercourse, breast tenderness and nausea, or morning sickness can indicate pregnancy.
- Stress.
- Heavy exercise.
- Severe weight loss; poor eating.

What to Do

1. If pregnancy is likely, see "Pregnancy and Wilderness Travel—General Considerations" later in this chapter.
2. A missed period usually requires no treatment. Consult a doctor if periods do not occur for 3 months.

▶ Heavy or Prolonged Vaginal Bleeding

Heavy or prolonged bleeding can occur after a missed period or in a woman who has irregular periods.

What to Look For

- Length of time since the woman's last period
- Recent history of unprotected sex to suggest risk of pregnancy

- Amount and duration of bleeding
- Pale skin, nails, and lips
- Weakness
- Signs and symptoms of shock

What to Do

1. Have the woman rest until bleeding decreases to a normal menstrual flow.
2. Give the victim generous amounts of fluids to drink.
3. Seek medical care if:
   - Bleeding saturates a pad every 3 hours or less over a 24-hour period.
   - The woman becomes pale and weak.

▶ Vaginal Bleeding While on Hormonal Contraceptives

Irregular, light bleeding is common in women who are on low-dose birth control pills. Erratic bleeding with birth control pills is normal. If no pills were missed, have the woman continue taking them daily as directed. If a pill was missed, give her two the next day, and make sure the woman uses condoms or abstains from sex until she has taken the rest of the pills in the pack as scheduled.

▶ Vaginal Bleeding During Pregnancy

Bleeding in a pregnancy of less than 12 weeks suggests possible miscarriage. Bleeding in a pregnancy of more than 12 weeks occurs with miscarriage, labor, and abnormalities of the placenta.

What to Look For

- Length of time since the victim's last period. If more than 4 weeks, the woman may be pregnant.
- Amount of bleeding: spotting or free-flowing.
- Low abdominal pain.
- Signs and symptoms of shock.

What to Do

If a woman is less than 12 weeks pregnant and bleeding remains light and painless, have her avoid physical exertion until the bleeding stops. She should abstain from sex until 3 weeks after the bleeding stops.

Seek medical care or evacuate if:

1. There is heavy bleeding.
2. Tissue (purple and spongy) passes vaginally.

3. There is low abdominal pain.

4. Pregnancy is longer than 12 weeks.

5. The victim becomes weak or pale, or her mental status is altered.

▶ Low Abdominal Pain

Low abdominal pain in women arises in the pelvic organs, intestines, or urinary tracts. A precise cause cannot be determined in the wilderness, so if the symptoms do not subside or if the woman is obviously sick and becoming worse, seek medical care.

▶ Pain Due to Infections

What to Look For

- Low abdominal pain
- Fever
- Nausea and vomiting
- Diarrhea

What to Do

1. When pain coincides with fever, nausea, vomiting, and diarrhea, give the victim as much fluid as tolerated.

2. If the woman has increasing or constant pain, fever, nausea, and vomiting, seek medical care. Meanwhile, maintain hydration with frequent sips of water.

▶ Pain With Internal Bleeding From Ruptured Cyst or Ectopic Pregnancy

Normally, a fertilized egg will travel down the fallopian tube to the uterus, where it attaches and develops. If the egg becomes lodged in the fallopian tube, an ectopic pregnancy results. As the ectopic pregnancy grows, it can rupture and cause severe internal bleeding. Rupture usually occurs within 6 weeks of the first missed period.

Cysts can form in the ovaries. If these rupture, abdominal pain, internal bleeding, and signs of peritonitis can result.

What to Look For

- Low or generalized abdominal pain
- Nausea
- Signs of blood loss or shock, including pale color, weakness, dizziness on standing, rapid pulse, and confusion

What to Do

1. Keep the woman lying at rest
2. Have her walk out of the area if she is capable and there is no possibility of timely help
3. If she is unable to walk, send for help and evacuate

▶ Pain Associated With Pregnancy

What to Look For

- Time since the woman's last period
- Recurring pains
- Signs of blood loss or shock

What to Do

1. If cramping is mild and not associated with bleeding, make sure the victim is well-hydrated and allow her to rest.
2. For pain with bleeding in pregnancy, follow the advice given for bleeding only.
3. If the woman is more than 5 months pregnant and she experiences cramps that last roughly 30 seconds every 15 minutes, have her drink a quart of water over 20 minutes. She may be having preterm contractions, and hydration tends to reduce them. If the contractions do not subside over the next hour, evacuate her to medical care.

Emergency Delivery

The delivery of a baby is a natural process that will occur safely and normally in most cases without interference **Figure 14-2A-D**. The mother's natural instincts usually will take over. Provide her with a clean, safe place to deliver, and give support and encouragement.

What to Look For

- Advanced pregnancy, beyond 6 months
- Regular contractions occurring every 4 minutes
- Mother feels urge to push, or to move her bowels
- Baby's head or other body part is visible

What to Do

1. Have the mother lay or squat in a clean area.
2. Mother and rescuers should wash their hands, if possible.
3. Have the mother push with contractions and rest in between.

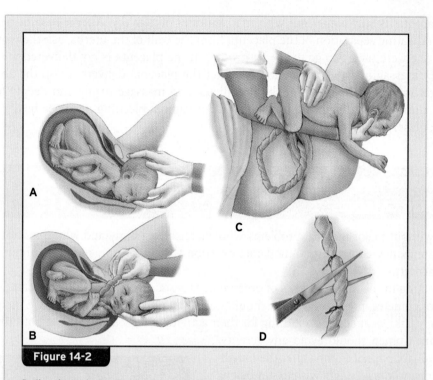

Figure 14-2

Delivering a baby. **A.** Apply gentle pressure to the baby's head to control the speed of delivery and avoid large tears of the mother's perineum. If the head is still enveloped in the sac of amniotic fluid that is bulging out, nick or tear the sac to release the fluid. **B.** If the cord is wrapped around the baby's neck, gently unloop it. **C.** Tilt the baby's head down and rub the baby dry to stimulate breathing. Pat the baby on the back if necessary to stimulate crying. Wrap the baby in clothing to keep him or her warm and place the baby on the mother's stomach. **D.** Tie the cord in two locations. Cut between the ties. After the placenta delivers, massage the lower abdomen firmly. The uterus should feel firm through the abdominal wall.

4. When baby's head starts to come out, have the mother stop pushing.
5. Apply gentle, firm pressure to the baby's head with the palm of your hand to prevent sudden expulsion of the baby. Do not try to hold the baby in.
6. If the umbilical cord is wrapped around the baby's head, unloop it.
7. If any body part besides the head comes out first, evacuate immediately.
8. After the infant is delivered, tie off the umbilical cord with a broad or flat cord, such as a shoelace, in two places. Do not use any material that can cut into the cord, such as wire.
9. Hold the baby facedown with the face lower than the body to allow drainage of fluids from the airways.
10. Dry the baby and keep him or her warm.

The placenta usually comes out within 15 minutes of delivery. After a gush of blood (½ to 1 cup), indicating separation of the placenta from the wall of the uterus, ask the woman to push (as if she were trying to go to the bathroom). If the placenta is not delivered within 30 minutes, try massaging the lower abdomen. After the placenta delivers, grasp the abdomen over the uterus at about the level of the umbilicus, and massage firmly and deeply for 1 to 2 minutes, until the uterus feels like a firm ball. If vaginal bleeding becomes heavy, repeat the uterine massage.

Pregnancy and Wilderness Travel—General Considerations

A woman without major medical problems who exercises regularly and who does not have a high-risk pregnancy can continue moderate exertion throughout pregnancy without risk to herself or her fetus.

Overheating in the first 12 weeks of pregnancy is associated with abnormal fetal development. In hot climates, pregnant women should maintain adequate hydration, pace themselves appropriately, and wear suitable clothing for their activities. They should avoid hot tubs.

Pregnant women should avoid any activity with a risk of abdominal trauma after the fourth month. Pregnant women might wish to stay below 16,000 feet because of a possible association of higher altitudes with birth defects **Figure 14-3**. They should not travel to the wilderness within 3 weeks of the due date because of the risk of labor, and they should refrain from scuba diving, as it is dangerous to the fetus.

Water treated with iodine is safe to drink for a few weeks during pregnancy. An alternative method using chlorine, filtration, or heat for disinfection must be used for a longer wilderness stay (see the appendix *Field Water Disinfection*).

A pregnant woman planning international travel must get advice from her doctor about vaccinations and medications that are contraindicated in pregnancy.

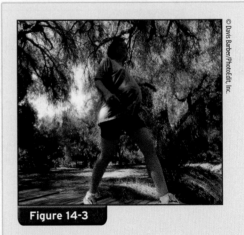

Figure 14-3

Exercise at moderate altitude is safe in pregnancy if there is no risk of trauma to the fetus.

© Davis Barber/PhotoEdit, Inc.

Problems Specific to Men

Genitourinary problems in men are rarely life threatening but are likely to be uncomfortable or worrisome enough that the victim will want to see a doctor.

▶ Problems With Urination

Painful urination or burning during urination usually indicates an infection.

What to Look For

- Frequent, painful urination with only small amounts of urine, usually indicating an infection in the bladder.
- Yellow or white pus at the end of the penis, seen before urination in the morning or as stains on the underwear; indicates a possible infection or irritation of the urethra. Causes include sexually transmitted diseases and chemical irritation from birth control cream.

What to Do

1. For bladder/urinary tract infection, see Frequent Urination (below).
2. For sexually transmitted disease, have the man avoid sex and seek medical care.

▶ Bloody Urine

Blood in the urine can be frightening, but it is not generally an emergency. Causes include problems with any part of the urinary system. The most common problems are kidney stones and bladder infections.

What to Look For

- Pink or red urine
- Severe back or flank pain, suggesting a kidney stone or infection
- Fever, suggesting an infection
- Inability to urinate, possibly resulting from a blood clot in the bladder

What to Do

1. Give the victim several extra quarts of water per day unless the victim is unable to urinate.
2. Have the victim walk out of the wilderness if there is no pain or fever.
3. Evacuate if there is a high fever with flank pain, which suggests a kidney infection.

▶ Frequent Urination

This might be a symptom of infection, urinary obstruction, or diabetes with elevated blood sugar.

What to Look For

- Fever, chills, flank pain, and/or burning during urination, indicating an infection.
- Constant thirst and drinking and urinating large volumes, suggesting diabetes.
- Frequent small amounts of urine with a sense that the bladder cannot be emptied completely and fullness in the lower abdomen, suggesting infection or urinary obstruction.

What to Do

1. Increase intake of water and fruit juices unless there is possible obstruction.
2. Give the victim vitamin C (500 mg three times daily), which makes the urine acid and slows bacterial growth. Juices such as cranberry may be helpful.
3. If infection is likely and the affected person has an antibiotic, he should take it.
4. Seek medical care (see Guidelines for Evacuation of Genitourinary Problems).

▶ Inability to Urinate

Obstruction occurs in older men with enlarged prostates and often is induced by prolonged sitting during travel or by medications such as antihistamines and cold remedies. It can occur in young men with prior surgery on the urinary tract or after pelvic injury.

What to Look For

- Painfully full bladder
- Inability to pass any urine or frequent dribbling of small amounts of urine without relief

What to Do

1. Stop any medications for allergies, congestion/colds, stomach cramps, and motion sickness; stop over-the-counter sleep medication.
2. Limit fluid intake.
3. Have the man listen to running water, place his hand in a pot of warm water, or have him sit in warm water.
4. If the victim is still unable to urinate, evacuate.

▶ Testicular Pain

Sudden onset of pain and swelling in the testicle of a young man (less than 25 years old) usually means it is twisted (torsion). If it cannot be untwisted, surgery is required within 24 hours to prevent damage to the testicle. Gradual onset of pain and swelling in an adult older than 25 years likely indicates infection (epididymitis).

> ### ADVANCED PROCEDURE
>
> **Twisted Testicle**
> The testicle can sometimes be untwisted by hand. Try rotating the testicle 180°, first in one direction then the other, while exerting gentle traction in a vertical axis with the man standing. If relief is obtained, it will be rapid.

What to Look For

- Severe pain in a testicle, often spreading to the groin or lower abdomen on the same side; can cause vomiting
- The affected testicle is firm and swollen
- Urine can pass but can be hard to start due to pain

What to Do

1. If torsion is suspected, try untwisting (see Advanced Procedure box).
2. If pain does not resolve within a few minutes, evacuate.
3. If epididymitis is suspected, use warm compresses and give antibiotics, if available.

▶ Pain and Swelling of Foreskin

In uncircumcised men or boys, the foreskin can become inflamed and it may become impossible to move the foreskin back and forth over the end of the penis.

What to Look For

- Redness, swelling, and pain of the foreskin; inability to retract or extend the foreskin freely.
- Signs of infection such as pus or whitish mucus under the foreskin or redness and swelling that extends toward the base of the penis.

What to Do

1. Have the man gently compress the swollen tissue and try to move the foreskin.
2. Have him wash the area daily with mild soap, cleaning beneath the foreskin as well.
3. Have him dry the area, and then apply an antifungal cream and/or antibiotic ointment.
4. Administer an antibiotic if available, in cases in which infection is suspected.
5. If the man is unable to urinate or to relieve the pain and swelling, seek medical care.

▶ Kidney Stone

A kidney stone is one of the most common causes of sudden severe flank and abdominal pain.

What to Look For

- Sudden onset of pain in the flank on one side, often spreading to the lower abdomen, groin, or testicle
- Severe pain causing restlessness and vomiting
- Bloody urine

What to Do

1. Administer pain medication.
2. Increase fluid intake.
3. Evacuate the victim if there is severe pain or fever.

Guidelines for Evacuation of Genitourinary Problems

Evacuate for:

- Urinary obstruction with inability to urinate.
- Urinary symptoms with fever, chills, and back pain.
- Sudden testicular pain.
- Swelling, redness, and pain around the shaft of the penis or scrotum.

No evacuation is necessary (the victim may walk) for:

- Bloody urine.
- Frequent urination without fever.
- Pus discharge from or sores on the genitalia.

▶ Emergency Care Wrap-up

What to Look For	What to Do
Problems Specific to Women	
Vaginitis • Vaginal soreness, burning or itching, redness • Increased vaginal discharge • Pain with urination	1. Wear cotton underwear and loose-fitting pants. 2. Irrigate the vulva with clean water several times daily. 3. Use vaginal antifungal medication.
Vulvar Irritation • Vaginal soreness, burning, or itching • Vulvar redness • Pain with urination	1. Avoid further contact with the irritating substance. 2. Wash the vulva with clean water and mild soap. 3. Apply hydrocortisone cream.
Painful Urination • Frequent, burning urination • Low abdominal pain, cramping, and burning with urination • Cloudy or bloody urine • Foul-smelling urine	1. Have the victim drink a lot of water. 2. Have the victim drink acidic fluids or juices. 3. Have the victim take vitamin C to acidify the urine. 4. Have the victim avoid sexual intercourse.
Missed Menses • A history of unprotected intercourse, breast tenderness and nausea, or morning sickness • Stress, heavy exercise • Severe weight loss; poor eating	1. A missed period usually requires no treatment.
Heavy or Prolonged Bleeding • Length of time since last period • Recent history of unprotected sex to suggest risk of pregnancy • Amount and duration of bleeding • Pale skin, nails, lips • Weakness • Signs and symptoms of shock	1. Have the woman rest until bleeding decreases to a normal menstrual flow. 2. Give generous amounts of fluids to drink. 3. Seek medical care.

What to Look For	What to Do
Bleeding With Pregnancy • Length of time since last period • Amount of bleeding • Low abdominal pain • Signs and symptoms of shock	1. Avoid physical exertion until the bleeding stops. 2. Seek medical care if the bleeding is uncontrollable.
Pain Due to Infections • Low abdominal pain • Fever • Nausea and vomiting • Diarrhea	1. If the pain has caused vomiting or diarrhea, give as much fluid as tolerated. 2. If the pain increases, seek medical care.
Ectopic Pregnancy or Ruptured Cyst • Low or generalized abdominal pain • Nausea • Signs of blood loss or shock	1. Keep the woman lying at rest. 2. Have her walk out if capable. 3. If she is unable to walk, send for help and evacuate.
Pain Associated With Pregnancy • Time since last period • Recurring pains • Signs of blood loss or shock	1. Mild cramping in pregnancy without bleeding does not require treatment. 2. For pain with bleeding in pregnancy, follow the advice given for bleeding. 3. A woman who is more than 5 months pregnant who has cramps lasting about 30 seconds every 15 minutes may be in labor.

Problems Specific to Men

Bloody Urine • Pink or red urine • Severe back or flank pain • Fever • Inability to urinate	1. Give several extra quarts of water per day unless the victim is unable to urinate. 2. Have the victim walk out if he has no pain or fever.

What to Look For	What to Do
Frequent Urination • Fever, chills, and back pain with burning on urination • Constant thirst, drinking and urinating large volumes • Frequent small amounts of urine with a sense that the bladder cannot be emptied completely and fullness in the lower abdomen	1. Increase intake of water and fruit juices unless there is possible obstruction. 2. Give vitamin C. 3. If infection is likely, give antibiotics. 4. Seek medical care.
Inability to Urinate • Painfully full bladder • Inability to pass any urine • Frequent dribbling of small amounts of urine	1. Stop any medications for allergies, congestion/colds, stomach cramps, and motion sickness; stop over-the-counter sleep medication. 2. Limit fluid intake. 3. If he is still unable to urinate, evacuate.
Testicular Pain • Severe pain in testicle • Testicle is firm and swollen • Urination may be difficult to begin	1. Try rotating the testicle 180°. 2. If no relief is felt, evacuate immediately.
Pain and Swelling of Foreskin • Redness, swelling, and pain of the foreskin • Inability to retract or extend the foreskin freely • Pus or whitish mucus under the foreskin	1. Have the man gently compress the swollen tissue and try to move the foreskin. 2. Have him wash the area daily with mild soap, cleaning beneath the foreskin as well. 3. Have him dry the area, then apply an antifungal cream and/or antibiotic ointment. 4. Administer an antibiotic, if appropriate. 5. If the man is unable to urinate or to relieve the pain and swelling, seek medical help.
Kidney Stone • Sudden onset of pain in flank on one side • Severe pain causing restlessness and vomiting • Bloody urine	1. Administer pain medication. 2. Increase fluid intake. 3. Evacuate if severe pain or fever.

15

Physical and Environmental Hazards

The environment and its effects on the body distinguish wilderness first aid from urban first aid. Altitude, cold, heat, wind, rain, lightning, soaking wetness, and parching dryness not only cause injuries and illnesses but also affect those that occur in the wilderness **Figure 15-1**. An injury that has little significance in the city becomes important if it stops a person from hiking and exposes him or her to a cold night outdoors. Both the severity of the elements and the length of time for which the injured person is exposed can affect the outcome. A night spent with a broken ankle, in mild temperatures with neither rain nor wind, will be uncomfortable and painful, but the victim ordinarily will survive. The same broken ankle experienced in winter at 10,000 feet on the windy slopes of a mountain, far from camp and with no way to call for help, could be fatal.

It is, therefore, important to understand both the management of individual injuries and the effects of the surrounding environment on an injured person. How will the temperature, altitude, and weather affect the outcome? How can you prevent further injury by protecting an injured person from the heat or cold, the wind or rain? What must you do to provide food and fluids to maintain the victim's strength? How can you improvise a shelter? The answers can mean the difference between life and death, but first you must understand how the environment affects the body.

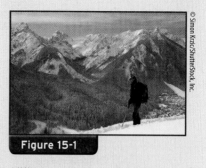

Figure 15-1

Altitude and temperature not only cause injuries, but affect the ones that occur as well.

Acclimatization

Acclimatization comprises the physiological changes in the body that compensate for hypoxia (low oxygen levels) at altitudes above 8,000 feet (2,500 meters) and allows humans to live, work, and exercise with what little oxygen is available **Figure 15-2**. It proceeds at different rates in different people. Acclimatization is best achieved through slow, progressive ascent with rest or descent if symptoms caused by hypoxia persist **Figure 15-3A-C**.

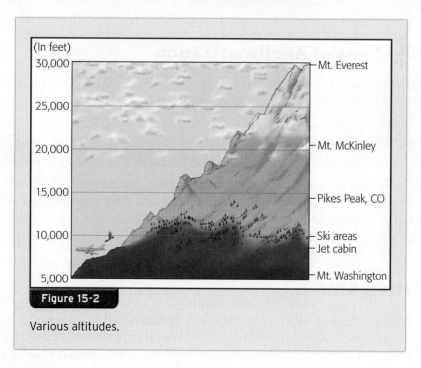

Figure 15-2

Various altitudes.

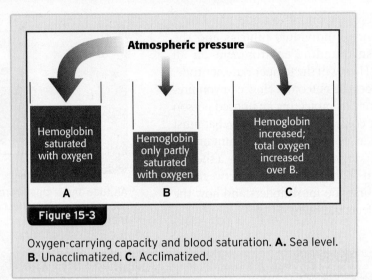

Atmospheric pressure

A	B	C
Hemoglobin saturated with oxygen	Hemoglobin only partly saturated with oxygen	Hemoglobin increased; total oxygen increased over B.

Figure 15-3

Oxygen-carrying capacity and blood saturation. **A.** Sea level. **B.** Unacclimatized. **C.** Acclimatized.

▶ Immediate Changes of Acclimatization

The rate and depth of breathing increase to improve oxygen delivery to the blood; the heart beats stronger and more quickly, increasing the flow of blood and transport of oxygen.

▶ Late Changes of Acclimatization

The bone marrow produces more red cells to carry oxygen. An increase in the number of capillaries improves oxygen supply to muscles and other tissues.

Acute Mountain Sickness

Going above 8,000 feet (2,500 meters) can produce one of several types of altitude illnesses due to lack of oxygen in the blood **Table 15-1**. One of these is acute mountain sickness (AMS). AMS affects those who ascend too high too fast and those who have not acclimatized to high altitude. AMS usually is relieved by descent to a lower altitude.

▶ Predicting AMS

No one can predict who will suffer from AMS, how severe it will be, or when it will occur. Those who have suffered AMS before are more likely to suffer it again, and at a similar altitude. Fitness and training guarantee no protection and both sexes are affected equally. Although no age is exempt, the young seem more prone to AMS, regardless of fitness and rate of ascent.

Table 15-1   Characteristics of Altitude Illnesses

	AMS	HAPE	HACE
Elevation	Above 8,000 ft (2,500 m)	Usually above 10,000 ft (3,000 m)	Above 12,000 ft (3,500 m)
Time after ascent	1-2 days	3-4 days, possibly later	4-7 days, possibly later
Symptoms	Result from hypoxia and include headache, sleep disturbance, fatigue, shortness of breath, dizziness, loss of appetite, nausea with or without vomiting	Caused by pulmonary fluid and include shortness of breath, dry cough, mild chest pain, weakness, insomnia, rapid pulse, cyanosis, rales (crackles) or gurgling sounds	Caused by swelling of the brain and include severe headache (unrelieved), vomiting, Cheynes-Stokes breathing (irregular breathing pattern followed by breathing stops), staggering gait, inability to balance, unconsciousness
First aid	• Stop ascending or go down • Drink fluids • Rest • Give the victim aspirin or ibuprofen • Give the victim acetazolamide	• Descend at least 2,000 ft (600 m) • Seek medical care immediately.	• Descend as soon as possible; 1,000 ft (300 m) minimum, 3,000 ft (900 m) if possible or until symptoms disappear. • Seek medical care immediately.

Notes: AMS = acute mountain sickness; HAPE = high-altitude pulmonary edema; HACE = high-altitude cerebral edema.
HAPE and HACE occur when reduced oxygen causes capillary leakage and body-tissue swelling. Both conditions are life threatening.

▶ Prevention of AMS

Climbers should allow ample time to acclimatize at various levels of ascent. AMS is more likely to occur the higher, the faster, the harder, and the longer the climb. Cold and wind, fear, fatigue, dehydration, strenuous exercise soon after ascent, and upper respiratory infections all predispose to AMS.

- *Gradual ascent.* Limiting the number of feet (meters) gained per day is a highly effective way of preventing acute altitude illness. The altitude at which someone sleeps is considered more important than the altitude reached during waking hours.

- *Medication.* Medications are not necessary for those with no prior history of altitude illness and those climbing to 9,000 feet (2,800 meters) and taking more than 2 days to arrive at 8,000-10,000 feet (2,500-3,000 meters) with later increases in sleeping elevation of less than 1,500 feet (500 meters) per day. Above an altitude of 10,000 feet (3,000 meters), individuals should not increase the sleeping elevation by more than 1,500 feet (500 meters) per day and should include a rest day every 3 to 4 days. Medication in the form of Diamox (acetazolamide) should be considered for those with a past history of AMS and ascending to 8,000-9,000 feet (2,500-2,800 meters) in 1 day, those with no history of AMS but who are ascending to 9,000 feet (2,800 meters) in 1 day, and all those sleeping at an increased 1,500 feet (500 meters) than the night before. Acetazolamide requires a medical prescription.

▶ High-Altitude Climbing

Mild symptoms of AMS can develop at 6,000 feet (1,800 meters), but are more likely above 8,000 feet (2,500 meters). Above 13,000 feet (4,000 meters), climbers and trekkers on multiday trips should reach sleeping altitude at about 1,000 feet (300 meters) higher than the previous day. The motto is, "Climb high, sleep low."

Climbers who become sick and do not improve with rest must descend 1,000 to 3,000 feet (300 to 900 meters) as quickly as possible. Be aware of climbers who acclimatize poorly.

Climbers should drink 4 to 5 quarts or liters of fluid daily, enough to produce clear, copious urine. Dark (concentrated) urine usually indicates an inadequate fluid intake.

Alcohol, sedatives, and sleeping pills depress respiratory ventilation at night and increase the likelihood of disturbed sleep. Climbers should eat a high-calorie, high-carbohydrate diet.

Groups traveling above 10,000 feet (3,000 meters) should consider carrying a portable hyperbaric chamber, supplemental oxygen, and medications.

▶ AMS

Mild AMS has vague, ill-defined symptoms but can drift subtly into severe altitude sickness, which can result in death. Signs and symptoms of mild AMS occur within 6 to 48 hours of arrival at high altitude. Similar symptoms often are the result of dehydration, exhaustion, hypoglycemia, hypothermia, or hyponatremia.

What to Look For

- A generalized headache that often develops during the night and is present on waking; by day, the victim might feel light-headed
- Unusual tiredness out of proportion to the activity
- Appetite loss and nausea
- Restless sleep with irregular breathing

- Shortness of breath with exertion
- A swollen face, with bags under the eyes; rings on the victim's fingers feel tight

What to Do

- *Descend.* Descending remains the single best treatment for AMS. However, it is not necessary in all cases. Victims should descend until symptoms resolve, unless impossible due to terrain. Victims should not descend alone.
- *Medications.* Diamox (acetazolamide) will help treat AMS, but it works better for prevention than for treatment.
  Decadron (dexamethasone) is more effective than Diamox in treating AMS. It can be given by mouth, which is easier to give than by injection. It requires a medical prescription.
- *Portable hyperbaric chambers.* These devices are effective for treating severe altitude illness but require constant tending by health care providers and are difficult to use with claustrophobic or vomiting victims. On most mountain-climbing trips, these chambers will not be available.

Mild AMS can progress into severe altitude sickness. Life-threatening symptoms can develop within hours and frequently do so at night, when descending is more difficult. It is better to take precautions early.

▶ High-Altitude Pulmonary Edema

In high-altitude pulmonary edema (HAPE), the lungs become waterlogged, hindering the passage of oxygen into the blood. Victims can drown in their own fluid. HAPE usually starts above 10,000 feet (3,000 meters) but can occur at lower altitudes; it begins 36 to 72 hours after arriving at high altitude and is relieved by descent.

What to Look For

- Shortness of breath, which occurs with slight exertion and is even present at rest. The victim needs to sit up to breathe comfortably
- Cough, at first dry, then producing frothy, pink (blood-stained) sputum
- Rattling or crackling and moist breathing and coughing
- Cyanosis (the lips, face, and fingernails look blue at rest; compare the victim's color to a fit companion or yourself in natural light, not in a tent)
- Rapid pulse, more than 100 beats per minute at rest

What to Do

1. Descend at least 1,000 to 1,500 feet (300 to 500 meters); this is the single best treatment for HAPE.

2. Give the victim oxygen, if available.

3. Commence treatment in a portable hyperbaric chamber (but this should not delay descending).

4. Administer acetazolamide and/or nifedipine in accordance with pre-arranged instructions. If traveling to high altitude, discuss treatment plans with a physician ahead of time, and prepare equipment and medications as described in the appendix *First Aid Equipment and Supplies*.

> **NOTE**
>
> Ataxia and fatigue also occur in other conditions such as hypothermia (check the temperature), alcohol intoxication (smell the breath), and opiate drug abuse (look for pinpoint pupils).

▶ High-Altitude Cerebral Edema

High-altitude cerebral edema (HACE) usually occurs above 12,000 feet (3,500 meters). It can accompany HAPE and can kill quickly. Symptoms of HACE and HAPE can overlap. HACE is caused by fluid collecting within the brain, which increases pressure on the brain until it fails to function properly and results in death.

What to Look For

- Severe, constant, throbbing headache, like a bad toothache or migraine; no relief from acetaminophen, codeine, or a night's rest.
- Loss of coordination (ataxia); the victim staggers as if drunk, fumbles fine movements, and cannot walk a straight line with the heel of one foot against the toes of the other. If ataxia is severe, the victim cannot sit upright without support.
- Extreme fatigue that is not reversed by rest. The affected person won't talk, eat, or drink and is apathetic and isolated, irritable, and confused. The person can hallucinate, hear voices, or see nonexistent companions.
- Vomiting; combined with the inability to drink, this can lead to severe dehydration. Urine becomes scant and dark yellow.
- Coma; the affected person becomes unarousable and unresponsive and may die.

What to Do

1. Take the victim to a lower altitude as soon as possible **Figure 15-4**. This usually cures severe altitude sickness rapidly. Do not delay descent because of night, inconvenience, trying drugs or oxygen, or in expectation of a mountain rescue team or helicopter—unless descending through difficult terrain in the dark will cause unwarranted danger to the whole party. The victim should descend at least 1,000

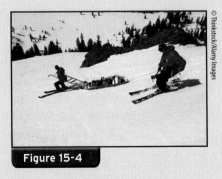

Figure 15-4

Take the victim to a lower altitude.

to 3,000 feet (300 to 900 meters) and must be accompanied or even carried. Even a modest descent can save a life. The greater and faster the descent, the swifter the recovery. Once down, the victim should stay at the lower elevation.

2. If descent is not feasible, supplemental oxygen or a portable hyperbaric chamber (Gamow bag) should be considered if available. Treat the victim for several hours in a portable hyperbaric bag, such as a Gamow bag, if available **Figure 15-5**. This can be lifesaving under extreme circumstances and might buy time while a rescue operation is being mounted. Climbing parties going to extreme altitudes should consider equipping themselves with one of these bags.

3. Have the victim sit propped up to improve breathing. Keep the afflicted person warm and relaxed; cold and anxiety aggravate AMS.

4. Have the victim drink at least 4 to 5 quarts or liters of fluid daily to maintain a copious flow of clear urine.

5. The medically prescribed drug Decadron should be given in small doses; however, you should never rely on drugs to avoid the need for a rapid descent.

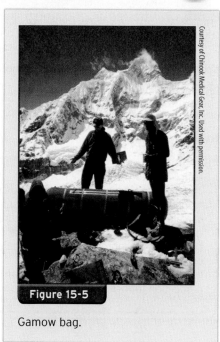

Courtesy of Chinook Medical Gear, Inc. Used with permission.

Figure 15-5

Gamow bag.

Cold Injury

Cold injuries include hypothermia, frostbite, cold immersion injury, and chilblains. Hypothermia is a general cooling of the body core and develops when the body's temperature drops more than 2°F to about 95°F (35°C) . Frostbite is local freezing of the skin and flesh. Prolonged immersion of an extremity in cold, but not freezing, water causes a unique injury, often referred to as "trench foot" but more accurately referred to as "cold immersion injury."

▶ Hypothermia

Hypothermia occurs when the body loses enough heat to cause the core body temperature to drop. Hypothermia is exacerbated by inadequate clothing and exhaustion. Anxiety, injury, drugs, poor nutrition, and alcohol consumption predispose people to hypothermia.

Wetness and wind are a lethal combination that chill a person more rapidly than dry, still air. Clothes that become wet, even from perspiration, are also a potent cause of heat loss. The conditions for hypothermia therefore exist in all seasons. The hiker exposed to a sudden summer hailstorm while wearing only a T-shirt and cutoff jeans is more likely to become hypothermic than a well-dressed cross-country skier in the winter. Changing into dry clothing can be the most important first step in the first aid of all cold victims.

Plan carefully, even for the shortest outdoor expedition, and carry a water/wind-repellent shell, a pile jacket, hat and mittens, matches, and an emergency blanket (a thin, packable, Mylar sheet with reflective coating) or tarp for shelter. If the weather changes, be prepared to abandon the original plan and take an easier, shorter route home, or bivouac.

PREVENTION

Watch for early signs of hypothermia, and act promptly to avert it. Gauge the day's activity to the party's weakest member. Being exhausted, hungry, dehydrated, or demoralized prevents a proper response to cold and hastens the onset of hypothermia. After exertion stops, body temperature can plummet, because heat loss continues while heat production decreases sharply. Evaporation of sweat is the most important source of heat loss during exercise; therefore, avoidance of sweating with appropriately ventilated clothing is important to maintain comfort and avoid excessive heat loss.

Children and adolescents lose heat faster than adults, because their surface area is large in proportion to their weight, and, generally, they have less subcutaneous fat.

The windchill factor shows the cooling effects of wind at any given temperature and wind speed **Figure 15-6**. Wearing windproof clothing and covering the face with a mask and goggles can reduce or eliminate the effects of windchill, except under the most severe circumstances.

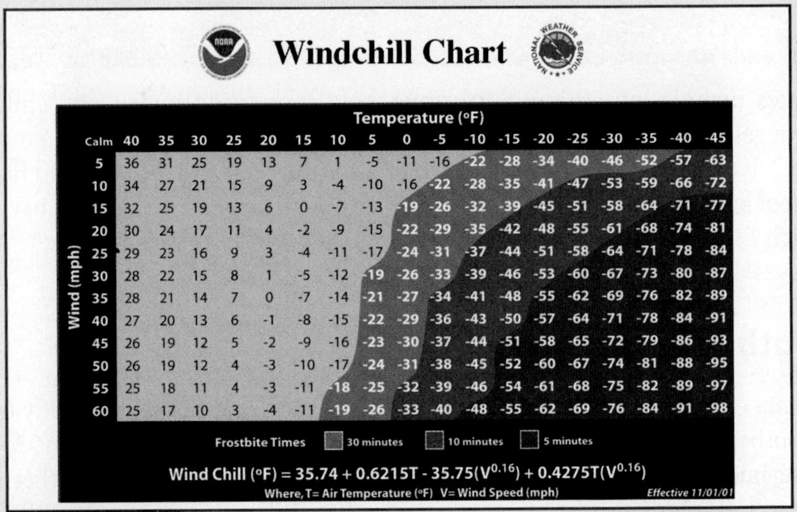

Courtesy of NWS/NOAA

Windchill Chart

Wind (mph)	Temperature (°F)																		
Calm	40	35	30	25	20	15	10	5	0	-5	-10	-15	-20	-25	-30	-35	-40	-45
5	36	31	25	19	13	7	1	-5	-11	-16	-22	-28	-34	-40	-46	-52	-57	-63
10	34	27	21	15	9	3	-4	-10	-16	-22	-28	-35	-41	-47	-53	-59	-66	-72
15	32	25	19	13	6	0	-7	-13	-19	-26	-32	-39	-45	-51	-58	-64	-71	-77
20	30	24	17	11	4	-2	-9	-15	-22	-29	-35	-42	-48	-55	-61	-68	-74	-81
25	29	23	16	9	3	-4	-11	-17	-24	-31	-37	-44	-51	-58	-64	-71	-78	-84
30	28	22	15	8	1	-5	-12	-19	-26	-33	-39	-46	-53	-60	-67	-73	-80	-87
35	28	21	14	7	0	-7	-14	-21	-27	-34	-41	-48	-55	-62	-69	-76	-82	-89
40	27	20	13	6	-1	-8	-15	-22	-29	-36	-43	-50	-57	-64	-71	-78	-84	-91
45	26	19	12	5	-2	-9	-16	-23	-30	-37	-44	-51	-58	-65	-72	-79	-86	-93
50	26	19	12	4	-3	-10	-17	-24	-31	-38	-45	-52	-60	-67	-74	-81	-88	-95
55	25	18	11	4	-3	-11	-18	-25	-32	-39	-46	-54	-61	-68	-75	-82	-89	-97
60	25	17	10	3	-4	-11	-19	-26	-33	-40	-48	-55	-62	-69	-76	-84	-91	-98

Frostbite Times ▨ 30 minutes ▨ 10 minutes ☐ 5 minutes

Wind Chill (°F) = 35.74 + 0.6215T - 35.75($V^{0.16}$) + 0.4275T($V^{0.16}$)

Where, T= Air Temperature (°F)　V= Wind Speed (mph)　Effective 11/01/01

Figure 15-6

Windchill chart.

Means of Heat Loss

- *Convection.* Heat is carried away from the body by currents of air or water.
- *Conduction.* There is a direct transfer of heat from the body to a colder object (such as wet clothes or cold ground).
- *Evaporation.* Sweat or water evaporates from the surface of the skin.
- *Radiation.* This is the loss of heat from a warm body to a surrounding colder environment. This is independent of wind or contact. Radiative heat loss is significant on cold, dark, cloudless nights.

Sources of Heat Gain

- *Radiation.* Heat comes from the sun or a fire.
- *Exercise.* About 75% of muscular energy is produced as heat; exercise, therefore, rewarms the body.
- *Shivering.* Shivering can increase body metabolism fivefold but consumes energy and oxygen in achieving this.
- *Food.* Food provides calories for basic body functions and exercise. Carbohydrates provide energy quickly; protein provides greater energy, but more slowly and at the expense of more body energy used for digestion.
- *Blood vessel constriction.* Skin blood vessels constrict, thereby keeping warm blood circulating in the core, where it is most needed by the vital organs (brain, heart, liver, and kidneys), and reducing heat loss through the skin.
- *Insulation.* This prevents heat loss but does not by itself produce heat. Water, an excellent heat conductor, reduces the insulating value of most fabrics. Wool, polypropylene, and pile insulate well by trapping air in the interstices of the fibers, which do not collapse when wet. The more layers of clothing, the better the insulation. Windproof, water-repellent fabrics worn as an outer layer of clothing trap warm air in the inner layers and diminish heat loss by convection, conduction, and evaporation.

▶ Mild Hypothermia

In mild hypothermia, the core temperature of the body will range from 95°F to 91°F (35°C to 33°C).

What to Look For

- Shivering, the first sign of body cooling. Shivering later becomes uncontrollable.
- Uncharacteristic behavior. The affected person can still talk but grumbles and mumbles about feeling cold. Such behavior might be obvious only to someone who knows the victim. Inappropriate

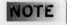

Putting a rescuer in a sleeping bag with the victim is not always the best thing to do. Having another person in the sleeping bag warms the skin. Warming the skin stops shivering, which is the most effective internal method of rewarming. Provide maximum shelter, and allow shivering to do the rewarming. It might be better to have one person in two sleeping bags than two people in one bag.

excitement or lethargy, poor judgment, and poor decision making are common. The victim becomes confused and might hallucinate.
- Stiff muscles and cramps. These cause uncoordinated movements, so the victim fumbles and stumbles and might not be able to walk along a straight line for 50 to 100 feet (15 to 30 meters).
- Cold, pale, and blue-gray skin caused by constricted blood vessels.

What to Do

1. Find shelter out of the wind.
2. Light a fire or stove, change or remove the victim's wet clothes, add dry layers to increase insulation, and give the victim some food and a hot drink.
3. If the victim is shivering strongly, allow shivering to continue inside a sleeping bag, keeping the victim well insulated from the ground.
4. Give the victim warm, sweet liquids.
5. Do not delay providing rest and warmth. If the victim responds to rest and warmth, he or she might be able to descend to a camp or hut to be thoroughly warmed.
6. Never leave a hypothermic victim alone.

▶ Severe Hypothermia

With severe hypothermia, the body's core temperature falls below 90°F (32°C). Because few people carry a low-reading thermometer in the wilderness, a more practical way of differentiating between mild and severe hypothermia is to classify victims as shivering and nonshivering. A victim who is responsive and shivering is mildly hypothermic. A barely conscious victim who is no longer shivering is severely hypothermic.

What to Look For

- No shivering.
- Behavior changing from erratic to apathetic to unresponsive.
- Stiff muscles and uncoordinated movement.
- Weak, slow, irregular pulse.
- Slow breathing.
- Coma, with dilated pupils. (It can be difficult to determine if the victim is alive or dead.)

What to Do in the Field

Rewarming a victim in the field is very difficult, if not impossible; concentrate your efforts on reducing further heat loss **Table 15-2**.

1. The leader or most-competent person in the group must take charge. Do not endanger other members of the party.

Table 15-2	**Field Management of Hypothermia**
Assessment	Victim: Severity of hypothermia
	Group: Number, condition, strength, available equipment
	Circumstances: Weather, time of day, distance from help, and the like
Plan	Rewarming
	Shelter
	Communications/logistics
Action	Evacuation
	Shelter, clothing, food, heat sources, contacting help, preparation for stay or evacuation
	Treatment of associated injuries or illnesses

2. Shelter the victim and the rest of the group from wind, rain, and snow and keep everyone out of danger from avalanche or rock fall. Erect a tent, dig a snow hole, or build a lean-to.

3. Stop further heat loss. Remove wet or freezing clothing and dress the victim in dry clothes. Put the hypothermic person in a sleeping bag, bivouac sack, or a strong polyethylene bag and insulate him or her well from the cold ground.

4. Provide heat to the victim's trunk during the first half hour after rescue by whatever means are available: body-to-body contact, hot water bottles, chemical heating pads, or hot rocks wrapped in clothing. Place the heat sources in the groin and armpits and alongside the neck. Always have clothing between a heat source and the skin.

5. Cover the victim's head with a wool cap to reduce heat loss.

What to Do (Rescue)

1. Leave at least one person to look after the victim. Send the strongest, most-competent members of the party for help. Provide the location and the condition of the victim in a written message.

2. If you have decided to stay put and await rescue, do not change your plan even if the victim improves. If you are forced to carry the hypothermic person, insulate him or her well, because cooling can continue during transportation.

3. If you must descend, choose the safest route that avoids ridges and windy places. If the victim is on an improvised stretcher or sled, handle it gently; rough handling can induce ventricular fibrillation in a hypothermic victim (a fatal abnormality of heart rhythm). Carry the victim with the head downhill to maintain blood pressure but keep him or her in a horizontal position as much as possible to avoid pooling of blood in the legs.

What to Do (Base Camp)

1. If rescue is impossible or is days away, use all available means to rewarm the victim slowly in a sleeping bag.
2. If the victim has become hypothermic over hours or days due to exposure, do not try rapid rewarming in a bath or in front of a fire.
3. Give the affected person plenty of warm, sweet liquids when he or she is able to drink. Hypothermic victims are often dehydrated and their energy is depleted. You cannot expect to provide enough heat in warm drinks to rewarm a hypothermic person, but the hydration and usable energy are valuable, and the warmth will help build morale in the victim.
4. Be careful not to place warm objects (hot water bottles, chemical heating pads, and the like) directly on the victim's skin. Hypothermic skin burns at low temperatures.

▶ Deep Hypothermia

With deep hypothermia, the body's core temperature falls below 82°F (28°C). The victim might appear dead, but declare a victim of hypothermia dead only after warming has been attempted. The person's pupils can be dilated and fixed, the limbs stiff, and the skin icy. Profoundly hypothermic persons cannot generate enough metabolic heat to rewarm themselves, despite good shelter and insulation. They cannot be rewarmed in the field, but, once rescued, all hypothermic victims in whom there appears even a remote chance of recovery should be resuscitated. Protect and insulate a victim during transportation to prevent further heat loss. The only sure sign of death is failure to revive with rewarming. Victims have survived after several hours of CPR.

▶ Immersion Hypothermia

Immersion hypothermia differs from exposure hypothermia in its rapid onset and even faster rate of cooling. Heat is lost 25 times faster in water than in air, because water is an excellent conductor of heat. The victim can drown in addition to becoming hypothermic.

Most people can swim less than 0.6 mile (1 km) in water at 50°F (10°C). Energetic swimming increases heat loss, while floating in a fetal position minimizes it. A personal flotation device (PFD) prolongs survival time threefold. Clothes decrease heat loss; wool insulates better than other materials when wet, and covering the head reduces heat loss by half.

It is safer to stay with an overturned boat than to strike out for shore **Figure 15-7**. A person will stay warmer out of the water, clinging to an overturned boat—despite wind and rain—than staying immersed. Staying with the boat increases the chance of rescue. Unfortunately, despair is the overwhelming emotion among shipwreck victims, who often fail to use the simple survival skills that can tip the balance from death to life.

In water colder than 45°F (7°C), hypothermia can develop in less than an hour, but clothing may slow the onset of hypothermia. Many victims drown because of a combination of cold, which reduces their ability to swim or float, and submersion. The heat escape lessening position (HELP) or huddle position can minimize heat loss and increase chances of survival **Figure 15-8A-B**.

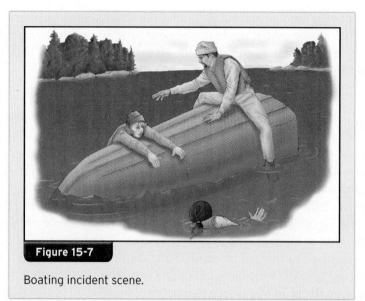

Figure 15-7

Boating incident scene.

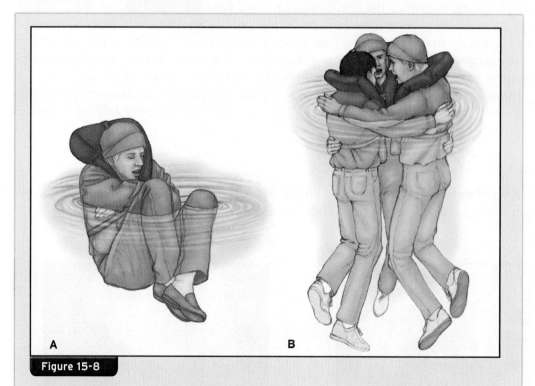

A   B

Figure 15-8

HELP or huddle. **A.** A person wearing a flotation device can minimize heat loss and increase chances of survival by assuming the heat escape lessening position, or HELP, in which the knees are pulled up to the chest and the arms crossed. **B.** Groups of two or more can conserve heat by wrapping their arms around one another and pulling into a tight circle.

If CPR is warranted, it must be started as soon as possible after the victim is removed from the water. If the victim is very cold, it might not be possible to restart the heart until the person has been rewarmed in a hospital; however, rescue efforts should continue until this has been done or there is clearly no hope of recovery.

▶ Frostbite

Freezing cold injuries can occur whenever the air temperature is below freezing (32°F, or 0°C). Freezing limited to the skin surface is frostnip **Figure 15-9**. Freezing that extends deeper through the skin and into the flesh is frostbite.

Frostbite happens only in below-freezing temperatures. Tissue is damaged in two ways: (1) actual tissue freezing, which results in the formation of ice crystals within the tissue (the ice crystals expand as they freeze, damaging cells), and (2) the obstruction of the blood supply to the tissue, which causes sludged blood clots and further prevents blood from flowing to the tissues. The second type of tissue damage is more extensive than the first. In severely cold temperatures, flesh can freeze in less than a minute.

Frostbite affects mainly the feet, hands, ears, and nose **Figure 15-10** and **Figure 15-11**. These areas do not contain large heat-producing muscles and are some distance from the body's heat-generation sources. The most severe consequences of frostbite occur when tissue dies (gangrene), and the affected part might have to be amputated. The longer the tissue stays frozen, the worse the injury. Check for hypothermia in any frostbitten victim.

Factors contributing to frostbite include wetness, contact with metal, prolonged exposure, dehydration, poor nutrition, and extremely cold temperatures. In severe cold, or if there is contact with metal, frostbite can occur in a minute.

What to Look For

The severity and extent of frostbite are difficult to judge until hours after thawing. Before thawing, frostbite can be classified as superficial or deep.

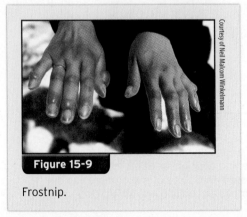

Figure 15-9

Frostnip.

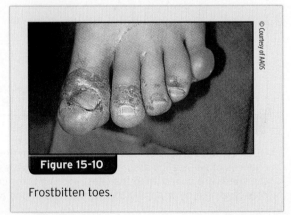

Figure 15-10

Frostbitten toes.

The signs and symptoms of *superficial frostbite* include:

- The skin is white, waxy, or grayish yellow.
- The affected part feels very cold and numb. There might be tingling, stinging, or an aching sensation.
- The skin surface feels stiff or crusty and the underlying tissue feels soft when depressed gently and firmly.

These signs and symptoms indicate *deep frostbite*:

- The affected part feels cold, hard, and solid and cannot be depressed—it feels like a piece of wood or frozen meat.
- The affected part has pale, waxy skin.
- A painfully cold part suddenly stops hurting.

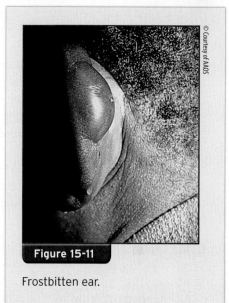

© Courtesy of AAOS

Figure 15-11

Frostbitten ear.

After thawing, frostbite can be categorized by degrees, similar to the classification of burns.

- First-degree: The affected part is warm, swollen, and tender
- Second-degree: blisters form minutes to hours after thawing and enlarge over several days.
- Third-degree: blisters are small and contain reddish blue or purplish fluid. The surrounding skin can be red or blue and might not blanch when pressure is applied.

What to Do

All frostbite injuries require the same first-aid treatment.

1. Get the victim out of the cold and to a warm place. If possible, the victim should not use a frozen extremity until medical care is reached.
2. Remove any wet clothing and constricting items, such as rings, that could impair blood circulation.
3. Do not attempt to thaw the part if: (a) medical care is less than 2 hours away; (b) the affected area has thawed, (c) if shelter, warm water, and a container are not available, or (d) there is a risk of refreezing.
4. If: (a) more than 2 hours from medical care, (b) there is no possibility of refreezing the affected area, and (c) shelter, warm water, and a container are available, use the following wet, rapid rewarming method. While rapid rewarming is recommended, slow thawing may be unavoidable and should be allowed if it is the only method available. Do not rub the affected area.

Place the frostbitten part in warm (100 to 104°F, or 38 to 40°C) water. Do not use other heat sources (i.e., fire, space heater, oven). If you do not have a thermometer, you can put your hand into the water for 30 seconds to test that it is warm, not hot enough to burn. Maintain water temperature by adding warm water as needed. Rewarming usually takes 20 to 40 minutes or until the part becomes soft and pliable to touch and takes on a red/purple appearance. Air dry the area—do not rub. To help control the severe pain during rewarming, give the victim ibuprofen. For ear or facial injuries, it is best, but may be difficult, to apply warm, moist cloths, changing them frequently.

5. After thawing:
   - If the feet are affected, treat the victim as a stretcher case—the feet will be impossible to use after they are rewarmed unless only the toes are affected.
   - Protect the affected area from contact with clothing and bedding.
     - Place bulky, dry, clean gauze to the affected part and between the toes and the fingers to absorb moisture and keep them from sticking together.
     - Slightly elevate the affected part above heart level to reduce pain and swelling.
     - Apply aloe vera gel to promote skin healing.
     - Give the victim ibuprofen to limit pain and inflammation.
     - Do not allow the tissues to refreeze, because this will result in greater damage (ie, gangrene).
6. Fluids can be given if the victim is alert, can swallow, and has no gastrointestinal problems.
7. Seek medical care immediately.

| **CAUTION** |

DO NOT
- Rub the affected part with snow.
- Break blisters.
- Allow a thawed part to refreeze.
- Warm the affected part in front of a fire or heater. A burn can add to the damage. Rewarming can be very painful.

| **PREVENTION** |

To avoid frostbite, those who are outdoors should:

- Wear windproof, water-repellent clothing.
- Avoid wetness or handling metal with bare hands.
- Avoid tight clothes, boots, and crampons.
- Wear gaiters to keep snow out of boots.
- Pull a plastic bag over the foot next to the skin to act as a vapor barrier.
- Change socks frequently to keep feet dry.
- Carry spare dry socks that double as mittens.
- Warm feet or hands as soon as they begin to feel cold or lose feeling.
- Wear mittens rather than gloves, with a silk or polypropylene liner.
- Watch each other's faces for white patches of frostnip.
- Jump up and down, wiggle their toes, flex their ankles, clap their hands, and swing their arms if their feet or hands are becoming cold. If possible, place cold feet against the trunk of a warm companion.

▶ Frostnip

Frostnip is caused when water on the skin surface freezes. Frostnip should be taken seriously, because it could be the first sign of impending frostbite.

What to Look For

It is difficult to tell the difference between frostnip and frostbite. Signs of frostnip include:

- Yellowish to gray colored skin
- Frost (ice crystals) on the skin
- Tingling at first and later can be painful

What to Do

1. Seek shelter.
2. Gently warm the affected area by placing it against a warm body part (ie, put bare hands under the armpits) or by applying a warm chemical heat pack covered by a cloth. For the nose, breathe with cupped hands over the nose.
3. Do not rub the area.

▶ Immersion (Trench) Foot

Immersion foot is a nonfreezing cold injury caused by prolonged exposure (average 3 days) to cold and wet, but without freezing. Mild numbness can progress to swelling, loss of feeling, and burning pain. Blisters develop in severe cases. The injury can occur in people rafting or kayaking in very cold water or in sailors stranded for days in a life raft and unable to keep their feet out of the water.

Prevent injury by keeping feet warm and dry, with frequent sock changes and foot hygiene. Rubber boots do not necessarily protect the feet since cold sweat can have the same effect as water.

Treat victims by elevating the feet and exposing them to the air. The burning feeling is relieved by cool air. Give victims analgesics as necessary. In very severe cases, walking can be impossible due to pain, and evacuation of the victim is mandatory.

▶ Chilblains

Chilblains result from repeated exposure of bare skin to moisture, wind, and cold; the result is red, itchy, tender, swollen skin, usually on the fingers. Chilblains are not a severe problem and can be prevented by wearing gloves.

Heat Illness

The body balances heat loss against heat gain to keep the core body temperature within narrow limits. Evaporation of sweat is the most important means of dissipating heat when exercising. With strenuous exercise in hot climates, heat gain can exceed loss **Figure 15-12**. Core temperature can rise, sometimes to dangerous levels.

Dehydration, factors that limit the ability to sweat (certain skin diseases, extensive prior burns, some medications), and pre-existing cardiovascular problems can predispose people to heat illness.

Acclimatization to heat produces physiologic changes in the body over the course of 3 to 10 days. These changes allow greater comfort and ability to exercise or work in the heat. Acclimatization is stimulated by 1 to 1.5 hours of exercise in the heat, per day.

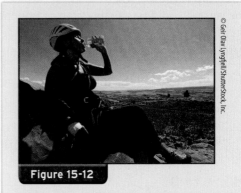

Figure 15-12

Replenish fluids lost through heat exposure.

▶ Heat Exhaustion

Heat exhaustion is caused by water and electrolyte loss from sweating and develops over hours or days. The symptoms are nonspecific and often referred to as "summer flu" because of the resemblance to viral illness. These symptoms include headache, dizziness, fatigue, nausea, and vomiting.

PREVENTION

To avoid heat illness, anyone who is active in hot weather should drink when exercising, before feeling thirsty, and continue to drink after thirst is satisfied. Such people should drink water or a sports electrolyte solution every hour, enough to produce clear urine regularly during the day. For exercise lasting 2 to 3 hours, salt and glucose should be replaced after the exertion. For sustained exertion in the heat, glucose and salt must be replaced during exercise; this is best done by eating in addition to drinking (see the appendix *Fluid and Electrolyte Replacement*). Salt food liberally or include salty snacks.

- Avoid heavy exercise in high temperatures and high humidity.
- Wear light-colored clothes that fit loosely and cover all sun-exposed skin surfaces.
- Avoid alcohol and caffeine; both increase the loss of fluid.
- Be aware of the early symptoms of dehydration—headache, nausea, and muscle cramps.

What to Look For

- Inability to continue exercise or work due to symptoms
- Headache, nausea, dizziness, and weakness
- Rapid pulse
- Thirst and profuse sweating
- Gooseflesh, chills, and pale skin
- Possible fainting

What to Do

1. Have the victim rest in the shade and maximize air circulation.
2. Have the victim remove excess clothing.
3. Wet the victim with cold water to increase evaporation.
4. Have the victim drink fluids.
5. For more severe cases, add 0.25 teaspoon (1.25 milliliters) salt and 6 teaspoons (20 milliliters) sugar to 1 quart or liter of water.
6. If body temperature is above 102°F (39°C), seek medical care.

▶ Heatstroke

Heatstroke is a life-threatening condition in which the body becomes dangerously overheated. Heatstroke can occur in otherwise healthy, fit people of any age who undertake heavy exertion in hot climates (such as military training and warfare, endurance races and sporting events, and strenuous occupations).

The condition also can occur without exercise when victims are exposed to high temperatures for several days (usually in people with chronic medical or psychiatric illness). Heatstroke results in sudden collapse with extreme elevation of body temperature, decreased mental status, and circulatory shock. It is a medical emergency and can be fatal. See   Table 15-3   and   Table 15-4 .

What to Look For

- Extremely hot skin when touched—usually dry, but can be wet from sweating related to strenuous work or exercise.
- Altered mental status ranging from slight confusion, agitation, and disorientation to unresponsiveness.
- Temperature (preferably taken rectally) above 106°F (41°C). Do not attempt to take an oral temperature in a confused or combative person.

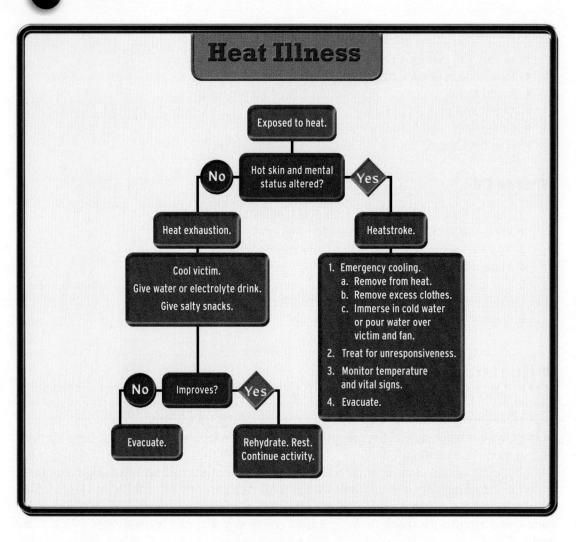

Heat Illness

Exposed to heat.

Hot skin and mental status altered?

No →

Heat exhaustion.

Cool victim.
Give water or electrolyte drink.
Give salty snacks.

No | Improves? | **Yes**

Evacuate.

Rehydrate. Rest.
Continue activity.

Yes →

Heatstroke.

1. Emergency cooling.
   a. Remove from heat.
   b. Remove excess clothes.
   c. Immerse in cold water
      or pour water over
      victim and fan.
2. Treat for unresponsiveness.
3. Monitor temperature
   and vital signs.
4. Evacuate.

What to Do

Heatstroke is a medical emergency and must be treated rapidly! Every minute delayed increases the likelihood of serious complications or death. Do the following:

1. Remove the victim from the hot environment to a cool, shaded area.
2. Remove clothing down to the victim's underwear.
3. The only way to prevent serious complications or death is to cool the victim quickly and by any means possible. In some remote locations, prompt cooling might be difficult. Controversy exists about the best cooling method. In no way should cooling of the heatstroke victim be delayed if any of the below methods are available. Cooling methods include the following:
   - Spray the victim with water and then fanning. This method is not as effective in high-humidity conditions (greater than 75%).

- Apply cool, wet sheets or cloths.
- Place ice packs against the large veins on the groin, armpits, and sides of the neck; this cools the body, regardless of humidity.
- Immerse the victim's body in a stream, pond, or lake. Using this method or the next two methods can be dangerous because of a chance of drowning.
- Place the victim in an ice bath; this cools a victim quickly, but it requires a great deal of ice—at least 80 pounds (about 36 kilograms)—to be effective. The need for a big enough tub also limits this method.

Table 15-3   Fallacies about Heatstroke and Heat Illness

- The skin is always hot and dry.
- It always takes several days of heat stress for heatstroke or heat illness to develop.
- Sports drinks will keep electrolytes normal.
- One should not drink too much water during exercise or performance will suffer.
- People can train themselves to go with less water.
- Physical fitness prevents heat illness.

Table 15-4   Heat Exhaustion Versus Heatstroke

	Heat Exhaustion	Heatstroke
Mental state	Mild, brief confusion.	Confusion progresses to coma and does not resolve quickly.
Temperature	Normal to moderate elevation.	Extreme elevation–above 105°F (41°C).
Temperature regulation	Heat-regulating mechanisms intact; temperature will fall with rest in shade and intake of fluid.	Heat-regulating mechanism fails and requires aggressive cooling measures.
Skin	Often cool and clammy.	Hot; might be moist or dry.
Pulse	Mild elevation (100-120).	Markedly elevated (120-140).
Injury to other organs	No underlying damage.	Can lead to liver or kidney damage.
Evacuation	Treat in the field; the victim can continue activity when he or she is feeling better.	The victim must be evacuated rapidly for further treatment and monitoring.

- Placing the victim in a cool water bath (less than 60°F, or 15°C) can be successful if the water is stirred to prevent a warm layer from forming around the body. This is the most effective method in high-humidity conditions (greater than 75%).
4. Do not give aspirin or acetaminophen, because they are ineffective for heatstroke.
5. Stop cooling when the rectal temperature falls to 102°F (39°C) or when mental status improves. Rectal thermometers are seldom found or used in remote locations.
6. Monitor the victim frequently because high temperatures can rise after cooling.
7. Evacuate to medical care immediately.

▶ Heat Cramps

Heat cramps occur alone or accompany heat exhaustion and also are caused by salt and water depletion during physical activity.

What to Look For

Look for cramps in the calf, thighs, or abdomen, usually beginning after exercise has stopped.

What to Do

1. Stretch the affected muscles.
2. Give the victim salted fluids; do not give the victim salt tablets (except 1–2 tablets dissolved in 1 quart or liter of water).

▶ Other Heat Illnesses

Less serious heat illnesses include heat syncope, heat edema, and prickly heat.

- Heat syncope, in which a person becomes dizzy or faints after exposure to high temperatures, is a self-resolving condition. Victims should lie down in a cool place and, if not nauseated, drink water. Syncope may be associated with heat exhaustion.
- Heat edema, which is also a self-resolving condition, causes the ankles and feet to swell from heat exposure. It is more common in women who are not acclimatized to a hot climate. It is related to salt and water retention and tends to disappear after acclimatization. Wearing support stockings and elevating the legs could help reduce the swelling.
- Prickly heat, also known as a heat rash, is an itchy rash that develops because of moisture on skin wet from sweating. Treat by drying and cooling the skin.

Lightning Injury

The electric discharge of lightning during a thunderstorm is very powerful (30 million volts and 250,000 amps) but very short lived (1 to 100 milliseconds Figure 15-13). Lightning kills by stopping the heart and breathing; external injury and both superficial and deep burns occur but are uncommon. General protection and support of the victim can be the most important first aid to give.

▶ Lightning Safety Guidelines

To reduce the chance of being struck by lightning, those who are outdoors while lightning is striking should avoid:

- Isolated tall trees, hilltops, power lines or pylons, and small exposed shelters.
- Tents, because the poles and wet fabric act as conductors.
- Hill ridges and summits (if this is unavoidable, those on the ridge should seek the lowest point).
- Rock walls—everyone should stay 10 feet (3 meters) away to avoid side flashes.

▶ Injuries Caused By Lightning

One third of all people struck by lightning die. Some recover spontaneously and begin breathing within seconds.

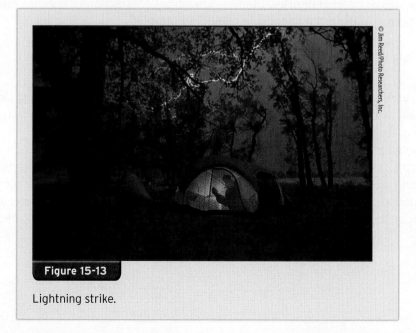

Figure 15-13

Lightning strike.

© Jim Reed/Photo Researchers, Inc.

PREVENTION

During a thunderstorm, people who are outdoors should:

- Find shelter in a stone or brick building or in a car (the metal body, not the rubber tires, affords protection).
- Squat on their heels to avoid being the highest object around and to keep ground currents from passing through the body.
- Stay in thick bush or among low trees, if in a forest.
- Separate from others in a group; everyone should remain 100 feet from the nearest person.
- Avoid metal conductors, such as ice axes.

What to Look For

- Loss of responsiveness. Victims may be confused after regaining responsiveness.
- Cardiac arrest. This is usually what kills lightning victims.
- Lightning can enter by the eyes (and cause later cataracts and blindness) or ears (rupturing the drum or mastoid and causing later deafness).
- Superficial steam burns. These occur in moist areas in linear, rosettelike, or feathery patterns. Deep burns are rare.
- Clothing that has been blasted apart and shredded.
- Bare feet. When someone is standing when struck by lightning, the energy can flow up one leg and down the other, literally blowing the shoes and socks off.
- Blue, mottled limbs caused by intense blood-vessel spasm.
- Fractures or internal injuries. Intense generalized contraction of muscles can throw the person to the ground, causing secondary injuries.

What to Do

1. Ensure scene safety. Rescuers are at risk if thunderstorms are in the area. Do not be afraid to touch lightning-strike victims; they do not store an electrical charge that can affect the rescuer **Table 15-5**.
2. Check for breathing, and, if the victim is not breathing, begin CPR. If more than one victim has been struck by lightning at the same time, the care of victims differs from other situations with multiple-injured victims. Rather than ignoring the victims who appear dead and giving priority to those who are still alive, go to the quiet and motionless victim first to check for breathing, and, if absent, begin CPR. "Resuscitate

Table 15-5 **Lightning Fallacies**
• A lightning strike is always fatal.
• You cannot be hit if you have heard the thunder.
• Lightning only strikes during a storm.
• You are totally safe inside a building.
• If there is no external injury, there is no internal injury.
• Someone struck by lightning is dangerous to touch and is still charged.
• If you are not killed by the lightning, you will be okay.
• Lightning never strikes twice in the same place.

the dead" is the rule in lightning incidents. If the victim has not started to breathe within 30 minutes of starting CPR, stop CPR—the rescuer should not feel guilty about stopping.

3. Because spinal injuries can occur with lightning strikes, precautions should be taken to stabilize the spine.
4. Check for other injuries and treat them accordingly.
5. Evacuate all victims to medical care.

▶ Emergency Care Wrap-up

What to Look For	What to Do
Altitude Illnesses	
Acute Mountain Sickness (AMS) • A generalized headache • Unusual tiredness • Appetite loss and nausea • Restless sleep with irregular breathing • Shortness of breath with exertion • Facial swelling • Rings on fingers feel tight	1. Rest and do not go any higher. 2. Wait and see. 3. Give Diamox for the prevention and treatment of mild AMS symptoms. 4. Give Decadron for severe headache. Decadron is more effective than Diamox. 5. Drink at least 4 to 5 quarts or liters of fluid daily, enough to maintain a copious flow of clear urine.
High Altitude Pulmonary Edema (HAPE) • Shortness of breath • Productive cough • Rattling or crackling and moist breathing or coughing • Cyanosis • Rapid pulse	1. Descend. 2. Give oxygen if available. 3. Commence treatment in a portable compression chamber. 4. Administer Diamox and/or nifedipine in accordance with prearranged instructions.
High Altitude Cerebral Edema (HACE) • Severe, constant, throbbing headache, like a bad toothache or migraine; no relief from acetaminophen, codeine, or a night's rest • Loss of coordination (ataxia) • Extreme fatigue • Vomiting • Coma	1. Descend. 2. If descent is not feasible, treat for several hours in a Gamow bag. 3. Have the victim sit propped up to improve breathing. 4. Give Decadron in small doses.

What to Look For   **What to Do**

Cold Injuries

What to Look For	What to Do
Mild Hypothermia • Shivering • Uncharacteristic behavior • Stiff muscles and cramps • Cold, pale, and blue-gray skin	1. Find shelter out of the wind and cold. 2. Light a fire or stove, change the victim's wet clothes, add layers to increase insulation. 3. If the victim is shivering strongly, remove wet clothing and allow shivering to continue inside a sleeping bag. 4. Give warm, sweet liquids. 5. Do not add anything warm to the skin; let shivering rewarm the body. 6. Never leave a hypothermic victim alone.
Severe Hypothermia • No shivering • Unresponsive behavior • Stiff muscles and uncoordinated movement • Weak, slow, irregular pulse • Slow breathing • Coma	1. Shelter everyone in the group and stop further heat loss. 2. Leave at least one person with the victim, and send the strongest, most competent members of the party for help. 3. Do not move if you have sent someone for help. 4. Do not rewarm unless in a very remote location.
Frostbite • White, waxy skin that has no feeling and is wooden to the touch • Possible thawing	1. Avoid a freeze-thaw-refreeze cycle. 2. If you are more than 8 hours from help, allow the part to thaw. 3. Keep the part clean. 4. Cover the part with a dry, protective dressing. 5. Elevate the limb above the level of the heart. 6. Do not massage or rub the area. 7. Evacuate as soon as possible.

What to Look For

What to Do

Heat Illness

What to Look For	What to Do
Heat Exhaustion • Inability to continue exercise or work • Headache, nausea, dizziness, and weakness • Rapid pulse • Thirst and profuse sweating • Gooseflesh, chills, and pale skin • Normal or moderately raised temperature	1. Have the victim rest in the shade and maximize air circulation. 2. Have the victim remove excess clothing. 3. Wet the victim with cold water to increase evaporation. 4. Have the victim drink fluids. 5. For more severe cases add $\frac{1}{4}$ teaspoon salt and 6 teaspoons sugar to 1 quart or liter of water.
Heatstroke • Altered mental status from slight confusion, agitation, disorientation to unresponsiveness • Rapid pulse • Dry or wet-moistened extremely hot skin when touched • Temperature above 106°F (41°C)	1. Remove the victim from heat. 2. Remove all of the victim's clothing down to the underwear to accelerate cooling. 3. Quickly use water or cold packs to cool the victim. 4. Monitor the victim's temperature frequently. 5. Evacuate after cooling.
Heat Cramps • Cramps in the calf, thighs, or abdomen	1. Stretch the affected muscles. 2. Give salted fluids; do not give salt tablets.

Poisons, Toxins, and Poisonous Plants

We are constantly encountering chemicals and plants whose toxic properties are unknown to us. Commonly used medications, pesticides, insect repellents, and sunscreens can be toxic to some people even when used appropriately, and they can be toxic to anyone if used inappropriately. The danger of misuse and overdosage is particularly likely in small children.

Chemical poisons are not common in the wilderness, and those most likely to be ingested are medications. You cannot be expected to know the antidote to every chemical. However, you should learn the simple principles used to treat most poisonings.

Few of us are expert in the identification of toxic plants and mushrooms. Nettle stings can result in trivial irritation for a short time, while eating a dangerous mushroom can result in death. As in so many areas of wilderness first aid, some knowledge of what we might encounter—what is dangerous and what is safe—is extremely important. The safest policy is never to touch or eat a plant unless you know, with certainty, that it is safe.

chapter
at a glance

▶ Carbon Monoxide Poisoning

▶ Toxic Plants and Poisons

▶ Plant-Induced Dermatitis

▶ Carbon Monoxide Poisoning

In the wilderness, the most likely causes of gas poisoning are carbon monoxide inhalation due to a faulty heater or stove or cooking on a stove in a tightly closed tent or snow cave 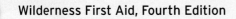 , or prolonged use of a car heater with the motor idling. Beware of the possible accumulation of a toxic gas as the cause of unresponsiveness in a confined space.

Victims of inhaled poisons are often unaware of the presence of a toxic gas. The symptoms of inhaled poisons worsen or improve, depending on the victim's proximity to the source—the closer to the source, the worse the symptoms. Do not become a victim yourself. Many people have been overcome while attempting to rescue another individual from a confined space.

What to Look For

- Flu-like symptoms without low-grade fever, generalized aching, or swollen glands.
- Similar symptoms in others exposed.
- Sick pets.
- Difficulty with breathing.
- Headache.
- Ringing in the ears (tinnitus).
- Chest pain (angina).

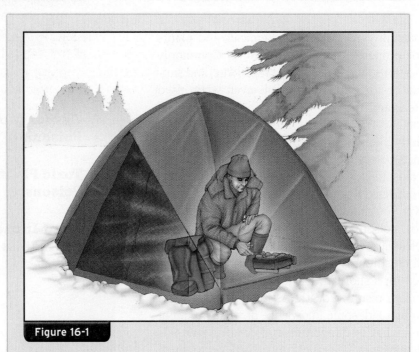

Figure 16-1

Cooking in a closed tent is dangerous and can lead to carbon monoxide poisoning.

- Muscle weakness.
- Nausea and vomiting.
- Dizziness and blurred or double vision.
- Altered mental status.
- Cardiac arrest.
- In the terminal stages of carbon monoxide poisoning, bright-pink skin (as opposed to victims of other forms of asphyxia, in whom the skin will be bluish-gray).

What to Do

1. Do not move into an enclosed space where someone has already collapsed without first trying to determine the cause of the problem.
2. When the site is safe, move the victim into fresh air immediately.
3. Check breathing, and if the victim is not breathing, initiate CPR.
4. Give the victim oxygen, if available.
5. Call for rescue; evacuate the victim as soon as possible.

▶ Toxic Plants and Poisons

Fortunately, most poison ingestions happen with products or plants of low toxicity or with amounts so small that severe poisoning rarely occurs. However, the potential for severe or fatal poisoning is always present.

Swallowed poisons usually remain in the stomach only a short time, and the stomach absorbs only small amounts. Most absorption takes place after the poison passes into the small intestine.

Do not eat plants you cannot identify. Never eat mushrooms unless you are absolutely certain that they are safe. In the rare event that someone in a wilderness setting far from medical help eats a potentially lethal mushroom, it may be necessary to induce vomiting. A teaspoonful of liquid soap in a cup of water may be the only agent available to induce vomiting, and it is frequently effective.

What to Look For

- Abdominal pain and cramping
- Nausea or vomiting
- Diarrhea
- Burns, odor, and stains around and in the mouth
- Drowsiness or unresponsiveness
- Poison containers or evidence of poisonous plants nearby

What to Do

1. Determine critical information, including the following:
   - Age and size of the victim
   - What was swallowed

CAUTION

DO NOT give water, milk, or other liquid to dilute poisons other than caustic or corrosive substances (acids and alkalis). They can dissolve a dry poison more rapidly allowing faster absorption.

DO NOT try to induce vomiting by any of these methods:

- gaging or tickling the back of the victim's throat with a finger or spoon handle.
- giving dish soap or raw eggs.
- giving syrup of ipecac.

DO NOT try to neutralize a poison.

DO NOT think there is a universal antidote for all poisons nor believe that most poisons have a specific antidote. An antidote is a substance that counteracts a poison's effects.

DO NOT give activated charcoal.

- How much was swallowed (for example, a taste or a handful)
- When it was swallowed

2. Place the victim on the left side to position the end of the stomach where it enters the small intestine straight up. Gravity will delay by as much as 2 hours advancement of the poison into the small intestine. The side position also helps prevent inhalation into the lungs if vomiting occurs.

3. Evacuate the victim as soon as possible.

4. If the poison is from a plant that you cannot identify, take a specimen for identification by an expert.

The treatment of severe poisoning in the wilderness might be impossible because antidotes such as activated charcoal likely will not be available. Evacuate all victims of suspected poisoning, preferably to a hospital, as soon as possible.

▶ Plant-Induced Dermatitis

Poison ivy, oak, and sumac are the three most common causes of contact dermatitis in the United States. Poison ivy can be found in every state except Hawaii and Alaska **Figure 16-2**. It is the most widespread of these three poisonous plants. Poison oak **Figure 16-3** occurs in two forms—western and southern. Poison sumac **Figure 16-4** is found in the swamps of the East and South.

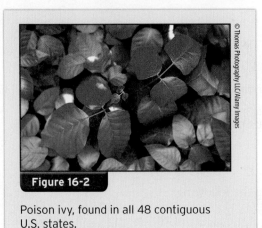

Figure 16-2

Poison ivy, found in all 48 contiguous U.S. states.

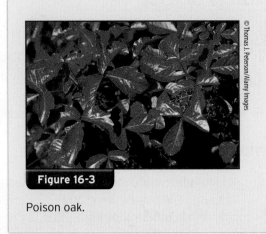

Figure 16-3

Poison oak.

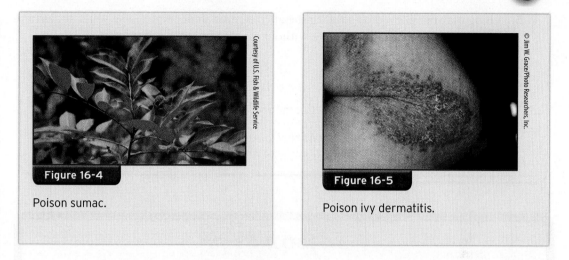

Figure 16-4

Poison sumac.

Figure 16-5

Poison ivy dermatitis.

The cause of the allergy is contact with a resin (urushiol) in the plant stalk and leaves. Nearly 50% of people in the United States are sensitive to the resin. A reaction called poison ivy dermatitis **Figure 16-5** develops within 8 to 48 hours after exposure, first as a line of small blisters where the skin brushed against the plant, followed by redness, swelling, and larger blisters. The blister fluid does not contain the irritant.

Resin can be transferred by clothing and the fur of animals. A pet can be the source of contact. The resin spreads soon after contact by the hands of the victim through scratching or during personal hygiene. Washing the hands after contact prevents further spread.

What to Look For

- Itching, redness, swelling, and blisters on skin exposed to the resin.
- Reactions starting 8 to 48 hours after exposure. The reaction can continue to erupt in different areas for several days.

What to Do

1. Wash the exposed body parts thoroughly with soap and water as soon as possible after known contact. The resin is firmly fixed to the skin within 30 minutes and then cannot be washed off except with special solutions. Many victims are unaware of their contact until the itching and rash begin, several hours or days later.
2. For mild, localized contact, apply calamine lotion or hydrocortisone ointment or cream, 1.0%.
3. For a more severe, generalized eruption, apply calamine as an immediate treatment, but seek medical care for treatment with prescription corticosteroids.
4. As a temporary measure, apply hydrocortisone ointment or cream, cover with a transparent plastic wrap, and lightly bind with an elastic or self-adhering bandage.

5. Itching may be relieved by soaking the affected area in hot water. The water should be as hot as the victim can tolerate without causing burns.

PREVENTION

- Those entering a wilderness area should learn to recognize dangerous plants, especially poison ivy, poison oak, and poison sumac.
- After hiking through infested areas, hikers should wash hands, clothes, and any accompanying pets. Barrier creams can be useful for preexposure prevention.

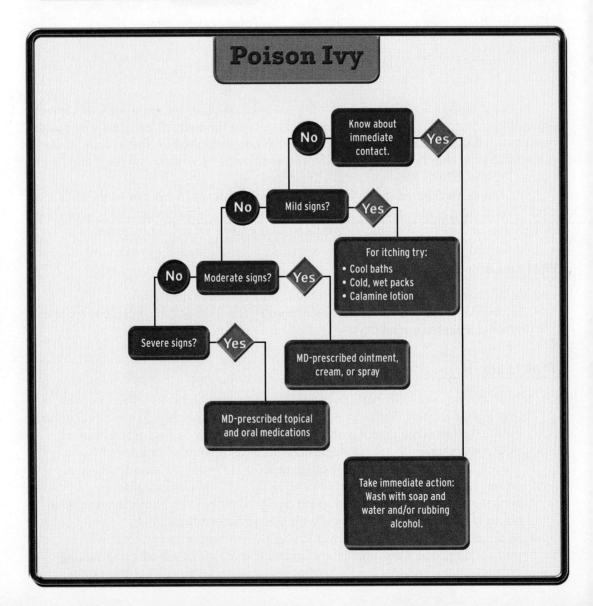

▶ Emergency Care Wrap-up

What to Look For	What to Do
Carbon Monoxide Poisoning • A complaint of winter flu • Similar symptoms in others exposed • Sick pets • Difficulty with breathing • Headache • Ringing in the ears • Chest pain • Muscle weakness • Nausea and vomiting • Dizziness and blurred vision • Altered mental status • Cardiac arrest • Bright-pink skin (late sign)	1. Do not enter an enclosed space where someone has already collapsed. 2. Move the victim into fresh air. 3. Check breathing, and if not breathing initiate CPR. 4. Give oxygen, if available. 5. Call for rescue. 6. Evacuate as soon as possible.
Toxic Plants and Poisons • Abdominal pain and cramping • Nausea or vomiting • Diarrhea • Burns, odor, stains around the mouth • Drowsiness or unresponsiveness • Poison containers or evidence of poisonous plants nearby	1. Determine critical information (age and weight of the victim, what was ingested, how much was ingested, time of ingestion). 2. Place the victim on the left side. 3. Evacuate as soon as possible. 4. Take a specimen of the plant with you if possible.
Plant-Induced Dermatitis • Itching, redness, swelling, and blisters on skin • Reactions starting 8 to 48 hours after exposure	1. Wash the exposed body parts thoroughly with soap and water as soon as possible after known contact. 2. For mild, localized contact, apply calamine lotion or hydrocortisone ointment or cream, 1.0%. 3. For a more severe, generalized eruption, apply calamine as an immediate treatment, but seek medical care for treatment with prescription corticosteroids.

17 Animal Bites, Human Bites, and Snake Bites

The wilderness traveler is sure to encounter animals; the species will depend on the geography. Animals vary in size and ferocity, but large and obviously aggressive animals are not the only ones that present danger. A small, rabid skunk is far more dangerous than a placid grizzly bear that turns and runs at the first sign of a human scent.

First aid providers should be aware of the animals they are likely to see, their appearance and identifying marks, and their habits and habitats. An attacking animal will not likely remain in the area, and the victim may be too frightened to give a coherent account and description. If the animal is large and has horns or antlers, precise identification of the animal is not as important as the injuries suffered. If, however, the animal is potentially venomous, identification can be critical in deciding whether to evacuate the victim.

Animal Bites

▶ Wild Animals

In Asia and Africa, attacks by elephants, hippos, lions, tigers, crocodiles, and snakes kill thousands of people every year. Snake bites alone cause 30,000 to 50,000 deaths per year in Asia, but fewer than 10 deaths per year in the United States and, in some recent years, no deaths.

In North America, the wild animals most likely to attack humans are bears, bison, moose, cougars, and alligators. Not all injuries are bites. Severe injuries result from victims being thrown in the air, gored by antlers, butted, or trampled on the ground. Injuries include puncture wounds, bites, lacerations, bruises, fractures, rupture of internal organs, and evisceration. Many small animals such as squirrels and chipmunks bite people trying to feed them; these bites are seldom serious. The dangers of infection and rabies are discussed later in the chapter.

> **PREVENTION**
>
> Prevention of animal attacks is the best treatment. Never approach or attempt to feed or touch a wild animal, even if it appears docile or other people are doing it. In bear country, every member of the party should carry bear repellant spray and make lots of noise so the bears will hear you. Wild animals will usually flee if they hear you coming. Attacks are more common if the animal is surprised.

▶ Domestic Animals

Most animal bites in the United States are inflicted by dogs (4 million bites yearly) and by cats. Dog bites can be severe and may even be fatal **Figure 17-1**. The simple bites tend to be puncture wounds; more severe bites are tearing lacerations.

Cat bites also should be treated seriously. The fangs of a cat are short and sharp and inflict puncture wounds that frequently become infected. Most cat bites occur on the hands and can puncture tendons and joints.

What to Do

The principles of treatment are the same for injuries inflicted by domestic or wild animals.

1. If the wound is not bleeding heavily, irrigate it with water for 5 to 10 minutes. Remove any foreign material. Only the superficial entrance of a puncture wound can be cleaned; extensive scrubbing cannot clean the depths of a puncture wound. Control bleeding with pressure.

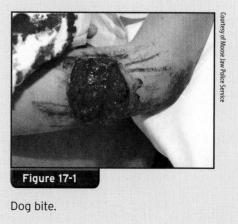

Courtesy of Moose Jaw Police Service

Figure 17-1

Dog bite.

2. If there is a possibility of rabies, wash the wound with soap and water or with benzalkonium chloride. Povidone-iodine may not be as effective but can be used.

3. After a large-animal attack, examine the victim for internal injuries.

4. Cover wounds with a sterile dressing. Do not close wounds, because this could trap bacteria, leading to an infection.

5. Evacuate the victim for further wound cleaning and closure and possible tetanus or rabies care.

▶ Rabies

Rabies is a viral infection of the brain that can follow the bite of a rabid animal. The disease only affects warm-blooded animals, and it can be fatal.

In North America, strict rabies-control programs in domestic animals have made the disease rare Figure 17-2 . The reservoir of rabies in wild animals, however, remains large. Animals

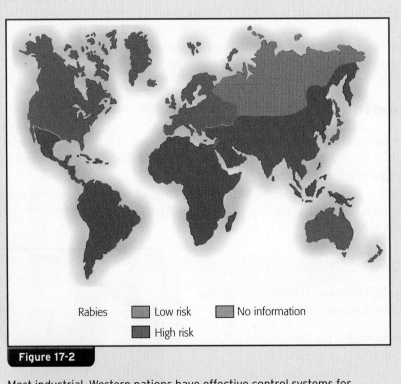

Rabies   ▢ Low risk   ▢ No information
         ▢ High risk

Figure 17-2

Most industrial, Western nations have effective control systems for domestic animals, but South and Central America, Africa, and Asia have poor controls and a high incidence of rabies in dogs. Some island countries, such as Britain and New Zealand, have eliminated rabies through strict quarantine regulations.

most commonly infected are skunks, raccoons, and bats. Foxes occasionally are found to be rabid, but rodents only rarely. In a recent year, only 148 domestic dogs in the United States were found to be infected.

Rabies is found in all climes but not in all countries. There are thousands of cases per year in many countries, but in the United States, there have been fewer than four human cases per year since 1980. All cases resulted from dog and bat bites, and the victims were mostly bitten outside the United States but developed rabies after returning home.

Consider rabies in the following situations:

- In an area or country where rabies is endemic.
- If a bite by a dog, cat, skunk, raccoon, or fox is unprovoked and the skin is broken.
- If the victim was bitten by a bat.
- If the victim was bitten by a large carnivore.
- If an already open wound or abrasion is licked by a potentially rabid animal.

Rabies vaccines and serum are effective even if given after exposure. The sooner antirabies serum is given after a bite, the better the chance of recovery. Because there is no other treatment, the correct management after exposure is very important.

What to Do

1. Wash the bite vigorously with a strong solution of soap and water or irrigate the bite marks with benzalkonium chloride. Iodine solutions are not as effective, but, in the absence of other agents, use povidone-iodine.

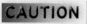

CAUTION

DO NOT
- Try to capture the animal yourself.
- Approach the animal.
- Kill the animal unless it is wild and likely to escape. If it is killed, protect the head and brain from damage for examination for rabies. Transport the dead animal intact to prevent exposure to potentially infected tissues or saliva. Refrigerate, but do not freeze, animal remains.

PREVENTION

Preventive immunization is recommended for veterinarians, zoologists, and biologists who handle wild animals.

- Bats are a common reservoir of rabies. Spelunkers who explore caves heavily occupied by bats should be immunized.
- In countries where rabies is common, travelers should take great care in approaching village dogs or cats, monkeys, or any wild animals.

2. The brain of an infected animal must be examined to make an exact diagnosis. Therefore it may be necessary to capture or kill the animal based on the following conditions:

- Domestic animals: Report the incident to the local health and animal control authorities. The animal will then be kept for 10 days to see if signs of rabies become obvious.
- Wild animals: It might be difficult or impossible to capture a wild animal. Kill or capture the animal only if feasible without risk of being bitten. Deliver the body to the local health authority for diagnostic examination.

Human Bites

Any contact between the teeth and saliva of one human that causes an open wound on another is, technically, a bite (for example, a hand injury caused by hitting another person's teeth during a fist fight is a bite). Wound infections are more common after human bites than animal bites.

▶ Treating Human Bites

What to Do

1. If the wound is not bleeding heavily, wash it with soap and water for 5 to 10 minutes. Rinse liberally with water under pressure from a faucet or irrigation syringe.
2. Control bleeding with pressure.
3. Cover the wound with a sterile dressing. Do not close the wound, because it could trap bacteria and lead to an infection.
4. Seek medical care and tetanus immunization, if needed. All tooth wounds over a joint should receive medical care as soon as possible.

Snake Bites

This section deals only with snakes found in North America **Figure 17-3** . Travelers to other areas should consult appropriate authorities for local information.

Only two snake families in the United States are poisonous: pit vipers (rattlesnakes, copperheads, and water moccasins) and coral snakes. Pit vipers have a triangular, flat head, wider than the neck; vertical, elliptical pupils (like a cat's eye); and a heat-sensitive pit located between the eye and nostril **Figure 17-4** , **Figure 17-5** , and **Figure 17-6** .

The coral snake is small and very colorful, with a series of bright red, yellow, and black bands that go all the way around its body **Figure 17-7** . Every other band is yellow, the red and yellow bands touch, and the snout is black. The color banding is similar to the nonvenomous king snake, but on the king snake the yellow and red bands are separated by black bands, and the snout is red. Remember the saying: "Red on yellow kill a fellow; red on black, venom lack."

The venom of young snakes is as toxic as that of adults, but the larger volume injected by adults usually causes a more-severe reaction.

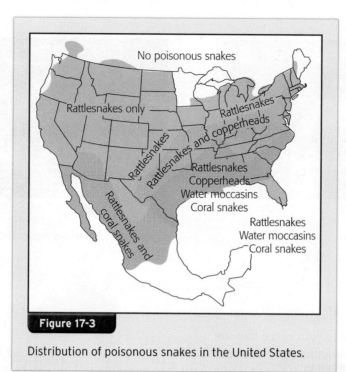

Figure 17-3

Distribution of poisonous snakes in the United States.

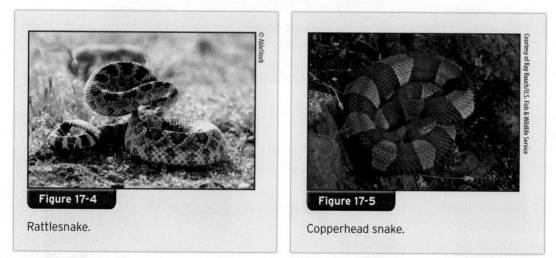

Figure 17-4

Rattlesnake.

Figure 17-5

Copperhead snake.

▶ Pit Viper Snake Bite

Rattlesnakes inflict about 65% of all venomous snake bites and cause nearly all snake-bite deaths in the United States. There are fewer than 15 snake-bite deaths per year in the United States.

About 25% of rattlesnake bites are dry; no venom is injected. There can be a fang mark, but no local or systemic symptoms.

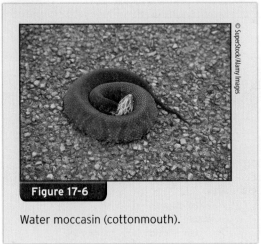

Figure 17-6

Water moccasin (cottonmouth).

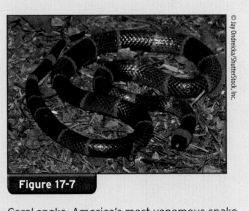

Figure 17-7

Coral snake, America's most venomous snake.

What to Look For

- Severe burning pain at the bite site.
- Two small puncture wounds about 0.25" to 1.5" apart (some cases have only one fang mark) **Figure 17-8** . If the snake has struck several times, there can be more than two fang marks.
- Swelling, starting within 5 minutes and progressing up the extremity in the next hour. Swelling can continue to advance up the limb for several hours.
- Discoloration after 2-3 hours and blood-filled blisters in 6-10 hours **Figure 17-9** .
- In severe cases: nausea, vomiting, sweating, weakness, bleeding, coma, and death.

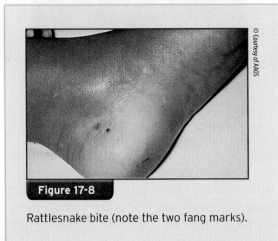

Figure 17-8

Rattlesnake bite (note the two fang marks).

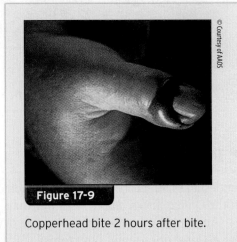

Figure 17-9

Copperhead bite 2 hours after bite.

What to Do

1. Get the victim and bystanders away from the snake. Snakes have been known to bite more than once. Pit vipers can strike from about one-half of their body length. Be careful around a decapitated snake's head or what appears to be a dead snake—it is able to bite reflexively for as long as 90 minutes after death.

2. Do not attempt to capture or kill the snake. It wastes valuable time, and there is a risk of additional bites. Identification of the snake is not usually needed because the same antivenom is used for all pit viper bites.

3. If there are immediate, severe symptoms, keep the victim quiet. Activity increases venom absorption.

4. If there is no immediate reaction, start to walk slowly with the victim to the trailhead or source of transportation. Carrying the victim may minimize exertion but requires more rescuers than may be available and may be slower. Sending for help can take longer than walking for help. If evacuation is prolonged and there are no symptoms after 6 to 8 hours, there has probably been no envenomation.

5. Gently wash the bitten area with soap and water. Any ring(s) or jewelry on a bitten extremity that might reduce blood circulation if swelling occurs should be removed.

6. Stabilize the bitten extremity (arm or leg) against movement with an arm sling or a splint as you would for a fracture.

NOTE

Snake Bite First Aid Controversy

For North American pit viper (rattlesnake, copperhead, and cottonmouth) bites, the American Heart Association/American Red Cross (AHA/ARC) recommends applying a pressure immobilization bandage to slow the dissemination of venom by slowing lymph flow.

The American College of Medical Toxicology's position statement [*Journal of Medical Toxicology*. 2011 Dec;7(4):324-326] disagrees with the AHA/ARC recommendation of applying a pressure immobilization bandage as a treatment for North American pit viper snake bites.

The main concern in North American pit viper envenomations is not death but tissue damage. Since most North American pit viper snake bite victims do not die, using a pressure immobilizer may result in increased tissue damage (necrosis). Applying an elastic bandage as a pressure immobilizer may be compared to a constriction bandage or tourniquet, which have been long discouraged for pit viper bites because they sequester venom in a small area, increasing the likelihood of greater tissue damage. Additionally, studies have shown that pressure immobilization bandages are commonly applied incorrectly, even in a simulated setting after receiving instruction and training.

In the past, many first-aid measures have been promoted and used in treating snake bites (ie, ice packs, cutting-and-sucking, electric shock, constriction band, suction devices), but none have been shown to be effective. (See the CAUTION box of DO NOTs.)

7. Keep the extremity at or slightly below heart level despite the fact that swelling might occur. Mark the progression of swelling up the extremity by drawing a line on the skin and writing the time with a pen to help a physician determine if antivenom should be given.

8. Evacuate to the nearest medical facility as soon as possible. Use the fastest means available. This is the most important thing to do for the victim. Antivenom is only available at hospitals and is most effective within 4 hours of the bite (not every venomous snake bite requires antivenom) but can be given a day or more following the bite and still be beneficial.

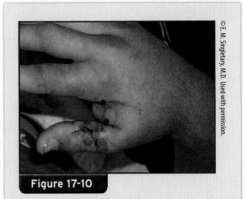
© E. M. Singletary, M.D. Used with permission.

Figure 17-10

Do not incise a snake bite.

CAUTION

DO NOT

- Use cold or ice, which does not inactivate the venom and poses a frostbite hazard.
- Use the cut-and-suck method, which can damage blood vessels and nerves **Figure 17-10**.
- Use mouth suction; your mouth is filled with bacteria, and you can infect the wound.
- Use electric shock; no medical studies support this method.
- Use a tourniquet, which can cause serious damage if it is too tight.
- Give alcohol, which dilates vessels and enhances shock.
- Use aspirin, which increases bleeding.

▶ Coral Snake Bite

The coral snake is America's most venomous snake, but it rarely bites humans. It is nocturnal and not aggressive. Its fangs are short, and it tends to hang on and chew venom into the victim rather than strike and release like a pit viper.

What to Look For

- Respiratory depression.
- Double vision.
- Difficulty in swallowing.
- Several hours can pass before the onset of these symptoms. Local, immediate signs are minimal. The absence of immediate symptoms is not evidence of a harmless bite.

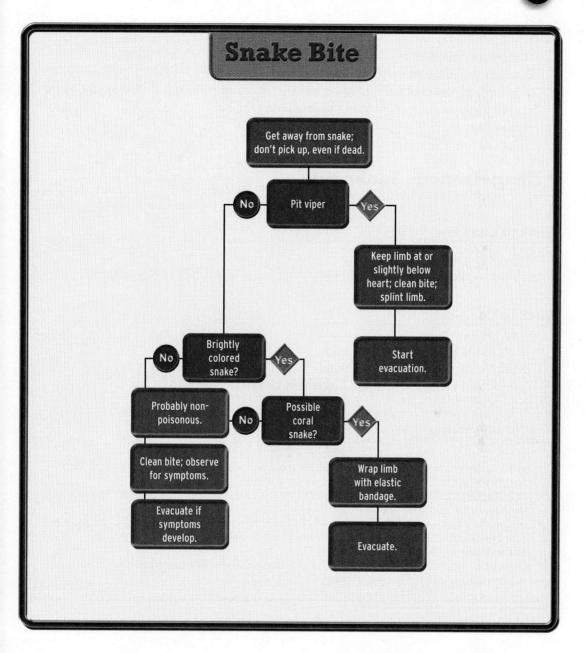

Snake Bite

Get away from snake; don't pick up, even if dead.

Pit viper

Yes → Keep limb at or slightly below heart; clean bite; splint limb. → Start evacuation.

No → Brightly colored snake?

Brightly colored snake? **Yes** → Possible coral snake?

Possible coral snake? **Yes** → Wrap limb with elastic bandage. → Evacuate.

Brightly colored snake? **No** → Probably non-poisonous. → Clean bite; observe for symptoms. → Evacuate if symptoms develop.

Possible coral snake? **No** → Probably non-poisonous.

What to Do

1. Keep the victim calm.
2. Clean the bite with soap and water.
3. Wrap a bitten limb with an elastic bandage, starting at the bite and wrapping along the length of the arm or leg and back again to the bite.
4. Evacuate the victim to a hospital for medical care.

▶ Nonpoisonous Snake Bite

What to Look For

- Horseshoe-shaped tooth marks
- Some swelling and tenderness but no evidence of significant envenomation

What to Do

1. Clean the bite with soap and water.
2. Care for the bite as a minor wound.
3. Seek medical care; a tetanus booster may be needed.

PREVENTION

- Make noise as you walk. Shuffle your feet or use a walking stick to thump the ground. Most snakes will flee if they hear you and usually only strike if surprised.
- At night, carry a flashlight and watch where you step. Most snakes are nocturnal and hide from the heat in the middle of the day.
- During the day, do not step into places where you cannot see; do not reach up to ledges or put your hands down holes. Wear high boots. If you see a snake, do not try to catch or kill it. Stand still and let it move away.
- If someone has been bitten, try to get one good look at the snake, and then leave it alone—avoid having additional victims to evacuate.

▶ Emergency Care Wrap-up

What to Look For	What to Do
Animal Attacks	
Domestic Animal Wounds • Puncture wounds • Lacerations • Bites or scratches from a dog or cat	1. If the wound is not bleeding heavily, irrigate it with water for 5 to 10 minutes. 2. Remove any foreign material. 3. Control bleeding with pressure. 4. If there is a possibility of rabies, wash the wound with soap and water or with benzalkonium chloride. 5. After a large animal attacks, examine the victim for internal injuries. 6. Cover wounds with a sterile dressing. 7. Evacuate the victim.
Rabies Consider rabies possible: • In an area or country where rabies is endemic • If a bite by a dog, cat, skunk, raccoon, or fox is unprovoked and the skin is broken • If bitten by a bat • If bitten by a large carnivore • If an already open wound or abrasion is licked by a potentially rabid animal	1. Wash the bite vigorously with soap and water or with benzalkonium chloride. 2. It may be necessary to capture or kill the animal.
Human Bites	
Human Bite • Any contact between the teeth and saliva of one human that causes an open wound on another	1. Wash the wound with soap and water. 2. Control bleeding with pressure. 3. Cover the wound with a sterile dressing. 4. Seek medical care.

What to Look For   **What to Do**

Snake Bites

What to Look For	What to Do
Pit Viper Bite • Severe burning pain at the bite site • Two small puncture wounds about $1/4$" to $1^1/_2$" apart • Swelling • Discoloration and blood-filled blisters • Nausea, vomiting, sweating, weakness, and bleeding	1. Get the victim away from the snake. 2. Do not attempt oral suction or incising the skin. 3. If there are immediate, severe symptoms, keep the victim quiet. 4. To be effective, antivenom is best given within 4 to 6 hours after the bite. 5. Start to evacuate all victims at once. 6. Use a sling or a splint to immobilize the limb loosely.
Coral Snake Bite • Local, immediate signs are minimal • Respiratory depression • Double vision • Difficulty in swallowing	1. Keep the victim calm. 2. Clean the bite with soap and water. 3. Wrap with an elastic bandage. 4. Evacuate to a hospital for medical care.
Nonpoisonous Snake Bites • Horseshoe-shaped tooth marks • Swelling or tenderness	1. Clean the bite with soap and water. 2. Care for the bite as a minor wound. 3. Seek medical care; a tetanus booster may be needed.

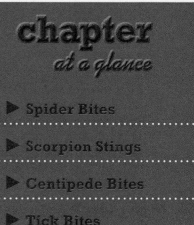

Insect and Arthropod Bites and Stings

Wilderness travelers generally worry about insects and take precautions to avoid being bitten. Most bites and stings are merely annoying; others can give rise to dangerous diseases, such as the bites of some ticks and mosquitoes.

This chapter discusses the more common bites and stings that occur in North America and does not discuss the dozens of species in other countries around the world that give painful or sometimes lethal bites. Travelers leaving North America should become familiar with the local insects and the diseases those insects carry. Information is available from state health departments or the Centers for Disease Control and Prevention.

Spider Bites

Many spiders are venomous, but few have either venom that is dangerous to humans or fangs long enough to penetrate human skin. Exceptions in North America include the black widow, brown recluse, hobo spider, and tarantula. Death from a spider bite is rare in North America.

▶ Black Widow Spider

The black widow spider is found throughout the world **Figure 18-1**. Only the female is dangerous; she has a glossy black body with a red spot (often in the shape of an hourglass) on the abdomen. Identification of a black widow spider bite is difficult because the spider itself is usually not seen.

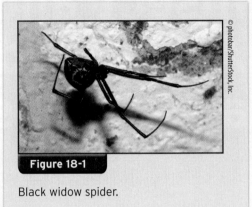

Figure 18-1

Black widow spider.

© photobar/ShutterStock, Inc.

What to Look For

- Possibly, a sharp pinprick sensation with no visible mark. However, some victims are unaware of being bitten.
- Faint red bite marks, which appear later.
- Muscle stiffness and cramps affecting the bitten limb and ascending to the abdomen and thorax.
- Headache, chills, fever, heavy sweating, dizziness, nausea, vomiting, and severe abdominal pain occurring later.

What to Do

1. If possible, catch the spider for identification. Save the body, even if it is crushed.
2. Clean the bitten area with soap and water.
3. Relieve pain with an ice pack on the bite. Administer pain medication orally.
4. Monitor breathing.
5. Seek medical care immediately.

▶ Brown Recluse Spider

The brown recluse is a nondescript spider with a brown, sometimes purplish, violin-shaped figure on its back **Figure 18-2**. It is generally found in the southern United States but has been identified as far north as Wisconsin.

The brown northwestern hobo spider can be mistaken for the brown recluse; it is similar in appearance but does not have a violin-shaped marking. Its bite can be painful, but it is not as dangerous as that of

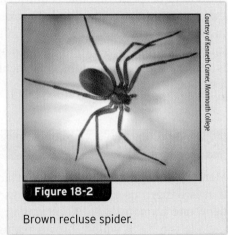

Figure 18-2

Brown recluse spider.

Courtesy of Kenneth Cramer, Monmouth College

the brown recluse. The two spiders are found in widely separate geographic locations. Find out which spiders are located in your travel area. The brown recluse should not be implicated only from an initial skin lesion, because other spider bites and even some insect bites can also result in a large area of redness with a central blister or small ulcer.

What to Look For

- During the early stages, a bite with a bull's-eye appearance—a central white core surrounded by red, ringed by a whitish or blue border **Figure 18-3**. A blister at the site, along with redness and swelling, appears 1 to 2 days after the bite.
- Local pain, which can remain mild but can become severe. It then subsides, to be replaced by aching and itching.
- Fever, weakness, vomiting, joint pain, and a rash may occur.

What to Do

1. Capture or kill the spider for identification.
2. Clean the bite with soap and water.
3. Relieve pain with an ice pack on the bite; give pain medication.
4. Seek medical care immediately.

▶ Tarantula

The North American variety of the tarantula—a large, hairy spider—has a frightening appearance but is almost always harmless **Figure 18-4**. There is moderate pain at the site of the bite but few later symptoms. In some areas other than North America, tarantulas are dangerous. Know the local species.

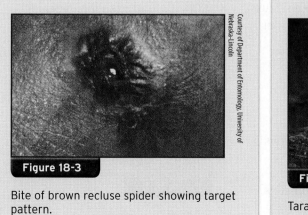

Courtesy of Department of Entomology, University of Nebraska-Lincoln

Figure 18-3

Bite of brown recluse spider showing target pattern.

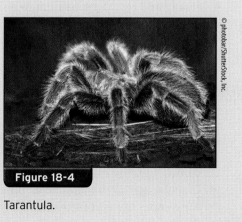

© photobar/ShutterStock, Inc.

Figure 18-4

Tarantula.

What to Do

1. Clean the bite with soap and water.
2. Relieve pain with an ice pack and pain medication.
3. Evacuate the victim if the species is known to be dangerous.

To care for a victim with embedded tarantula hairs:

1. Remove the hairs from the skin with sticky tape, repeating as necessary.
2. Wash the area with soap and water.
3. Apply hydrocortisone cream.
4. Give pain medication and an antihistamine.

Scorpion Stings

Scorpions are found worldwide in desert and semiarid regions ▬Figure 18-5▬. Dangerous species exist in both hemispheres. In the southwestern United States, the bark scorpion is potentially lethal to small children and the elderly if in poor health. Be aware of its appearance and distribution.

▶ Recognizing a Scorpion and Its Sting

Scorpions look like miniature lobsters; they have pincers and a long, upturned tail with a poisonous stinger. The sting causes immediate local pain and burning, followed by numbness or tingling. Symptoms include paralysis, muscle spasms, or breathing difficulties.

What to Look For

- Instant local pain and burning (all bites)
- Blurred vision, difficulty swallowing, slurred speech, numbness and tingling, occasional paralysis, muscle spasms, and breathing difficulties (severe bites)
- Jerking and twitching (similar to a seizure)
- More severe symptoms in children than adults

What to Do

1. Monitor the victim's breathing.
2. Clean the sting site with soap and water.
3. Put an ice pack on the sting to relieve pain.
4. Evacuate the victim as soon as possible. Antivenom use is controversial, largely due to its high price.

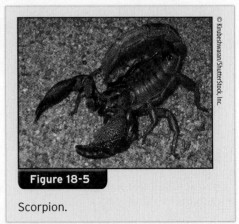

Figure 18-5

Scorpion.

Centipede Bites

Centipedes have small fangs and venom glands. If the fangs are long enough to penetrate skin, there can be local envenomation. Burning pain, swelling, and redness can last up to 3 weeks.

▶ Assessing and Treating Centipede Bites

What to Do

Most bites will get better without treatment.

1. Clean the wound with soap and water.
2. Apply an ice pack.
3. Give pain medication.
4. If symptoms persist, give antihistamine (Benadryl) or apply hydrocortisone ointment on the bite site.
5. Seek medical care for severe reactions.

Tick Bites

Tick bites are painless, and a tick can remain attached to someone for days without the victim being aware of its presence. See **Figure 18-6** and **Figure 18-7**. Some ticks can transmit serious diseases (including Lyme disease, Rocky Mountain spotted fever, and tick paralysis), but most tick bites are harmless. It is important to understand the difference between a blacklegged ("deer") tick and other types of ticks, such as Rocky Mountain wood and American dog ticks, because the medical treatment of their bites differs. Deer ticks are the main carriers of Lyme disease and are very small, usually the size of a pinhead. Most other ticks are larger, about 1/4 inch in length. If the tick is engorged with blood (round rather than flat), the victim should be evaluated by a physician for treatment with preventative antibiotics.

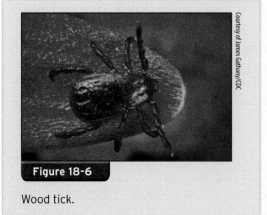

Courtesy of James Gathany/CDC

Figure 18-6

Wood tick.

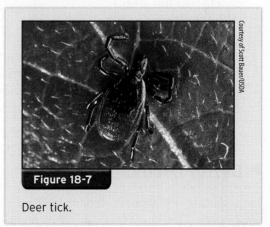

Courtesy of Scott Bauer/USDA

Figure 18-7

Deer tick.

▶ Assessing and Treating Tick Bites

What to Look For

- Tick on skin, not moving and not easy to brush off means it is imbedded
- Red area around tick means it has punctured skin and is feeding
- Engorgement, which increases the risk of infection
- Rash

What to Do

Ticks are difficult to remove because they secrete a cement that anchors them to the skin. Improper or partial removal can lead to local infection.

1. Use tweezers or a specially designed tool for tick removal, if available **Figure 18-8** .
   Grasp the tick close to the skin surface and lift the tick slightly upward. Hold in this position for at least one minute or untill the tick releases. If the tick does not release after one minute, pull up until the tick cames off. If the head is still embedded in the skin, remove it with a needle as you would a splinter.
2. Wash the bite with soap and water.
3. Put an ice pack on the bite to reduce pain.
4. Apply calamine lotion to relieve itching.
5. If the tick is engorged, seek medical advice. If medical advice is not available, such as during long, remote trips, consider starting preventative antibiotics. Discuss this with a physician before travel into high-risk areas.
6. Watch for signs of local infection or unexplained symptoms of tickborne illness (severe headache, fever, or rash) appearing 3 to 30 days after discovery of the tick. If symptoms appear, seek medical care.

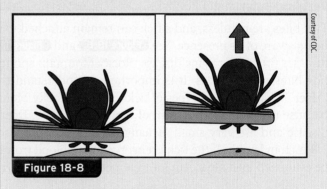

Courtesy of CDC.

Figure 18-8

Removing a tick with tweezers.

> **CAUTION**
>
> **DO NOT** use petroleum jelly, fingernail polish, rubbing alcohol, a hot match, petroleum products, or gasoline to remove ticks. They are ineffective.

▶ Lyme Disease

Lyme disease, a potentially serious tickborne infection, affects the joints, skin, heart, and nervous system. The disease is caused by a corkscrew-shaped bacterium that is transported by

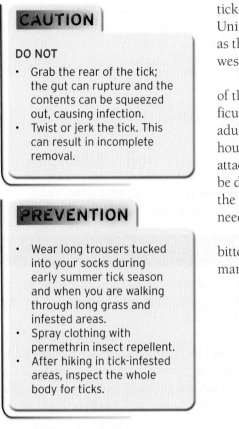

CAUTION

DO NOT

- Grab the rear of the tick; the gut can rupture and the contents can be squeezed out, causing infection.
- Twist or jerk the tick. This can result in incomplete removal.

PREVENTION

- Wear long trousers tucked into your socks during early summer tick season and when you are walking through long grass and infested areas.
- Spray clothing with permethrin insect repellent.
- After hiking in tick-infested areas, inspect the whole body for ticks.

ticks from deer and mice to humans. In the northeastern United States, the black-legged tick, commonly known as the deer tick, is the main carrier; in the West, it is the western black-legged tick.

Most infections are transmitted by the nymph form of the tick, which is about as big as a period (.) and difficult to see. Only 20% of infections are transmitted by adult ticks. The tick might have to be attached for 24 hours before transmitting infection; the longer a tick is attached, the greater the chance of infection. Since it may be difficult to know how long the tick has been attached, the best way to tell whether preventative antibiotics are needed is to see whether the tick is engorged.

Most victims of Lyme disease do not remember being bitten by a tick, because the disease might not become manifest until several weeks after the victim was bitten.

What to Look For

- In early stages (3 days to 1 month after the bite): a distinctive rash **Figure 18-9**, fatigue, fever, chills, weakness, headaches, stiff neck, muscle or joint pains.
- In later stages: one-sided paralysis, arthritis, meningitis, nerve or heart damage.

What to Do

If any symptoms develop within a month of a tick bite, seek medical care. Antibiotic treatment is usually curative, but is not necessary after every tick bite.

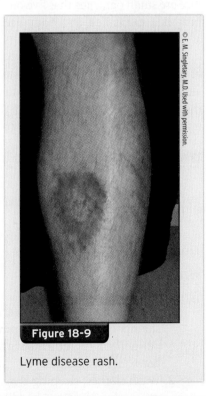

Figure 18-9

Lyme disease rash.

Mosquito Bites

Mosquitoes can carry many diseases, including West Nile virus, malaria, and yellow fever. Malaria and yellow fever have been eliminated from North America but are still common in other parts of the world. Travelers should know the local risks and take appropriate precautions. West Nile virus is a potentially fatal mosquitoborne disease that has recently spread to North America. There is no effective treatment for West Nile Virus. Prevention is critical for mosquitoborne illnesses. Travelers to areas of high mosquito density should use an effective repellant (DEET) as well as mosquito netting.

What to Do

1. Clean the wound with soap and water.
2. Apply an ice pack.
3. Apply calamine lotion or hydrocortisone ointment to decrease itching.
4. For a victim of numerous bites or a delayed allergic reaction, an antihistamine (Benadryl) every 6 hours or a physician-prescribed cortisone might be helpful.

Lice

Lice are small parasites that live on clothes, hair, or skin and drink blood. There are three types: head lice, pubic lice, and body lice. Body lice live on clothing, while head lice and pubic lice attach themselves to the hair shafts **Figure 18-10**. All cause itching.

Lice are passed from person to person by direct contact or through clothes, bedding, hats, or hairbrushes. Pubic lice are most likely passed by sexual contact. Head lice are very common among schoolchildren. Body lice usually accompany poor hygiene. Lice do not live outdoors in the wild, and lice discovered on a trip usually would have been brought from home or picked up in a dwelling. Lice live only 2 to 3 weeks off the body on clothes and sleeping bags.

What to Look For

- Small (1-2 mm) black lice attached to the hair shafts.
- Small white wormlike larvae (nits)
- Red rash or streaks
- Severe itching of affected area

What to Do

1. Treat victims with nonprescription lice shampoo or lotion containing permethrin, pyrethrins with piperonyl butoxide, or lindane.
2. Wash clothes, sleeping bags, pillowcases, or other bedding in soap and hot water.
3. Do not share clothes or hairbrushes.

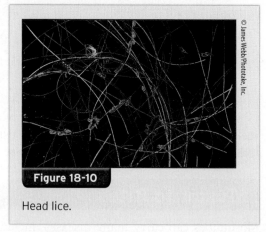

© James Webb/Phototake, Inc.

Figure 18-10

Head lice.

Insect Stings

More people die every year in the United States from bee, hornet, and wasp stings than from snake bites. The common stinging insects are the honeybee, bumblebee, hornet, wasp, and fire ant. A single sting to a severely allergic person can be fatal within minutes to an hour. Many people who die have had no previous history of severe reactions to stings. Multiple stings can kill, whether or not the victim is allergic to stinging insects. Massive attacks inflicting multiple stings are rare, but with the entrance of Africanized killer bees into the United States from South and Central America, multiple-sting cases are likely to increase. The venom of these bees is no more potent than that of the European type; however, killer bees earned their nickname from their aggressiveness and swarming attacks.

▶ Assessing and Treating Insect Stings

The sooner symptoms develop after the sting, the more serious the reaction. The responses of victims vary. One sting is not necessarily equivalent to another, even within the same species, because the amount of venom injected varies from sting to sting.

Stings to the mouth or eyes are more dangerous than stings to other body areas. The most dangerous stings in nonallergic individuals are those inside the throat, from accidentally swallowing an insect. Swelling in the airway—though not an allergic reaction—can cause serious obstruction to breathing.

Each wasp can sting multiple times, but each bee can only sting once. The bee stinger pulls off of the bee and pulls the venom sac with it. The venom sac can continue to pump venom into the skin for up to 3 minutes.

What to Look For

- A stinger may be visible, embedded in the skin.
- Local reactions: brief pain, redness and swelling around the sting site, itching, and heat.
- Generalized reactions: diffuse skin redness, hives, localized swelling of the lips or tongue, a tickle in the throat, wheezing, abdominal cramps, and diarrhea.
- Life-threatening reactions: inability to breathe due to swelling of the air passages and throat, bluish or gray skin color, seizures, and unresponsiveness.

CAUTION

DO NOT pull the stinger with tweezers or fingers because you can squeeze more venom into the victim from the attached venom sac.

What to Do

1. Look for a stinger, and, if found, remove it as soon as possible using any removal method (eg, brush it off with your hand or use a fingernail, credit card, or back of a knife). Do not squeeze the venom sac. Only bees leave their stinger embedded.

PREVENTION

DO NOT approach or disturb wasp, bee, and ant nests. Do not walk in grass with bare feet. Choose campsites with care.

Those who have had a serious reaction to an insect sting should carry with them a kit with self-injectable epinephrine at all times, wear a medical alert bracelet/necklace identifying them as allergic to insect stings, and see an allergist for desensitization.

2. Wash the sting site with soap and water.
3. Apply cold to the sting site for 15 to 20 minutes to relieve pain.
4. To relieve pain and itching, give the victim a pain medication (such as acetaminophen or ibuprofen) or use a topical medication. Use hydrocortisone cream and antihistamine pills to reduce local symptoms.
5. A paste made from baking soda and water may help absorb venom and relieve pain, except for wasp stings.
6. Observe victims for at least 60 minutes for signs of a serious allergic reaction.
7. If the victim develops hives or redness and swelling all over the body and difficulty breathing, immediately administer epinephrine if it is available. A large local reaction does not require epinephrine and does not indicate a risk of serious reaction after future stings.

Insect Repellents

Chemical insect repellents include natural repellents (citronella and lemon eucalyptus); synthetic repellents (DEET and dimethylphthalate); and insecticides (permethrin, deltamethrin, and alphamethrin).

Citronella and lemon eucalyptus provide 1 to 2 hours of protection. They are safe but not very effective and not recommended where serious protection is needed.

DEET (N, N-diethyl-m-toluamide) is the most widely used repellent. Allergic reactions can occur when DEET is applied to the skin in high concentrations. Although higher concentrations provide longer protection, new formulations have prolonged effect at lower concentrations. Some of the chemical is absorbed through the skin, and toxic reactions have been reported in small children. To avoid toxic effects, avoid using DEET on the lips, eyes, and broken skin. Do not use DEET on infants. On children, especially, use low concentrations (10%) applied more frequently rather than high concentrations applied infrequently. DEET can be applied to clothing but can damage some synthetic fabrics, including polyesters.

Permethrin is an effective repellent against ticks, chiggers, mosquitoes, fleas, and sand flies. It should be applied only to clothing, not to the skin. Clothing, sleeping nets, or tents can be impregnated with permethrin by spraying or soaking them in a solution. Permethrin does not stain, discolor, or degrade fabrics or plastics, and it maintains effectiveness on fabrics for weeks to months, even persisting through multiple washings.

In areas with mosquitoborne diseases, a permethrin-impregnated sleeping net is important protection. In addition, travelers should wear long-sleeved shirts and long pants during dusk and dawn, when mosquitoes are most active. The combination of DEET on skin and permethrin on clothing provides maximum protection.

▶ Emergency Care Wrap-up

What to Look For	What to Do
Spider Bites	
Black Widow Spider • A sharp pinprick may be felt • Faint red bite marks • Muscle stiffness and cramps • Headache, chills, fever, heavy sweating, dizziness, nausea, vomiting, and severe abdominal pain	1. If possible, catch the spider for identification. 2. Clean the bitten area with soap and water. 3. Relieve pain with an ice pack on the bite. 4. Administer pain medication orally. 5. Monitor breathing. 6. Seek medical care immediately.
Brown Recluse Spider • Bite with a bull's-eye appearance • Local pain • Fever, weakness, vomiting, joint pain, and a rash	1. Clean the bite with soap and water. 2. Relieve pain with an ice pack on the bite. 3. Give pain medication. 4. Capture or kill the spider for identification. 5. Seek medical care.
Tarantula • Moderate pain • Few later symptoms	1. Clean the bite with soap and water. 2. Relieve pain with an ice pack on the bite. 3. Evacuate the victim if the species is known to be dangerous.
Scorpion Stings	
• Instant local pain and burning • Blurred vision, difficulty swallowing, slurred speech, numbness and tingling, occasional paralysis, muscle spasms, and breathing difficulties • Jerking and twitching	1. Check breathing. 2. Clean the sting site with soap and water. 3. Relieve pain with an ice pack on the sting. 4. Evacuate the victim as soon as possible.
Centipede Bites	
• Burning pain • Swelling • Redness	1. Most bites will get better without treatment. 2. Administer antihistamines or apply hydrocortisone ointment on the bite if symptoms persist.

What to Look For	What to Do
Tick Bites	
Tick Bites • Embedded and engorged tick	1. Remove the tick using tweezers or a commercial tick removal device. 2. Wash the bite with soap and water. 3. Watch for signs of local infection. 4. If the tick is engorged, seek medical advice.
Lyme Disease • Distinctive rash, fatigue, fever, chills, weakness, headaches, stiff necks, muscle or joint pains • One-sided paralysis, arthritis, meningitis, nerve or heart damage	1. Seek medical care. 2. Antibiotic treatment is usually curative.
Lice • Small (1-3 mm long) insects attached to hair shafts or on clothing • Itching at infected areas	1. Treat with lice shampoo or lotion. 2. Wash clothes, sleeping bags, pillowcases, or other bedding in soap and hot water. 3. Do not share clothes or hairbrushes.
Insect Stings Bee, Hornet, and Wasp Stings • Brief pain, redness and swelling • Diffuse skin redness, hives, localized swelling of lips or tongue, tickle in throat, wheezing, abdominal cramps, diarrhea • Inability to breathe due to swelling of the air passages and throat, bluish or gray skin color, seizures, unconsciousness	1. Look for a stinger embedded in the skin and remove it immediately. 2. Wash the sting site with soap and water. 3. Apply a cold pack to the sting site for 15 to 20 minutes. 4. Give a mild analgesic or use topical medication. 5. Observe the victim for at least 60 minutes for signs of a serious allergic reaction.

Water Emergencies

© Photos.com

Submersion Incidents

Experts on the first World Congress on Drowning defined drowning as "the process of experiencing respiratory impairment from submersion/immersion in liquid."

Most submersion incidents are preventable. Teaching children to swim at a young age, close observation of toddlers around water, and minimizing drug and alcohol use around water would prevent the majority of incidents. For wilderness trips, general safety precautions, setting up of safety lines when crossing streams, and knowing the limits of your team and the hazards of the environment will help you minimize the risk of submersion incidents.

What to Look For

The victim is seen struggling in the water, floating motionless, or lying at the bottom of a body of water.

What to Do

The essentials of first aid for any water emergency are effecting a safe rescue, checking for breathing, and transporting the victim to the nearest medical facility.

1. Assess your resources and abilities before attempting a rescue. Rescue of a submerged or drowning victim can be dangerous.
2. Rescue the victim. Remember, do not become a victim yourself! The following guidelines are suggested for getting a victim safely out of the water: reach, throw, row, go **Figure 19-1** .
3. Treat the victim.
   - If the victim is unresponsive, check his or her breathing.
   - If there is no breathing, begin CPR.
   - If the first breath does not go in, retilt the head and try again. If the second breath does not go in, give the victim cycles of 30 chest compressions (just like CPR), check the victim's mouth for objects, and give the victim two breaths.
   - Protect the spine in unresponsive victims and in victims of diving and/or surfing accidents.
4. Perform resuscitation.
   - You need not start resuscitation if an adult is known to have been submerged more than 60 minutes in warm water.
   - Stop resuscitation after 30 minutes if there are no signs of life, unless the victim has been submerged in very cold water.

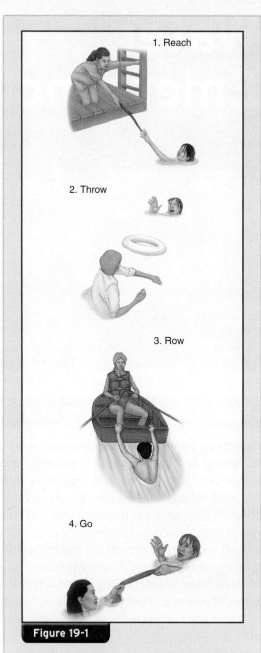

Figure 19-1

Water rescue sequence. Use all available techniques for water rescue before swimming to the victim. If you must swim, take something with you (such as a float, towel, or branch) that you can extend to the victim; this makes it harder for the victim to grab you as you attempt rescue.

- If submersion has been in very cold water, continue resuscitation for at least 60 minutes with concurrent attempts to warm the victim.
- If there is a heartbeat or a pulse, continue rescue breathing until spontaneous respirations resume or as long as possible.

5. Evacuate all victims who have been resuscitated. Assess the situation. Outside assistance may be required to transport the victim safely to the nearest medical facility or a higher level of care. Think about your resources and the best way to handle the situation while minimizing further risk to other members of the rescue team.

6. Victims not requiring resuscitation and whose only initial symptoms have been coughing or vomiting require close observation but not immediate evacuation; evacuate for medical evaluation if cough or shortness of breath increases.

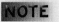

NOTE

Remember, immediate treatment by ventilation at the scene is the most important factor in survival.

Scuba Diving Injuries

Scuba (self-contained underwater breathing apparatus) divers should be familiar with the medical problems of diving from their certified training course **Table 19-1**. Those who do not dive should understand the basic problems that divers face and know how to begin appropriate treatment.

As a diver descends, water pressure on the body increases. For each 33 feet of descent, the pressure increases by 1 atmosphere (1 atmosphere [atm] = 14.7 pounds per square inch [psi]). Sea level = 1 atm; 33 feet = 2 atm; and 66 feet = 3 atm.

Table 19-1 Problems Associated with Scuba Diving	
Dysbarism	Environmental Problems
• barotrauma	• motion sickness
• air embolism	• near drowning
• decompression sickness	• hypothermia
Breathing-Gas Problems	• heat illness
• nitrogen narcosis	• sunburn
• oxygen toxicity	Miscellaneous Problems
• hypoxia	• hyperventilation
• carbon monoxide poisoning	• panic/anxiety
Hazardous Marine Life	

This changing pressure is exerted over the entire body and has two main effects. First, more gases can dissolve in the blood and tissues than at normal pressures. Second, pressure changes result in changes in the volume of gas in gas-containing areas of the body (lungs, ears, and sinuses). Increasing pressure during descent results in a decrease in gas volume, which reexpands upon ascent. If gas pressure cannot equilibrate, the compression upon descent or the expansion during ascent can cause pain and rupture of blood vessels, eardrums, or air sacs of the lung. If an air sac ruptures into one of the larger blood vessels, a large amount of air can suddenly enter the circulation, causing arterial gas embolism (AGE). Damage due to pressure changes is called barotraumas.

As the diver descends, more and more nitrogen dissolves in the blood and tissues. If ascent is too rapid, the nitrogen gas forms bubbles in the blood and tissue. Illnesses and injuries due to the mechanical effects of pressure changes are called dysbarism. Divers must monitor their total time under water and maximum depth, and adhere to precise schedules of ascent to avoid dysbarism.

▶ Breathing-Gas Problems

As depth and pressure increase, more gases are able to dissolve in the blood than at normal pressure. Even oxygen, when enough has dissolved in the blood, can cause toxic reactions such as visual changes, confusion, and seizures. Increased nitrogen can cause nitrogen narcosis ("rapture of the deep") leading to severe impairment of judgment, hallucinations, and unconsciousness. Hypoxia can occur when air for breathing is accidentally used up.

▶ Decompression Illnesses (Dysbarism)

The most serious dysbarisms are decompression sickness ("the bends") and AGE. AGE can cause sudden death and develops within 5 minutes of surfacing. Decompression sickness causes severe pain as bubbles form in the joints, nervous system, and other parts of the body. It can develop right after surfacing or it can be delayed hours to days. Confusion and death can also result from decompression sickness.

What to Look For

AGE

- Unconsciousness
- Paralysis or weakness
- Convulsions
- Cardiac/respiratory arrest
- Dizziness or visual problems

Decompression Sickness

- Joint or limb pain
- Paralysis
- Fatigue and weakness
- Breathing difficulty
- Numbness or tingling
- Rash

What to Do

Regardless of the cause, most diving injuries can be treated initially with similar measures **Figure 19-2**.

1. Evaluate the victim's breathing and resuscitate as needed. Barotrauma might have caused near drowning.
2. Give the victim 100% oxygen. Early administration of 100% oxygen is very important. Contact the local EMS as soon as possible.
3. Place the victim in the recovery position.
4. If the victim is conscious and alert, give him or her sips of water—no alcohol.
5. Protect the victim from excessive cold and heat.
6. If a seizure occurs, prevent injury and maintain the airway. Continue giving the victim 100% oxygen.
7. Evaluate the victim for other injuries, minor barotrauma problems, or environmental problems such as hypothermia.

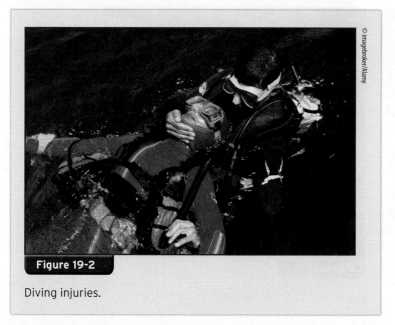

Figure 19-2

Diving injuries.

Table 19-2 Neurologic Examination

1. Is the diver oriented to person, place, and time?
2. Does the victim have normal vision and movement, and are the pupils equal? Is there any jerking motion in the eyes?
3. Is the victim able to smile, grit his or her teeth, and whistle? Is sensation in the face normal?
4. Does the victim have normal hearing?
5. Is the victim able to swallow?
6. Is the victim able to move his or her tongue in all directions?
7. Is the victim weak? Is muscle strength equal on both sides?
8. Does the victim have normal sensory perception on both sides? Is there any numbness or are there complaints of tingling?

8. Do a neurologic examination Table 19-2 .
9. Contact the local EMS and Divers Alert Network (DAN)—1-919-684-9111 (24-hour diving emergencies).
10. Get the victim with decompression sickness to recompression therapy in a hyperbaric (pressurized) chamber Figure 19-3 .

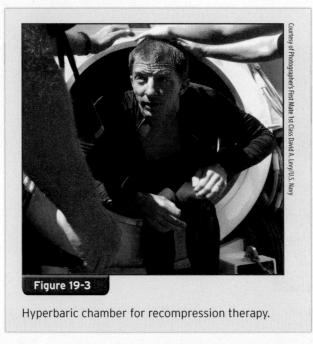

Courtesy of Photographer's First Mate 1st Class David A. Levy/U.S. Navy

Figure 19-3

Hyperbaric chamber for recompression therapy.

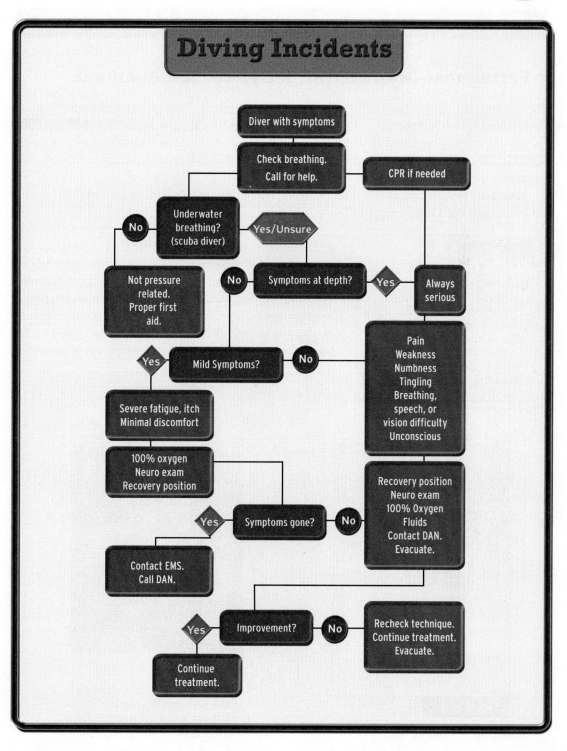

Marine Animal Stings

▶ Portuguese Man-of-War, Jellyfish, Sea Anemone

The Portuguese man-of-war and the jellyfish are two members of a large group of sea animals—coelenterates—with tentacles containing stinging organs called nematocysts **Figure 19-4**. Swimmers and divers who brush against nematocysts can receive serious, painful injuries **Figure 19-5**. When washed ashore or onto rocks, dead jellyfish or tentacle fragments can still sting for a long time.

Reactions to stings vary from mild to severe. Although most victims recover without medical care, some need it immediately.

Portuguese man-of-war stings cause well-defined, whiplike welts or scattered red blotches, which usually disappear within 24 hours. Jellyfish stings cause burning pain that lasts half an hour, severe muscle cramping, and multiple thin lines of zigzag welts that can disappear within a few hours. The severity of the reaction depends on the species, the number of nematocysts triggered, the age and health of the victim, and the extent of contact.

CAUTION

- For Portuguese Man-of-War stings, do not apply meat tenderizer, baking soda, alcohol, or papain.
- For all jellyfish stings, do not rub off the tentacles from the victim's skin—this activates the stinging cells.

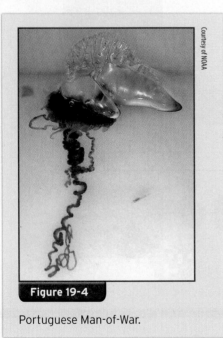

Courtesy of NOAA

Figure 19-4

Portuguese Man-of-War.

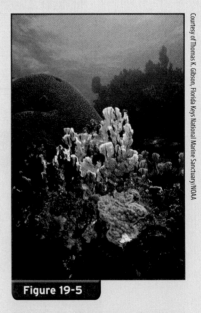

Courtesy of Thomas K. Gibson, Florida Keys National Marine Sanctuary/NOAA

Figure 19-5

Fire coral is in the same family as the Portuguese man-of-war. It has tiny nematocyst-bearing tentacles on the surface that cause the sting.

What to Look For

- Pain, varying in severity
- Whiplike streaks on the skin
- Blisters, welts, scattered red blotches within 24 hours
- In more severe cases, headache, dizziness, paralysis, and anaphylaxis
- Possible coelenterate poisoning in all cases of unexplained collapse in ocean swimmers

What to Do

A treatment useful for one jellyfish species may worsen an envenomation from another jellyfish species. This contributes to confusion about what treatment is best for stings.

1. **Immediately remove tentacles.** Tentacles may detach and stick to the skin. Remove them as soon as possible by washing the affected skin with seawater for at least 30 seconds. Avoid using fresh water because it may activate the venomous stingers (nematocysts) that are embedded in the skin. Do not touch the tentacles with your hands. Do not try to rub the tentacles off with a towel or clothing because it may cause the discharge of more venom. Removing tentacles with tweezers may also discharge more venom.
2. **Deactivate stingers.** Soak the affected skin with vinegar for 30 minutes. If vinegar is not available, apply a mixture of baking soda and water.
   Confusion exists about using vinegar. A review of 19 pertinent primary medical articles (*Annals of Emergency Medicine*. 2012;60:399-414) disagrees about using vinegar because it increases pain or nematocyst discharge in most jellyfish species and therefore should not be used.
3. **Relieve pain or irritation.** Use nonscalding hot water either by a shower or immersing for at least 20 minutes for all jellyfish stings in North America and Hawaii. Lidocaine, an over-the-counter medication, can be applied on the affected skin. However, these treatments are not always available at beach or diving sites.

The following remedies should be avoided because research does not support them or they have been shown to be ineffective: human urine, meat tenderizer, fresh water, alcohol, and pressure bandages. Be prepared to treat an allergic reaction with an antihistamine (Benadryl) or, if the reaction is life-threatening, help the victim administer his or her prescribed epinephrine available in a preloaded syringe.

Other Marine Life

Stingrays, sea urchins **Figure 19-6**, stonefish, and scorpion fish are found in temperate, subtropical, and tropical waters, generally in shallow, sheltered bays. When a person steps on a ray, the tail whips up and the stinging organ is thrust into the foot. The large tail barb can also cause a severe laceration; the venom causes intense burning pain at the site, and pieces of the barb can remain in the wound. Urchins and fish barbs can also break off in the victim.

Stonefish and scorpion fish venom is very toxic and can cause death.

What to Do

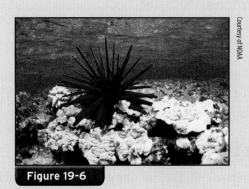

Courtesy of NOAA

Figure 19-6

1. Irrigate the injured part with water immediately to remove venom and relieve pain; soak in hot water for 30 to 90 minutes. The water must be as hot as the victim can tolerate.
2. Remove obvious pieces of the spine.
3. Treat as a puncture wound.
4. Seek medical care promptly. Pieces of spine can be embedded in the wound. Consider a tetanus booster.
5. If a poisonous fish is suspected (such as stonefish or scorpion fish), seek medical care immediately.

Sea urchin. Fish, ray, and urchin wounds can require exploration of the wound for embedded pieces of the spine.

▶ Emergency Care Wrap-up

What to Look For   **What to Do**

Submersion Incidents

Drowning

- The victim is seen struggling in the water, floating motionless, or lying at the bottom of a pool

1. Assess your resources and abilities before attempting rescue.
2. Rescue the victim. Remember Reach, Throw, Row, Go sequence.
3. Check breathing.
4. Perform CPR if needed.
5. Evacuate all victims who have been resuscitated.

Scuba Diving Injuries

Arterial Gas Embolism

- Unconsciousness
- Paralysis or weakness
- Convulsions
- Cardiac/respiratory arrest
- Dizziness or visual problems

1. Evaluate breathing, resuscitate as needed.
2. Give 100% oxygen.
3. Place victim in the recovery position.
4. If victim is conscious and alert, give sips of water.
5. Protect victim from excessive cold and heat.
6. If a seizure occurs, prevent injury and maintain the airway.
7. Evaluate for other injuries.
8. Contact the local EMS and DAN.
9. Get the victim with decompression sickness to recompression therapy in a hyperbaric chamber.

What to Look For	What to Do
Decompression Sickness • Joint or limb pain • Paralysis • Fatigue and weakness • Breathing difficulty • Numbness or tingling • Rash	1. Evaluate breathing, resuscitate as needed. 2. Give 100% oxygen. 3. Place victim in the recovery position. 4. If victim is conscious and alert, give sips of water. 5. Protect victim from excessive cold and heat. 6. If a seizure occurs, prevent injury and maintain the airway. 7. Evaluate for other injuries. 8. Contact the local EMS and DAN. 9. Get the victim with decompression sickness to recompression therapy in a hyperbaric chamber.

Marine Animal Stings

What to Look For	What to Do
Portugese Man-of-War, Jellyfish, and Sea Anemone Stings • Pain • Whiplike streaks on the skin • Blisters, welts, or scattered red blotches • Headache, dizziness, paralysis, anaphylaxis	1. Immediately remove tentacles by washing with seawater. 2. Deactivate stingers by soaking the area in vinegar or with mixture of baking soda and water. 3. Relieve pain or irritation using nonscalding hot water on the area for at least 20 minutes.
Other Marine Injuries • Stings to the foot • Severe lacerations • Intense burning at the site	1. Irrigate the injured part with water. 2. Soak in nonscalding hot water for 30 to 90 minutes. 3. Remove obvious pieces of the spine. 4. Treat as a puncture wound. 5. Seek medical care promptly.

CPR Basics

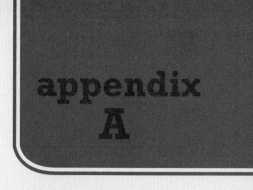

To obtain the skills necessary to resuscitate a person who has stopped breathing or is without circulation, you should take a course in cardiopulmonary resuscitation (CPR). This chapter will provide you only with the essentials required to start resuscitation until someone with more skill takes over or the situation becomes obviously hopeless.

CPR

▶ CPR in the Wilderness

CPR is effective only if it is started quickly and followed by advanced life support, which includes electrical defibrillation of the heart. In the wilderness, the chances of success with CPR alone are slight. You should therefore face the fact that few victims who require CPR in the wilderness will survive. But, in spite of that, you should be prepared to start CPR when necessary.

CPR has two parts: rescue breathing and chest compression.

▶ When to Start CPR

Start CPR on a motionless person in whom it is known that breathing has stopped. If the person is hypothermic, the delay in starting can be considerably longer, depending on the temperature of the victim.

What to Do for Adults (8 Years and Older) and Children (1 to 8 years)

1. Make sure the scene is safe before approaching the victim.
2. Tap the victim's shoulder and shout, "Are you OK?"
3. If the victim does not respond and is not breathing or is gasping, he or she needs CPR. You or someone else should call 9-1-1 and get an AED (automated external defibrillator), if available. Then roll the victim's head and body into a face-up position, if necessary **Figure A-1**.
4. Begin CPR with 30 chest compressions. Place the heel of your hand in the center of chest with the other hand on top and fingers interlaced. Push down at least 2 inches.

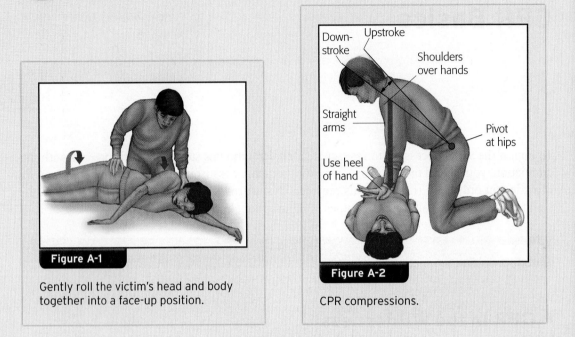

Figure A-1

Gently roll the victim's head and body together into a face-up position.

Figure A-2

CPR compressions.

The rate of compressions is faster than once per second (100 compressions a minute; use the beat of the Bee Gee's "Stayin' Alive" song). After each compression, let the chest come back up to its normal position **Figure A-2** .

5. Open the airway with the head tilt–chin lift maneuver.
6. Pinch the victim's nose and make an airtight mouth-to-mouth seal.
7. Give two rescue breaths with each lasting 1 second. Blow enough to make the chest rise. If the first breath does not go in and make the chest rise, the airway may be blocked. Retilt the head and give a second breath. If the second breath does not make the chest rise, begin CPR (cycles of 30 chest compressions and 2 breaths). Each time the airway is opened before giving the first breath, look for an object in the victim's mouth and, if seen, remove it **Figure A-3** . If the two breaths go in and make the chest rise, you do not need to look for an object before giving the first breath each time.
8. Continue CPR with 30 chest compressions and 2 breaths. See the section **When to Stop** for guidelines about how long to continue.

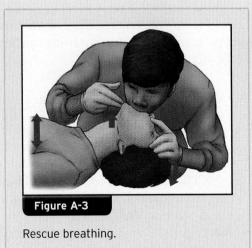

Figure A-3

Rescue breathing.

▶When to Give Prolonged CPR (longer than 30 minutes)

Give prolonged CPR when one of the following is present:

- The victim is hypothermic with a compressible chest.
- The victim has been submerged in cold water.
- There is cardiac arrest due to lightning or electric shock.

▶When Not to Start CPR

Do not start CPR when one of the following is present:

- The victim has a lethal injury—severe head injury, massive chest injury, or the like.
- There are signs that the victim has been dead for some time—rigor mortis, lividity (the purple color of blood as it sinks to the lowest part of a corpse).
- The known time from incident to resuscitation is too great for success, for example, 30 minutes since cardiac arrest; more than 1 hour of submersion of an adult in water.
- The victim is in cardiac arrest following severe trauma.
- The victim is hypothermic with a frozen, incompressible chest.
- The environment is unsafe and dangerous to the rescuers.

▶When to Stop CPR

Stop CPR when one of the following occurs:

- The victim revives.
- Another trained rescuer takes over.
- You are too exhausted to continue.
- The situation becomes unsafe for rescuers.
- A physician tells you to stop.
- CPR has been given for 30 minutes without signs of recovery, except when there are indications for prolonged CPR.

Infants

▶ CPR

The most likely wilderness incidents requiring the resuscitation of an infant are drowning, a lightning strike, or severe trauma such as a head injury.

What to Do for Infants

1. Make sure the scene is safe before approaching the infant.
2. Tap the infant's shoulder or bottom of a foot and shout, "Are you OK?"
3. If the infant does not respond and is not breathing or is only gasping, he or she needs CPR. If you are alone, give CPR described in Step 4 for 2 minutes and then make your call to 9-1-1. If someone else is available have them call 9-1-1 and get an AED (automated external defibrillator) if available.
4. Begin CPR with 30 chest compressions. Place 2 fingers, with one touching and one below the nipple line. Push down at least 1.5 inches. The rate of compressions is faster than once per second (100 compressions a minute; use the beat of the Bee Gee's "Stayin' Alive" song). After each compression let the chest come back up to its normal position.
5. Open the airway with the head tilt–chin lift maneuver. Do not tilt the head too far back.
6. Cover the infant's mouth and nose with your mouth, making an airtight seal. If this does not work, try either mouth-to-mouth or mouth-to-nose breaths **Figure A-4**.

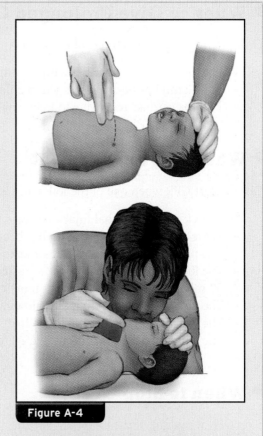

Figure A-4

Use two fingers for chest compressions on an infant. Give CPR to an infant with your mouth over both the victim's mouth and nose.

7. Give 2 rescue breaths with each lasting 1 second. Blow enough to make the chest rise. If the first breath does not go in and make the chest rise, the airway may be blocked. Retilt the head and give a second breath. If the second breath does not make the chest rise, begin CPR (cycles of 30 chest compressions and 2 breaths). Failure to make the chest rise is a sign of choking so each time the airway is opened before giving the first breath, look for an object in the victim's mouth and, if seen, remove it. If the two breaths go in and make the chest rise, you do not need to look for an object before giving the first breath each time.
8. Continue CPR with 30 chest compressions and 2 breaths. See the section, *When to Stop* for guidelines about how long to continue.

Airway Obstruction and Choking

Choking victims vary as to whether the victim has a mild airway obstruction or has a severe airway obstruction.

▶ Airway Obstruction in a Responsive Adult (8 Years and Older) or Child (1 to 8 Years)

A foreign body lodged in the airway can cause mild or severe airway obstruction. When a foreign body partially blocks the airway, it is considered to be minor, because good air exchange is usually present.

What to Look For

- Mild airway obstruction: The victim is still able to cough and make some sounds.
- Severe airway obstruction:
  - Cyanosis (blueness).
  - The victim is unable to speak, breathe, or cough.
  - The victim clutches his or her neck with one or both hands.

What to Do

1. For mild obstruction (victim is coughing forcefully), do not interfere with the victim's coughing or breathing efforts.
2. For severe obstruction, give the victim abdominal thrusts (the Heimlich maneuver) **Figure A-5**.
   - Stand behind the victim.
   - Wrap your arms around the victim's waist (do not allow your forearms to touch the victim's ribs).
   - Make a fist with one hand and place the thumb side just above the victim's navel and well below the lower tip of the breastbone.
   - Grasp your fist with your other hand.
   - Press your fist into the victim's abdomen, giving quick, upward thrusts. Each thrust should be a separate and distinct effort to dislodge the obstructing object.
3. Repeat abdominal thrusts until the victim coughs up the object. If the victim becomes unresponsive, perform CPR as previously discussed.

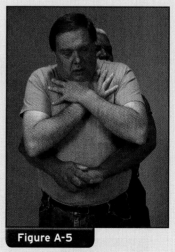

Figure A-5

Heimlich maneuver on responsive victim.

▶ Responsive Infant With Foreign Body Airway Obstruction (Choking)

The infant is responsive but cannot cough, cry, or breathe.

What to Do

1. Give the infant up to five back slaps **Figure A-6**.
   - Hold the infant's head and neck with one hand by firmly holding the jaw between your thumb and fingers.
   - Lay the infant face down over your forearm with the head lower than the chest. Support your forearm on your thigh.
   - Give the infant up to five back slaps between the shoulder blades with the heel of your hand.
2. Give up to five chest thrusts **Figure A-7**.
   - Support the back of the infant's head.
   - Sandwich the infant between your hands and forearms and turn the infant over onto his or her back with the head lower than the chest. If you are a small rescuer, you might need to support the infant on your lap.
   - Locate the proper chest position for thrusts (this is the same location as for chest compressions in CPR).
   - Give up to five separate and distinct thrusts with two fingers.
3. Check the mouth for a foreign object.
4. Repeat these steps until object is expelled or help arrives.
5. If the infant becomes unresponsive, begin CPR. Check the mouth for a foreign object before giving 2 breaths.

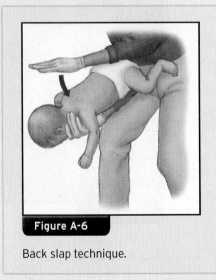

Figure A-6

Back slap technique.

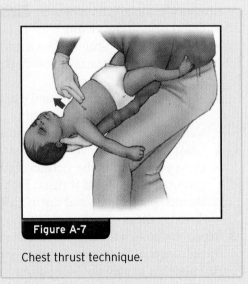

Figure A-7

Chest thrust technique.

First Aid Equipment and Supplies

Your wilderness first aid kit deserves careful planning. Consider trip duration, maximum time to medical care, space and weight available for the kit, activities and environmental conditions expected, age and preexisting health conditions of the group members, and the first aid knowledge and experience in the group. You may buy a prepackaged first aid kit or compile your own.

Carry the items in an easily recognized container such as a red or orange bag. If you anticipate water exposure (heavy rains, river crossings, boating), place individual items in resealable plastic bags and store the whole kit in a watertight container. Individual members of a group should carry their own kit with a few commonly used items in case they get separated.

Table B-1 and Table B-2 list useful first aid kit items for a short trip. Modify the list according to the specifics of your group and itinerary. Consult earlier sections of the text for information on additional items.

Table B-1 First Aid Items for a 3- to 4-Day Trip (for 2-3 Persons)

Topical antiseptic towelettes	10
Topical anesthetic cream	1 small tube, or pads
Antibiotic ointment	4 individual packs or 1 small tube
Aloe vera gel	1 small tube
Moleskin/molefoam	1 package
Irrigation syringe (20 mL)	1
Bandage strips	10-15 1" strips
Sterile gauze pads	4 @ 2" × 2", 6 @ 4" × 4"
Nonadherent pads	4
Self-adhering roller bandage	4" roll
Trauma pad	5" × 9" pad
Elastic bandage	3" roll
Tape	2" roll adhesive or duct tape
Safety pins	3 large
Pain and anti-inflammatory medication	10 acetaminophen tablets, 325 mg
	10 ibuprofen tablets, 200 mg
	10 aspirin tablets, 325 mg*

(continues)

Table B-1 First Aid Items for a 3- to 4-Day Trip (for 2-3 Persons) (continued)

Decongestant	6 tablets
Antihistamine	6 tablets
Hydrocortisone cream	1 small tube, 1%
Sunscreen	1 tube per person, minimum SPF 15
Lip balm (with sunscreen)	1 stick per person
Insect repellent with DEET	1 bottle, plus permanone spray if in tick country
Antacids	8-10 tablets
Antidiarrheal tablets	10 tablets
Povidone-iodine solution	1 oz, 10%
Triangular bandage	1
Scissors	1
Tweezers	1
Thermometer	1 (low-reading in cold climate)
Aluminum padded splint (SAM splint)	1
Non-latex disposable gloves	2-4
Pocket mask or microshield	1
Notebook/pencil	1 each

*Do not give aspirin to children.

Table B-2 First Aid Supplies: Wound Care

	Type/Brand/Size	Uses, Comments	Alternatives/Prevention
Blister care supplies	Moleskin, molefoam	Treat "hot spots" before blister formation. Pad painful blisters.	Wear a sock liner; break in hiking boots before trip; apply adhesive or duct tape over hot spot.
Irrigation syringe	10- or 20-mL syringe with 16-18 gauge catheter tip	High-pressure irrigation of wound to flush dirt and bacteria	Wash with topical antiseptics.
Topical antiseptic	Towelettes with benzalkonium chloride, and/or povidone iodine solution, 10%, 1 oz	Clean cuts, scrapes, and bites. Iodine solutions can be used for water disinfection.	Soap and water
Topical anesthetic	Ointment, solution, or cleansing pads with lidocaine	Provides some local numbing for cleaning dirt from abrasions and shallow cuts	Ice or cold water
Ophthalmic ointment	Polysporin	Conjunctivitis corneal abrasions	Do not use nonopthalmic ointments as alternatives.
Antimicrobial ointment	Triple antibiotic ointment Polysporin, Neosporin	Provides optimal healing environment, helps prevent skin infections associated with dirty cuts, scrapes, and bites. Makes nonstick dressings.	Does not replace meticulous wound cleansing
Aloe vera	100% gel or various creams with high concentration	Aloe can be used to soothe pain of thermal or sunburn and superficial frostbite.	Antibiotic ointment on burns Caution: some people develop sensitivity/reaction to aloe.

Table B-2 First Aid Supplies: Bandage Material

	Type/Brand/Size	Uses, Comments	Alternatives/Prevention
Adhesive bandages	Variety of sizes, including strips and "knuckle": Band-Aid	Cover minor wounds.	Improvise by cutting gauze pad and tape.
Steri-strips	¼" × 4" adhesive strips	Close certain minor, clean wounds.	Can fashion from regular tape; most wounds do not need closure in the wilderness.
Gauze pad dressings	2" × 2" and 4" × 4" sterile pads (individually wrapped packages of two pads)	Absorbent wound dressings; carry some sterile and some nonsterile. Nonsterile pads are adequate for most dressings, less expensive, and less bulky without packaging.	Cleanest available absorbent, lint-free material
Nonadherent gauze pads	Aquaphor, Xeroform, Adaptic, Telfa, Spenco Second Skin, Hydrogel	Nonadherent pads provide ideal protection for burns, blisters, and scrapes.	Antibiotic ointment on dry gauze or clean cloth creates a nonstick dressing.
Self-adhering gauze	2"–4" wide self-adhering roller gauze: Kerlex, Kling	Secure bandages and provide additional padding and barrier; easy to apply.	Clean cloth, elastic wrap
Sterile trauma pads	Highly absorbent pad 5" × 9", 8" × 10"	Dressing for large lacerations, abrasions, open fractures with substantial bleeding or oozing fluid.	Menstrual pads
Elastic bandage	3"–4" wide ACE Wrap	Provides compression to reduce swelling and minimal support for joint sprains; pressure dressing; bulky, but often useful.	Cloth strips, roller gauze, athletic tape for sprains
Tape	Porous cloth athletic tape and/or hypoallergenic "silk" tape, or waterproof tape	Secure bandages and splinting material in place; athletic tape useful for taping sprains.	Tie or pin gauze or elastic wrap; duct tape
Tincture of benzoin	Benzoin liquid 1/2 oz–1 oz or single-use ampules	Adhesive to enhance stickiness of wound closure strips or tape	Athletic tape or duct tape
Safety pins	1"–2" long	Create sling with bandana, cloth, shirttail or sleeve; hold dressings in place; drain blister; many other uses.	

Table B-2 First Aid Supplies: Nonprescription Medications

	Type/Brand/Size	Uses, Comments	Alternatives/Prevention
Analgesic antipyretics and nonsteroidal anti-inflammatory drugs (NSAIDs)	Acetaminophen(Tylenol), aspirin*, ibuprofen (Advil, Motrin), naproxen (Aleve, Naprosyn)	Treats fever, mild to moderate pain, and inflammation	
Decongestant tablets	Sudafed (decongestant); Actifed, Dristan, Contact, Dimetapp, others (decongestant/antihistamine)	Relieves nasal and upper respiratory congestion of viral "colds," allergies, and sinus infections, high-altitude runny nose	Nasal decongestant spray; let drip or blow nose
Antihistamine tablets	Diphenhydramine: Benadryl (best all-purpose); Chlorpheniramine, Dramamine, many others	Relieves allergy symptoms of watery eyes, nasal drainage, and hives. Treats itching and rash associated with poison ivy or oak. Reduces nausea and motion sickness. Causes drowsiness; induces sleep.	
Hydrocortisone cream, 1%	Cortaid, Lanacort, Cortizone	Soothes inflammation associated with insect bites, poison ivy, poison oak, and other allergic skin rashes.	Antihistamine tablets or cold compresses; calamine lotion
Antifungal cream	Clotrimazole, mycostatin: Lotrimin, Micatin, Nizoral	Treats athlete's foot and fungal and yeast infections of the groin and vagina. For longer trips, tropics, or susceptible persons.	Attempt prevention by avoiding long periods with wet feet and wet undergarments. Women may get a yeast infection if taking antibiotics.

(continues)

Table B-2   First Aid Supplies: Nonprescription Medications (continued)

	Type/Brand/Size	Uses, Comments	Alternatives/Prevention
Sunscreen	Lotion with sun protection factor (SPF) of at least 15, and/or opaque sunblock cream containing zinc oxide or titanium	Prevention of sunburn, windburn; especially important when traveling on snow or near water	Minimize sun exposure by wearing a wide-brim hat, light-weight long-sleeved shirt, and pants.
Lip balm	Sun protection factor of at least 15; Blistex SPF 15 or Chap Stick Sunblock 15	Prevents sunburn, chapping of lips; soothes cold sores	Opaque sunblock cream containing zinc oxide or titanium
Insect repellent	Those containing DEET; newer preparations longer-acting and contain about 30% DEET; Permanone for ticks	Reduces insect bites. For children, use no more than 10% DEET products. Permanone onclothes repels ticks.	Lightweight long-sleeved shirts, pants tucked into socks, daily tick inspection, mosquito nets
Antacids	Tablets to neutralize acid: Mylanta, Gelusil, Tums	Treats heartburn, acid indigestion	Avoid caffeine, sweets, chocolate, and spicy food; do not eat near bedtime.
Antidiarrheals	Loperamide: Imodium capsules, 1- or 2-mg capsules	Decreases diarrhea; victim must also maintain hydration.	Pepto-Bismol; diet change; antibiotic for traveler's diarrhea
Oral rehydration salts	WHO formulation: Oralyte; USA preparations: rehydralyte	When mixed with purified water, can help treat dehydration associated with diarrhea, vomiting, and heat exhaustion.	Sports drinks, water with salt and sugar, soup broth
Oral glucose gel (see Chapter 13)	Glucose paste or tablets	For victim who may be diabetic. Treats insulin shock. Carry if diabetic person in your group.	Hard candy or sugar if person is conscious

*Aspirin should not be given to children.

Table B-2 First Aid Supplies: Equipment

	Type/Brand/Size	Uses, Comments	Alternatives/Prevention
Water purification system	Iodine tablets or solutions, filters, chlorine tablets, or solutions	Removal of waterborne germs that can cause intestinal illness; iodine solutions can be used for wound cleaning	Boil water. Carry enough water with you from a known "safe" source.
Scissors	Bandage type with blunt ends; paramedic shears; small folding scissors available at sewing stores	Removing victim's clothing; modifying bandage material	Scissors or blade on pocket knife; seam ripper
Tweezers	Fine pointed, splinter forceps: Uncle Bill's Tweezers, Splinter Pickers, Swiss Army knife tweezers	Removing splinters and ticks	Fingernail, tip of knife, safety pin, needle from sewing kit
Splinting material	Malleable foam padded splint such as SAM splint, air splints, wire splints, portable traction splints also available	Immobilizing broken bone or severe sprain, emergency neck collar	Many materials for improvisation: boards, branches, ground pad, tent poles, metal stays, adjacent body parts
Thermometer	Usual thermometer ranges from 94°F–105°F; extended ranges (75°F–105°F) available	For diagnosis of fever; extended range for accurate reading in heatstroke or hypothermia. Carry in a protective case.	Oral temp-dot strips. Determine presence of fever by touch.
CPR mouth-to-mask barrier device	CPR Microshield, Pocket Mask	Provides "universal precaution" barrier between victim and first aid provider during rescue breathing	
Latex or vinyl gloves		Protects first aid provider from potentially infected blood and body fluids	Any barrier like gloves or plastic bags to avoid blood contact with skin; wash skin with soap if exposed.
Notebook		Recording information about injury or illness; sending detailed information to rescuers.	Blank page of guide book, first aid book, or paperback book
Writing utensil	Soft, waterproof pencil	Recording information about injury or illness. Pens may leak and do not work in cold.	
Emergency dental kit	Eugenol (oil of cloves) for pain relief. Cavit temporary filling (small tube, by prescription or from dentist); commercial kits available.	For repair of teeth or relief of pain from cracked tooth, lost fillings, or crowns	Candle wax

Table B-2 First Aid Supplies: Prescription Medications

These items should be considered for prolonged remote travel. They require more advanced first aid knowledge, special training, or instructions. The medications require a prescription from a doctor.

	Type/Brand/Size	Uses, Comments	Alternatives/Prevention
Asthma kit bronchodilating inhaler	Nonprescription–epinephrine: Primatene. Prescription–Ventolin, Proventil, Metaprel	Treatment of asthma attack or wheezing	Nonprescription tablets are available but are not as effective.
Antibiotic	Keflex, Bactrim, erythromycin, Augmentin, amoxicillin	Treatment of respiratory, skin, and urinary infections. May need more than one kind of antibiotic.	Many different antibiotics with specific indications. Need to discuss with health professional.
Antibiotic for traveler's diarrhea	Cipro, Bactrim, norfloxacin	For treatment of diarrhea acquired during travel in underdeveloped countries	Pepto-Bismol, Imodium, or Lomotil; fluid replacement
Prescription pain medication	Oral narcotics: acetaminophen with codeine (Vicodin)	Treatment of moderate to severe pain; helpful for long evacuations over difficult terrain	Intravenous pain medications administered by licensed provider
Altitude sickness medication	Diamox, Decadron, nifedipine	Prevention and treatment of symptoms of acute mountain sickness. Decadron is for cerebral edema (HACE). Nifedipine is for pulmonary edema.	Slow elevation gain to allow acclimatization; descent
Anaphylaxis kit	Injectable epinephrine (Epi-Pen, Ana-Kit)	Treatment of anaphylactic reaction to bee sting, insect bite, or other severe allergic reaction	Essential if responsible for group or history of previous reaction
Traction splint device	DABBS (National Ski Patrol) ski tip and tail adaptor for improvising traction from a ski; Kendrick traction device	Traction splinting of long bone fractures for evacuation.	Learn to improvise with paddle, ski poles, or non-traction splinting technique.
Communication equipment	Cellular phone, VHF radio, geographic (GPS) locator	Contact of search and rescue or other authorities.	

Water Disinfection

Waterborne disease is a risk for international travelers who visit countries that have poor hygiene and inadequate sanitation, and for wilderness visitors who rely on surface water in any country, including the United States. The list of potential waterborne pathogens is extensive and includes bacteria, viruses, protozoa, and parasitic helminths. Most of the organisms that can cause diarrhea in travelers can be waterborne. Where treated tap water is available, most travelers' intestinal infections are probably transmitted by food, but where untreated surface or well water is used and there is no sanitation infrastructure, the risk of waterborne infection is high. Microorganisms with small infectious doses can even cause illness through recreational water exposure, via inadvertent water ingestion.

Bottled water has become the convenient solution for most travelers, but in some places it may not be superior to tap water. Moreover, the plastic bottles create an ecologic problem because most developing countries do not recycle plastic bottles. All international travelers, especially long-term travelers or expatriates, should become familiar with and use simple methods to ensure safe drinking water. **Table C-1** compares benefits and limitations of different methods.

▶ Field Techniques for Water Treatment

Heat

Common intestinal pathogens are readily inactivated by heat. Microorganisms are killed in a shorter time at higher temperatures, whereas temperatures as low as 140°F (60°C) are effective with a longer contact time. Pasteurization uses this principle to kill foodborne enteric pathogens and spoiling organisms at temperatures between 140°F (60°C) and 158°F (70°C), well below the boiling point of water (212°F [100°C]).

Although boiling is not necessary to kill common intestinal pathogens, it is the only easily recognizable point that does not require a thermometer. All organisms except bacterial spores, which are not usually waterborne enteric pathogens, are killed in seconds at boiling temperature. Therefore, any water that is boiled for 1 minute (to allow for a margin of safety) should be adequately disinfected. Because the boiling point decreases with increasing altitude, water should be boiled for 3 minutes at altitudes above 6,562 ft (2,000 m). To conserve fuel, the same results can be obtained by bringing water to a boil and then turning off the stove but keeping the container covered for several minutes.

Comparison of Water Disinfection Techniques

Table C-1

Technique	Advantages	Disadvantages
Heat	• Does not impart additional taste or color • Single step that inactivates all enteric pathogens • Efficacy is not compromised by contaminants or particles in the water as for halogenation and filtration	• Does not improve taste, smell, or appearance of water • Fuel sources may be scarce, expensive, or unavailable • Does not prevent recontamination during storage
Filtration	• Simple to operate • Requires no holding time for treatment • Large choice of commercial product designs • Adds no unpleasant taste and often improves taste and appearance of water • Can be combined with halogens to remove or kill all pathogenic waterborne microbes	• Adds bulk and weight to baggage • Many do not reliably remove viruses • Channeling of water or high pressure can force microorganisms through the filter • More expensive than chemical treatment • Eventually clogs from suspended particulate matter and may require some maintenance or repair in the field • Does not prevent recontamination during storage
Halogens (chlorine, iodine)	• Inexpensive and widely available in liquid or tablet forms • Taste can be removed by simple techniques • Flexible dosing • Equally easy to treat large and small volumes	• Corrosive and stains clothing • Imparts taste and odor to water • Flexibility requires understanding of principles • Iodine is physiologically active, with potential adverse effects • Not readily effective against *Cryptosporidium* oocysts • Efficacy decreases with low water temperature and decreasing water clarity
Chlorine dioxide	• Low doses have no taste or color • Simple to use and available in liquid or tablet form • More potent than equivalent doses of chlorine • Effective against all waterborne pathogens	• Volatile and sensitive to sunlight: do not expose tablets to air and use generated solutions rapidly • No persistent residual concentration, so does not prevent recontamination during storage
Ultraviolet (UV)	• Imparts no taste • Portable devices now available • Effective against all waterborne pathogens • Extra doses of UV can be used for added assurance and with no side effects • Moderate benefit from solar UV exposure	• Requires clear water • Does not improve taste or appearance of water • Relatively expensive • Requires batteries or power source • Difficult to know if devices are delivering required UV doses • No persistent residual concentration, so does not prevent recontamination during storage

Courtesy of CDC.

If no other means of water treatment is available, a potential alternative to boiling is to use tap water that is too hot to touch, which is probably at a temperature between 131°F (55°C) and 140°F (60°C). This temperature may be adequate to kill pathogens if the water has been kept hot in the tank for some time. Travelers with access to electricity can bring a small electric heating coil or a lightweight beverage warmer to boil water.

Filtration and Clarification

Filter pore size is the primary determinant of a filter's effectiveness, but microorganisms also adhere to filter media by electrochemical reactions. Microfilters with "absolute" pore sizes of 0.1–0.4 µm are usually effective to remove cysts and bacteria but may not adequately remove viruses, which are a major concern in water with high levels of fecal contamination **Table C-2**. Filters that claim Environmental Protection Agency (EPA) designation of water "purifier" undergo company-sponsored testing that has demonstrated removal of 10^6 bacteria, 10^4 (9,999 of 10,000) viruses, and 10^3 *Cryptosporidium* oocysts or *Giardia* cysts. (EPA does not independently test the validity of these claims.) NSF International is a nonprofit, nongovernmental organization that develops standards and product certification for public health and safety. They are a designated collaborating center of the World Health Organization (WHO) for Food and Water Safety and Indoor Environment. They are accredited by the American National Standards Institute (ANSI), the International Accreditation Service (IAS), and the Standards Council of Canada (SCC) for third-party certification. Some water filtration units have been evaluated by NSF International under the NSF/ANSI Standard 53. A listing of certified water filtration products can be found at www.nsf.org/consumer.

New portable filter designs include hollow fiber technology, which is a cluster of tiny tubules with variable pore sizes that can remove virus-size particles **Figure C-1**. Reverse-osmosis filters can both remove microbiologic contamination and desalinate water. The high price and slow output of small hand-pump reverse-osmosis units prohibit use by land-based travelers; however, they are important survival aids for ocean voyagers.

Table C-2 Microorganism Size and Susceptibility to Filtration

Organism	Average Size (µm)	Maximum Recommended Filter Rating (µm Absolute)[1]
Viruses	0.03	Not specified (optimally 0.01)
Enteric bacteria (*Escherichia coli*)	$0.5 \times 3.0\text{-}8.0$	0.2-0.4
Cryptosporidium oocyst	4-6	1
Giardia cyst	$6.0\text{-}10.0 \times 8.0\text{-}15.0$	3.0-5.0

[1]NSF 53 rating on a filter certifies for cyst/oocyst removal.
Courtesy of CDC.

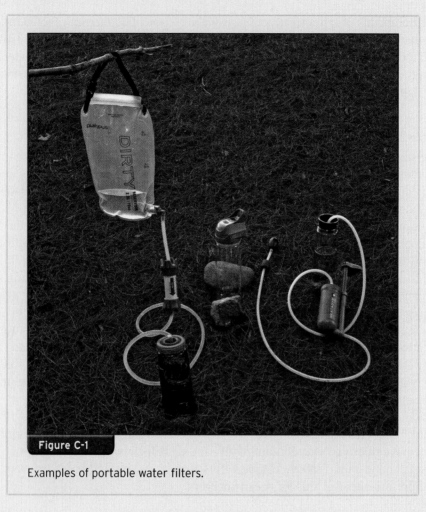

Figure C-1

Examples of portable water filters.

Coagulation-flocculation (CF) removes suspended particles that cause a cloudy appearance and bad taste and that do not settle by gravity; this process removes many but not all micro-organisms. CF is easily applied in the field. Alum, or one of several other substances, is added to the water, stirred well, allowed to settle, then poured through a coffee filter or fine cloth to remove the sediment. Tablets or packets of powder that combine flocculent and hypochlorite disinfection are available (commercial products such as Chlor-floc or PUR).

Chemical Disinfection

Halogens
The most common chemical water disinfectants are chlorine and iodine (halogens). World-wide, chemical disinfection with chlorine is the most commonly used method for improving

and maintaining the microbiologic quality of drinking water. Sodium hypochlorite, the active ingredient in common household bleach, is the primary disinfectant promoted by CDC and the WHO Safe Water System at a 1.5% concentration for household use in the developing world. Other chlorine-containing compounds, such as calcium hypochlorite and sodium dichloroisocyanurate, which are both solids, are also effective for household water treatment.

Given adequate concentrations and length of exposure (contact time), chlorine and iodine have similar activity and are effective against bacteria, viruses, and *Giardia* cysts. Because many factors in the field are uncontrolled, extending the contact time adds a margin of safety. However, some common waterborne parasites, such as *Cryptosporidium*, are poorly inactivated by halogen disinfection, even at practical extended contact times. Therefore, chemical disinfection should be supplemented with adequate filtration to remove these microorganisms from drinking water. Cloudy water contains substances that will neutralize disinfectant, so it will require higher concentrations or contact times or, preferably, clarification through settling or filtration before disinfectant is added. Tablets that combine flocculent and disinfectant are available.

Both chlorine and iodine are available in liquid and tablet form. Because iodine has physiologic activity, WHO recommends limiting iodine water disinfection to a few weeks of emergency use. Iodine use is not recommended for people with unstable thyroid disease or known iodine allergy. Iodine should not be used by pregnant women because of the potential effect on the fetal thyroid.

The taste of halogens in water can be improved by several means:

- Reduce concentration and increase contact time proportionately.
- After the required contact time, run water through a filter that contains activated carbon.
- After the required contact time, add a tiny pinch of ascorbic acid.

Iodine Resins

Iodine resins transfer iodine to microorganisms that come into contact with the resin, but leave little iodine dissolved in the water. The resins have been incorporated into many different filter designs available for field use. Most contain a 1-µm cyst filter, which should effectively remove protozoan cysts. Few models are sold in the United States because of inconsistent test results, but some models are still available for international use.

Salt (Sodium Chloride) Electrolysis

Passing a current through a simple brine salt solution generates oxidants, including hypochlorite, which can be used to disinfect microbes.

Chlorine Dioxide

Chlorine dioxide (ClO_2) can kill most waterborne pathogens, including *Cryptosporidium* oocysts, at practical doses and contact times. Tablets and liquid formulations are available to generate chlorine dioxide in the field for small-quantity water treatment.

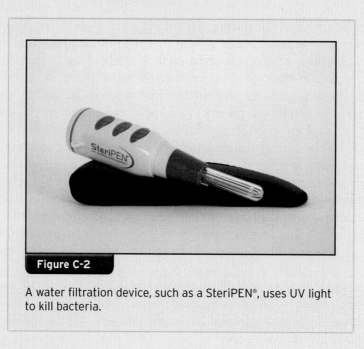

Figure C-2

A water filtration device, such as a SteriPEN®, uses UV light to kill bacteria.

Ultraviolet (UV) Light

Extensive data show that UV light can kill bacteria, viruses, and *Cryptosporidium* oocysts in water. The effect depends on UV dose and exposure time, and requires clear water because suspended particles can shield microorganisms from UV rays. These units have limited effectiveness in water with high levels of suspended solids and turbidity. They also have no disinfection residual. Portable battery-operated units that deliver a metered, timed dose of UV may be an effective way to disinfect small quantities of clear water in the field; however, more testing is needed for conclusive evidence **Figure C-2**.

Solar Irradiation and Heating

UV irradiation by sunlight in the UVA range can substantially improve the microbiologic quality of water. Recent work has confirmed the efficacy and optimal procedures of the solar disinfection technique. Transparent bottles (such as clear plastic beverage bottles), preferably lying on a dark surface, are exposed to sunlight for a minimum of 4 hours. UV and thermal inactivation are synergistic for solar disinfection of drinking water. Use of a simple reflector or solar cooker can achieve temperatures of 149°F (65°C), which will pasteurize the water after 4 hours. Solar disinfection is not effective on turbid water. If the headlines in a newspaper can't be read through the bottle of water, then the water must be filtered before solar irradiation is used. If more than half the sky is clouded over, then solar irradiation is not effective and should be repeated before using the water. Solar disinfection of drinking water may be acceptable for austere emergency situations.

Silver and Other Products

Silver ion has bactericidal effects in low doses and some attractive features, including absence of color, taste, and odor. The use of silver as a drinking water disinfectant is popular in Europe, but it is not approved for this purpose in the United States, because silver concentration in water is strongly affected by adsorption onto the surface of the container, and there has been limited testing on viruses and cysts. In the United States, silver is approved for maintaining microbiologic quality of stored water.

Several other common products have antibacterial effects in water and are marketed in commercial products for travelers, including hydrogen peroxide, citrus juice, and potassium permanganate. None have sufficient data to recommend them for water disinfection in the field.

▶ The Preferred Technique

The optimal technique for a person or group depends on personal preference, size of the group, water source, and the style of travel. Boiling is the most reliable single-step treatment, but certain filters, UV, and chlorine dioxide are also effective in most situations. Optimal treatment of highly contaminated or cloudy water may require CF followed by chemical disinfection. On long distance, oceangoing boats where water must be desalinated during the voyage, only reverse-osmosis membrane filters are adequate.

▶ Camp Hygiene

Proper hygiene prevents contamination of groundwater and limits the spread of illness among group members.

Waste Disposal in Areas Without Toilets or Group Latrines

- Dig a hole 8" to 10" deep to bury waste.
- Dig the hole at least 100 feet from surface water, and do not dig in natural drainages where the rain could wash waste into the water source.
- Burn or bury toilet paper with waste and stamp down or cover with a rock.
- For large groups or high-use areas, dig a common trench latrine. After each use, sprinkle a little dirt on the waste.
- Carry a small plastic spade or collapsible shovel or improvise with a stick or flat spade-shaped rock.

Personal Hygiene

Everyone should always wash their hands after going to the bathroom and before preparing food **Figure C-3** . Place a bucket of water, a dipper, and soap along the path to the latrine or next to the cooking area.

Group Hygiene

- Use utensils rather than hands to serve food.
- When washing dishes, add bleach to the final rinse water **Figure C-4**. Carry a few ounces of liquid or powder bleach (1 to 2 ounces should suffice for a small group for 1 week). Add enough to create a strong smell of chlorine. Allow dishes to air dry.

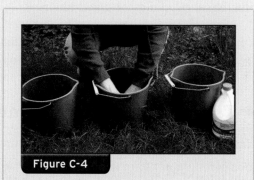

Figure C-4

Camp hygiene: put bleach in rinse water.

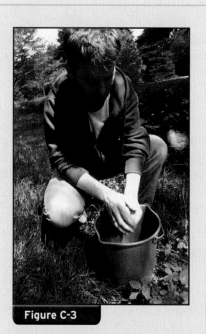

Figure C-3

Camp hygiene: handwashing.

Fluid and Electrolyte Replacement

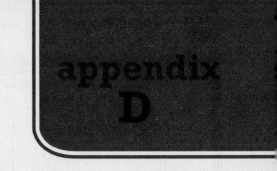

Oral rehydration/electrolyte solutions (ORS) are useful in four circumstances when fluids and electrolytes are lost in significant amounts: severe diarrhea and/or vomiting; treatment of mild to moderate heat illness; heavy, prolonged exercise with high-volume sweat loss; and injury with significant blood loss or fluid loss from burns **Figure D-1** .

▶ Replacement of Intestinal Fluid Losses

Diarrhea is the main reason for using oral electrolyte solutions. Most intestinal infections resolve by themselves, but they cause the loss of fluid and electrolytes and can result in dehydration. Even during severe diarrhea, the gut can absorb water and electrolytes when mixed with glucose.

The World Health Organization (WHO) has developed electrolyte salts specifically for diarrheal illness. The electrolyte salts contain sodium, potassium, chloride, bicarbonate or trisodium citrate, and glucose; these should be mixed with 1 quart or liter of disinfected water. Packets of these oral rehydration salts are distributed throughout the world by WHO and UNICEF, commonly under the name of Oralyte. In the United States, the WHO salts and rice-based solutions are hard to find. More expensive premixed solutions are available but impractical for wilderness or foreign travel.

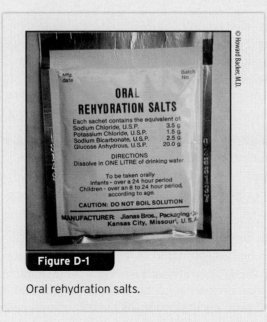

Figure D-1

Oral rehydration salts.

Table D-1 Recipe for ORS Powder

Add to 1 liter of disinfected water:

potassium chloride (KCl)	1.5 g
baking soda	2.5 g
salt (NaCl)	3.5 g
glucose	20.0 g

Table D-2 Home Sports Solution for Rehydration

Add to 1 Quart of Water	Resulting Concentration
3-4 tsp sugar	1%-2% solution, 50 kcal
0.5 tsp table salt	30 mEq/L

Notes: The teaspoon measurement is quite variable (3.5-5.0 grams/tsp), but the resulting concentration is fine in these solutions.
Milliequivalents (mEq) is a measure of substances related to both weight and electrical charge; 1.0 liter (L) = 1.05 quarts.

Cereal-based ORS contains complex carbohydrate molecules from rice or grains that are digested as simple glucose. Sports drinks and other clear liquids contain too little sodium and potassium and too much glucose for treating diarrhea-induced dehydration, but they can be better than plain water (see **Table D-1** and **Table D-2** for a homemade solution).

If premeasured salts are not available, a substitute recommended by the Centers for Disease Control and Prevention consists of alternating drinks of the following two fluids:

Glass 1: 8 oz fruit juice (apple, orange, lemonade, and the like)
          0.5 tsp honey or corn syrup
          1 pinch salt
Glass 2: 8 oz water (boiled or treated)
          0.25 tsp baking soda

Some ingredients may not be available in remote locations.

Plain salt-and-sugar solutions, similar to those used for heat/exercise replacement, can be used for mild dehydration but are not adequate for serious dehydration or replacing continuing high losses. For mild dehydration, partial maintenance, supplementation, or where nothing else is available, rice water, fruit juice, coconut milk, diluted cola drinks, or soup broth might suffice.

Guidelines for Fluid Replacement

Estimated fluid deficit should be replaced in about 4 hours. For mild dehydration, an adult should drink 8 ounces of ORS every 30 minutes for the first 4 to 6 hours. Children should drink 6 to 8 ounces of ORS per hour and as much water as they want. Give infants younger than 3 months a 4-ounce dose each hour, with every third dose replaced by plain water. To prevent vomiting, the dehydrated individuals should drink frequent small amounts slowly. Determine maintenance requirements by estimating or measuring stool losses plus normal maintenance requirements. Because this is not often possible in the field, give someone who is dehydrated at least 1 teaspoon (5 mL) per pound of body weight after each diarrheal stool.

Try to continue feeding. Basic grains and starches do not increase or prolong fluid losses. Rice-based ORS can reduce the illness associated with diarrhea. Most staple foods, such as cereals, bananas, lentils, potatoes, fruits, yogurt, and other cooked vegetables are well tolerated and can be continued during bouts of diarrhea. Avoid caffeine, alcohol, foods with high sugar concentrations, and fried or fatty foods. Intolerance to dairy products (gas, bloating, and persistent diarrhea) can follow an intestinal illness. Infants may continue breastfeeding. Dilute lactose formula 50% with water and observe for lactose intolerance.

Fluid Replacement During Exercise

Sweat losses of 1 quart per hour are common during moderate exercise in a hot, humid environment or heavy exertion in a temperate environment. Dehydration increases the risk of heat illness.

In high-altitude mountaineering, the scarcity of surface water, difficulty adjusting clothing to changing weather or levels of exertion, and respiratory fluid loss from hyperventilation in dry, cold air commonly create fluid needs of 7 to 8 quarts per day. Dehydration at high altitude increases the likelihood of altitude sickness, hypothermia, frostbite, and venous thrombosis.

During sustained hard exercise, especially in a hot environment, a person needs at least 16 ounces (1 pint) of fluid before exercising and 8 ounces every 20 minutes while exercising. The person should drink at every opportunity and gauge hydration by the volume and color of urine. Everyone should use only clean water for fluid replacement.

Sweat contains sodium, chloride, and small amounts of potassium (see **Table D-3** for electrolyte concentrations). In the wilderness, salt and other electrolyte needs are best replaced by regular meals and snacks, with fluid loss replaced with plain water. In addition, food will provide more calories than electrolyte solutions, and it will enhance fluid intake. Unfortunately, many hikers favor snack foods that are high in carbohydrates and fats (such as candy) but low in sodium. Some people, noting the swelling present in their hands and feet associated with heat or altitude exposure, mistakenly attempt to restrict their sodium intake.

Electrolyte supplements are advised in endurance events or sustained work/exercise longer than 6 hours; or for a shorter period, in a very hot environment with high sweat losses. Severe hyponatremia (low salt content in the body) that causes confusion and even seizures can occur in endurance athletes and recreational hikers in hot climates.

During exercise, a solution containing 2% to 6% glucose and 30 mEq/L sodium is palatable. Excessive sodium can cause nausea, and salt tablets swallowed whole cause gastric irritation

Table D-3 Concentrations of Electrolytes in Common Fluids

	Sodium, mEq/L	Potassium, mEq/L	Bicarbonate, mEq/L	Glucose, g/L
Blood	140	4.5	25	
Diarrhea	50-140	15-25	20-45	
Sweat	30-60	3-5		
Sports drink	10-25	3-5		60-70 (6%-7%)
WHO ORS	90	20	30	20 (2%)
U.S. ORS	45-75	20-25	30	20-25
Soft drinks	2-5	0		110
Orange juice	0-5	58		118

Note: Milliequivalents (mEq) is a measure of substances related to both weight and electrical charge; 1.0 liter (L) = 1.05 quarts.

and vomiting. Dissolve one or two tablets in a liter of water. Too much sugar can delay stomach emptying and cause diarrhea. Commercial sports drinks are available in powder form but simple substitutes can be made at home (see Table D-2).

Treatment of Mild Heat Illness

Oral electrolyte solutions are excellent for treating mild or moderate heat illness, such as heat syncope, heat cramps, and heat exhaustion. The victim must rest in the shade and sip 1 to 2 quarts or liters of fluids similar to exercise replacement fluids. Oral fluids cannot be used for treating heatstroke in victims who have altered responsiveness and are unable to swallow.

Fluid and Electrolyte Replacement for Blood Loss

The fluid lost with serious, continued bleeding cannot be replaced by mouth. But if sudden blood loss has occurred and subsequently stopped (such as a wound, nosebleed, or uterine bleeding), oral fluid replacement can help restore blood volume but will not replace lost blood cells. Victims of extensive skin burns lose large volumes of fluid. Give these victims fluids with salt, similar to diarrheal replacement fluids, until intravenous fluids are available.

Improving the Odds of Survival

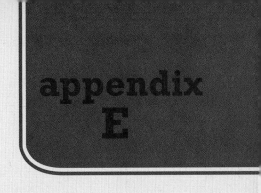

During any wilderness outing, you could be forced to spend an unexpected night out because of an unfamiliar trail, injury, illness, or sudden weather change. Good planning can turn a crisis into an adventure. In addition to skill, determination, and sound judgment, the items in **Table E-1** can improve the odds of survival; keep these items in your vehicle.

▶ Clothing

To prevent serious heat loss, always take at least the minimum amount of extra clothing for comfort in a bad storm. Layering clothing to preserve heat is crucial.

First Layer

Light to midweight synthetic long underwear provides warmth and absorbs or wicks moisture from skin. All materials lose insulating properties when they are wet, but cotton loses more than most.

Insulating Layers

Additional layers will be needed on top of the first layer to provide insulation. These layers could consist of pile or fleece jackets and vests, wool shirts and sweaters, and wool or pile pants.

Table E-1 Vehicle Survival Gear

Bottled water	Sleeping bag or blankets	Fire extinguisher
Flares	Jumper cables	Windshield scraper
Tools	Flashlight	Road maps
Short hose (to siphon gas)	Chains	Matches and cook pot
Nonperishable food	Tow cable	First aid kit
		Shovel and sand

Wind/Rain Layers

To keep dry, windproof, waterproof, and breathable layers are needed for both the upper and lower body. Uncoated nylon is sufficient only for wind and light precipitation.

Hats

To prevent heat loss via the head, as well as to prevent frostbite, bring a hat made of wool, pile, or waterproof material that covers the ears. A balaclava or ski hat and neck gaiter provide more warmth than a simple hat, and they protect the face from frostbite.

Mittens/Gloves

Mittens are warmer than gloves. Wear a synthetic liner as well as a wind/waterproof outer shell. Wool socks make a good substitute for mittens.

Footwear

Wear a polypropylene liner under wool or fleece socks. Boots should be ankle high, have a good traction sole, and be water repellent. Plastic bags between sock layers provide a vapor barrier that increases warmth but can also increase moisture.

▶ Shelter

To conserve heat beyond the insulation provided by clothes, make a shelter by finding a natural cave or windbreak, digging a snow cave or snow trench in a snowbank, or building a quinzhee hut (a snow shelter built by piling snow on a flat surface and tunneling into it). Carry a collapsible shovel to build snow shelters and for avalanche rescue. An effective shelter can be rigged up with rope, cord or wire, and a tarp, rainfly, or even a garbage bag. A tent is ideal but not always available. Bivouac sacks (also known as bivy sacks) provide a lot of warmth for their size and weight; two large garbage bags can function as a light bivy sack or rain suit. Putting the feet into a backpack offers some protection.

▶ Water and Food

Water

To melt snow you need a metal container, stove (and fuel if you are above the timberline), or campfire. A piece of aluminum foil, a black plastic garbage bag, or a space blanket can gather enough sunlight to melt snow and ice. A candle can be used for cooking and melting snow and for warmth in a snow cave. Carry a wide-mouth canteen filled with water. If possible, disinfect drinking water, but maintaining hydration takes precedence over disinfecting water.

Emergency Food Supply

Always carry emergency food rations. In general, it is best to take food that can be eaten without cooking to minimize preparation time and effort, but a cup of hot soup can do wonders for the psyche. Hard candy, energy bars, jerky, and bouillon cubes are compact and lightweight. Carry a pot and metal cup for cooking. Knowledge of edible native food sources will help.

▶ Heat

Know how to light a fire with minimal resources.

Stove and Fuel

A stove and fuel provide the best source of heat for glacier or desert travel, where wood is scarce. In a forest, fire starters and a folding saw can be useful.

Matches in Waterproof Container

Matches work better than a lighter, which cannot vaporize in the cold. Carry several sets in different waterproof containers.

Magnesium Fire Starters

An alternative to matches, magnesium fire starters can be scraped with a steel file or knife blade, producing sparks to ignite fine-grade steel wool, lint, moss, and the like.

Candle

A candle provides light and enough heat to melt snow or warm a drink.

Ground Insulation

To decrease conductive heat loss, do not sit or lie directly on cold ground. Sit on a foam pad (at least 18" square) or a self-inflating mattress, your backpack, or pine boughs to insulate yourself from the ground.

Toilet Paper

Toilet paper can be used as a fire starter. Otherwise, it is not necessary to survive, but it helps for comfort.

▶ Light

Flashlight

Carry fresh batteries and a spare bulb.

Headlamp

A headlamp provides light and frees your hands.

Candle

A candle provides minimal light by itself but can be used in a lantern for additional range. Emergency chemical light sticks can provide several hours of dim light. They have a limited shelf life and often do not work well in the cold.

▶ Route Finding and Navigation

Map and Compass

Carry a topographical map of the area in which you plan to travel. Know how to read the map and how to use a compass for finding your way and checking your location.

Altimeter

An altimeter is useful for positioning yourself on a topographical map based on the known elevation.

Global Positioning System

A global positioning system (GPS) can come in handy for expeditions and off-track remote vehicle travel. This is an advanced navigational tool that uses satellites to pinpoint your location on a longitude/latitude scale. It is generally very accurate; it can show your route and indicate the direction of travel to return to a previous location.

▶ Travel Aids

Snow and Ice Aids

If you plan to travel through a snowy area, take cross-country skis (wax and skins), snowshoes, crampons, an ice axe, and ropes.

Protection Devices

Depending on the type of travel, you should bring devices that protect you from rock, snow, or ice.

Avalanche Beacons and Rescue Equipment

General rescue equipment should include rope, harnesses, pulleys, carabiners, and ascenders. In the event of an avalanche, other tools should be considered. Shovel and probe poles are important tools for backcountry skiers and hikers traveling on an unstable or unknown snowpack. Also consider bringing surveyor's tape to mark a route if someone goes for help, to mark your location for an air search, and to use as a wind sock for a helicopter rescue.

▶ Tools and Repair Kit

Multifunction Knife

Carry a multifunction tool such as a Swiss Army knife or a Leatherman tool that includes pliers.

Duct Tape

Duct tape can be used to fix just about anything. Rather than carry a whole roll, wrap a supply around a ski pole, water bottle, or pencil.

Snare, Baling, or Picture Hanging Wire

Snare, baling, or picture hanging wire can be used for tying or fastening and for backpack repairs.

Safety Pins, Heavy-Duty Needle, and Carpet Thread

There are many uses for safety pins. Large sizes are preferred. A heavy-duty needle and thread will allow you to repair tears in clothing and your tent.

Braided Nylon Cord

Your pack should contain 50 feet (15 meters) of braided nylon cord. The cord has many uses.

First Aid Supplies

No wilderness outing should be attempted without a first aid kit. Various items in the kit can be used for treating illness or injury.

▶ Communication Equipment

Communication equipment is essential for contacting others for help or to notify them that all is well.

Whistle

A whistle is much more effective and efficient than shouting to alert others of trouble; the human voice carries only short distances in the outdoors and gives out quickly. Each member should carry a whistle around his or her neck. A whistle is especially useful for children.

Signal Mirror

Use a mirror to signal overhead aircraft or search parties Table E-2 .

Flares

Flares are also useful for signaling, but they are heavy.

Cellular Phone

A cellular phone is a compact and lightweight means of calling for help or notifying potential rescuers of your condition and whereabouts. However, a cellular phone works only where cellular phone networks are available.

VHF Radio

In remote areas, a VHF radio can provide a link with a telephone network or contact with authorities monitoring emergency bands. Check with local authorities regarding restricted frequencies.

Table E-2 Ground Signals for Aircraft

Search and rescue is commonly done by aircraft. Ground symbols can be used to signal aircraft so that the victims can remain in a shelter or proceed to find water or safer ground. Make markings in an open area, visible from above. Make designs 8 to 10 feet (2 to 3 meters) tall, and use items that contrast with the background. Three repetitive symbols indicates distress. An arrow indicates that you are traveling in that direction. A large **X** means that you are near that location and unable to proceed.

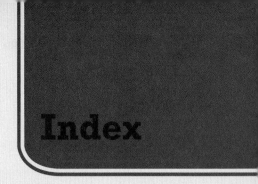

Index

Note: Page numbers followed by *f,* or *t* indicate material in figures or tables, respectively.